Frontiers in Vascular Stiffness

Frontiers in Vascular Stiffness

Editors

Paolo Salvi
Andrea Grillo

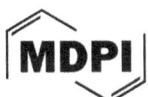 Basel • Beijing • Wuhan • Barcelona • Belgrade • Novi Sad • Cluj • Manchester

Editors
Paolo Salvi
Istituto Auxologico Italiano
Milan, Italy

Andrea Grillo
Azienda Sanitaria Universitaria Giuliano Isontina
Trieste, Italy

Editorial Office
MDPI
St. Alban-Anlage 66
4052 Basel, Switzerland

This is a reprint of articles from the Special Issue published online in the open access journal *Journal of Clinical Medicine* (ISSN 2077-0383) (available at: https://www.mdpi.com/journal/jcm/special_issues/vascular_stiffness).

For citation purposes, cite each article independently as indicated on the article page online and as indicated below:

Lastname, A.A.; Lastname, B.B. Article Title. *Journal Name* **Year**, *Volume Number*, Page Range.

ISBN 978-3-0365-9330-2 (Hbk)
ISBN 978-3-0365-9331-9 (PDF)
doi.org/10.3390/books978-3-0365-9331-9

© 2023 by the authors. Articles in this book are Open Access and distributed under the Creative Commons Attribution (CC BY) license. The book as a whole is distributed by MDPI under the terms and conditions of the Creative Commons Attribution-NonCommercial-NoDerivs (CC BY-NC-ND) license.

Contents

Ioana Mădălina Zota, Cristian Stătescu, Radu Andy Sascău, Mihai Roca, Larisa Anghel, Ovidiu Mitu, et al.
Arterial Stiffness Assessment Using the Arteriograph in Patients with Moderate–Severe OSA and Metabolic Syndrome—A Pilot Study
Reprinted from: *J. Clin. Med.* **2021**, *10*, 4238, doi:10.3390/jcm10184238 1

Ida Åström Malm, Rachel De Basso, Peter Blomstrand and Dick Wågsäter
Association of IL-10 and CRP with Pulse Wave Velocity in Patients with Abdominal Aortic Aneurysm
Reprinted from: *J. Clin. Med.* **2022**, *11*, 1182, doi:10.3390/jcm11051182 15

Jakub Baran, Anna Kablak-Ziembicka, Pawel Kleczynski, Ottavio Alfieri, Łukasz Niewiara, Rafał Badacz, et al.
Association of Increased Vascular Stiffness with Cardiovascular Death and Heart Failure Episodes Following Intervention on Symptomatic Degenerative Aortic Stenosis
Reprinted from: *J. Clin. Med.* **2022**, *11*, 2078, doi:10.3390/jcm11082078 25

Pengzhu Li, Guido Mandilaras, André Jakob, Robert Dalla-Pozza, Nikolaus Alexander Haas and Felix Sebastian Oberhoffer
Energy Drinks and Their Acute Effects on Arterial Stiffness in Healthy Children and Teenagers: A Randomized Trial
Reprinted from: *J. Clin. Med.* **2022**, *11*, 2087, doi:10.3390/jcm11082087 35

Paolo Salvi, Filippo Valbusa, Anna Kearney-Schwartz, Carlos Labat, Andrea Grillo, Gianfranco Parati and Athanase Benetos
Non-Invasive Assessment of Arterial Stiffness: Pulse Wave Velocity, Pulse Wave Analysis and Carotid Cross-Sectional Distensibility: Comparison between Methods
Reprinted from: *J. Clin. Med.* **2022**, *11*, 2225, doi:10.3390/jcm11082225 43

Maurizio Di Marco, Francesca Urbano, Agnese Filippello, Stefania Di Mauro, Alessandra Scamporrino, Nicoletta Miano, et al.
Increased Platelet Reactivity and Proinflammatory Profile Are Associated with Intima–Media Thickness and Arterial Stiffness in Prediabetes
Reprinted from: *J. Clin. Med.* **2022**, *11*, 2870, doi:10.3390/jcm11102870 57

Beáta Kovács, Orsolya Cseprekál, Ágnes Diószegi, Szabolcs Lengyel, László Maroda, György Paragh, et al.
The Importance of Arterial Stiffness Assessment in Patients with Familial Hypercholesterolemia
Reprinted from: *J. Clin. Med.* **2022**, *11*, 2872, doi:10.3390/coatings11030274 69

Andrea Grillo, Vincenzo Barbato, Roberta Maria Antonello, Marco Fabio Cola, Gianfranco Parati, Paolo Salvi, et al.
Arterial Stiffness in Thyroid and Parathyroid Disease: A Review of Clinical Studies
Reprinted from: *J. Clin. Med.* **2022**, *11*, 3146, doi:10.3390/jcm11113146 83

Michele Colaci, Luca Zanoli, Alberto Lo Gullo, Domenico Sambataro, Gianluca Sambataro, Maria Letizia Aprile, et al.
The Impaired Elasticity of Large Arteries in Systemic Sclerosis Patients
Reprinted from: *J. Clin. Med.* **2022**, *11*, 3256, doi:10.3390/jcm11123256 107

Davide Agnoletti, Federica Piani, Arrigo F. G. Cicero and Claudio Borghi
The Gut Microbiota and Vascular Aging: A State-of-the-Art and Systematic Review of the Literature
Reprinted from: *J. Clin. Med.* **2022**, *11*, 3557, doi:10.3390/jcm11123557 117

Paolo Salvi, Andrea Grillo, Sylvie Gautier, Luca Montaguti, Fausto Brunacci, Francesca Severi, et al.
Haemodynamic Adaptive Mechanisms at High Altitude: Comparison between European Lowlanders and Nepalese Highlanders
Reprinted from: J. Clin. Med. 2022, 11, 3843, doi:10.3390/jcm11133843 139

Michaela Kozakova, Carmela Morizzo, Giuli Jamagidze, Dante Chiappino and Carlo Palombo
Comparison between Carotid Distensibility-Based Vascular Age and Risk-Based Vascular Age in Middle-Aged Population Free of Cardiovascular Disease
Reprinted from: J. Clin. Med. 2022, 11, 4931, doi:10.3390/jcm11164931 151

Francesco Fantin, Anna Giani, Monica Trentin, Andrea P. Rossi, Elena Zoico, Gloria Mazzali, et al.
The Correlation of Arterial Stiffness Parameters with Aging and Comorbidity Burden
Reprinted from: J. Clin. Med. 2022, 11, 5761, doi:10.3390/jcm11195761 161

Afrah E. F. Malik, Alessandro Giudici, Koen W. F. van der Laan, Jos Op 't Roodt, Werner H. Mess, Tammo Delhaas, et al.
Detectable Bias between Vascular Ultrasound Echo-Tracking Systems: Relevance Depends on Application
Reprinted from: J. Clin. Med. 2023, 12, 69, doi:10.3390/jcm12010069 173

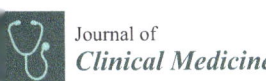

Article

Arterial Stiffness Assessment Using the Arteriograph in Patients with Moderate–Severe OSA and Metabolic Syndrome—A Pilot Study

Ioana Mădălina Zota [1], Cristian Stătescu [1], Radu Andy Sascău [1], Mihai Roca [1], Larisa Anghel [1], Ovidiu Mitu [1], Cristina Mihaela Ghiciuc [2,*], Daniela Boisteanu [3], Razvan Anghel [1], Sebastian Romica Cozma [4], Lucia Corina Dima-Cozma [1] and Florin Mitu [1]

[1] Department of Medical Specialties (I), Faculty of Medicine, Grigore T. Popa University of Medicine and Pharmacy Iași, 700115 Iasi, Romania; ioana-madalina.chiorescu@umfiasi.ro (I.M.Z.); cristian.statescu@umfiasi.ro (C.S.); radu.sascau@umfiasi.ro (R.A.S.); mihai.c.roca@umfiasi.ro (M.R.); larisa.anghel@umfiasi.ro (L.A.); ovidiu.mitu@umfiasi.ro (O.M.); razvan.anghel@umfiasi.ro (R.A.); cozma.dima@umfiasi.ro (L.C.D.-C.); florin.mitu@umfiasi.ro (F.M.)
[2] Department of Morpho-Functional Sciences (II), Faculty of Medicine, Grigore T. Popa University of Medicine and Pharmacy Iași, 700115 Iasi, Romania
[3] Department of Medical Specialties (III), Faculty of Medicine, Grigore T. Popa University of Medicine and Pharmacy Iași, 700115 Iasi, Romania; daniela.boisteanu@umfiasi.ro
[4] Department of Surgery (II), Faculty of Medicine, Grigore T. Popa University of Medicine and Pharmacy Iași, 700115 Iasi, Romania; sebastian.cozma@umfiasi.ro
* Correspondence: cristina.ghiciuc@umfiasi.ro

Abstract: Background: Both obstructive sleep apnea (OSA) and metabolic syndrome (MS) promote arterial stiffening. As a basis for this study, we presumed that arterial stiffness could be assessed using the Arteriograph (TensioMed, Budapest, Hungary) to detect early modifications induced by continuous positive airway therapy (CPAP) in reversing this detrimental vascular remodeling. Arterial stiffness is increasingly acknowledged as a major cardiovascular risk factor and a marker of subclinical hypertension-mediated organ damage. The aim of this pilot study was to evaluate the arterial stiffness changes in patients with moderate–severe OSA and MS after short-term CPAP use. Methods: We performed a prospective study that included patients with moderate–severe OSA and MS who had not undergone previous CPAP therapy. All subjects underwent clinical examination and arterial stiffness assessment using the oscillometric technique with Arteriograph (TensioMed, Budapest, Hungary) detection before and after 8-week CPAP therapy. Results: 39 patients with moderate–severe OSA were included. Eight weeks of CPAP therapy significantly improved central systolic blood pressure ($\Delta = -11.4$ mmHg, $p = 0.009$), aortic pulse wave velocity (aoPWV: $\Delta = -0.66$ m/s, $p = 0.03$), and aortic augmentation index (aoAix: $\Delta = -8.25\%$, $p = 0.01$) only in patients who used the device for a minimum of 4 h/night ($n = 20$). Conclusions: Arterial stiffness was improved only among CPAP adherent patients and could be detected using the Arteriograph (TensioMed, Budapest, Hungary), which involves a noninvasive procedure that is easy to implement for the clinical evaluation of arterial stiffness.

Keywords: arterial stiffness; Arteriograph; obstructive sleep apnea (OSA); continuous positive airway pressure (CPAP); metabolic syndrome (MS); adherence

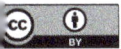

1. Introduction

Aging and cardiometabolic disease generates morphological and functional changes in the arterial wall, inducing endothelial dysfunction of the small vessels and stiffening of the larger arteries. The reduced compliance of the arterial wall leads to increased pulse wave travel velocities (PWV) and to an earlier reflection of the systolic pulse wave from peripheral bifurcation points [1]. PWV, the most direct measure of arterial stiffness [2], is generally associated with cardiovascular mortality in general and with all-cause mortality among subjects with arterial hypertension [3]. Carotid–femoral pulse wave velocity PWV (cfPWV) [4] is the reference technique for arterial stiffness assessment; however, measurements are time consuming and difficult to implement in routine clinical practice [5], resulting in arterial stiffness assessment being almost exclusively a research activity [4]. Consequently, the results using an oscillometric technique (Arteriograph, TensioMed, Budapest, Hungary) have been validated compared to an invasive method (cardiac catheterization) [5,6]. Studies that have compared the results using the Arteriograph (TensioMed, Budapest, Hungary) to those obtained using the standard arterial stiffness assessment methods showed similar Aix (augmentation index) and PWV (pulse wave velocity) values despite the fact that the techniques are not interchangeable [5,7,8]. The Arteriograph (TensioMed, Budapest, Hungary) calculates central (aortic) pulse wave velocity (aoPWV), aortic augmentation (aoAix), and central (aortic) systolic blood pressure (aoSBP). PWV and Aix are both cardiovascular risk factor predictors [5,9,10]. However, while PWV reflects only the studied arterial segment Aix is influenced by the characteristics of the entire arterial system that participates in pulse wave reflection [11].

Obstructive sleep apnea (OSA) is defined as a form of sleep-disordered breathing in which repetitive collapse of the upper respiratory airways induces iterative episodes of apnea and hypopnea, leading to micro-awakenings, fragmented sleep, depression, and a poor quality of life [12,13]. OSA is associated with altered intrathoracic pressure balance, overactivation of the sympathetic nervous system, and renin-angiotensin systems, along with pro-inflammatory status and oxidative stress [12,14–16], which promote and aggravate arterial stiffening [11,17], especially in patients with associated high blood pressure (HBP) or metabolic syndrome (MS) [11]. The impact of continuous positive airway pressure (CPAP) therapy on arterial stiffening in OSA patients remains conflicting [12,14,18–20], being dependent on OSA severity [21], daytime sleepiness [22], patient comorbidities [14,19], and CPAP adherence [21]. Several reports have shown a significant decrease in PWV after 1–6 months of CPAP therapy [20,23–25]. Information regarding the long-term effect of CPAP is scarce, with a previous study [26] showing that PWV decreases over the first 6 months before gradually increasing from 6 to 24 months (without exceeding baseline values) [23].

Metabolic syndrome is frequently associated with OSA [27,28], but it is also associated with an accelerated progression of arterial stiffening [29]. CPAP increases the chance of reversing arterial stiffening in patients with moderate–severe OSA [30], but Garleneau et al. [31] reported that arterial stiffening progression in obese OSA patients at 5-year follow-up was not influenced by CPAP adherence. Furthermore, a previous meta-analysis found that the proportion of adherent patients does not impact the benefit of CPAP on arterial stiffness [18].

There are debates on whether arterial stiffness improves under CPAP therapy in OSA patients with MS. The purpose of this pilot study was to use oscillometry (via Arteriograph (TensioMed, Budapest, Hungary) detection) to verify if there are differences in the progression of arterial stiffness in moderate–severe OSA patients with MS after receiving short-term (8 weeks) CPAP therapy. Second, we analyzed the relationship between OSA severity and arterial stiffness parameters.

2. Materials and Methods
2.1. Patients

Clinically stable patients with newly diagnosed moderate or severe OSA and MS, were prospectively recruited in the IIIrd Pneumology Clinic in Iași from January to December 2018, prior to the initiation of CPAP therapy. Moderate or severe OSA was diagnosed as having apnea–hypopnea Index (AHI) values of 15–30 events/h and >30 events/h, respectively. MS was diagnosed according to the American Heart Association/National Heart, Lung, and Blood Institute updated National Cholesterol Education Program—Adult Treatment Panel III criteria [32], which requires the presence of at least three of the following factors: fasting glucose ≥ 100 mg/dL or current treatment for diabetes, high blood pressure or current blood pressure-lowering treatment, abdominal obesity (waist circumference ≥ 102 cm for males and ≥ 88 cm for females), hypertriglyceridemia (TG levels > 150 mg/dL or current treatment for hypertriglyceridemia), high-density lipoprotein (HDL) cholesterol < 40 mg/dL for males and < 50 mg/dL for females or current treatment with statins. The 2018 European guidelines for the management of hypertension specifically recommend the use of ambulatory blood pressure monitoring (ABPM) in OSA patients [4]. As such, we defined high blood pressure as mean 24 h blood pressure (BP) ≥ 130/80 mmHg, mean daytime BP ≥ 135/85 mmHg, or mean nighttime BP ≥ 120/70 mmHg [4]. An OSA diagnosis was established by ambulatory or in-hospital six-channel cardiorespiratory polygraphy, using either a Philips Respironics Alice Night One or a DeVilbiss Porti 7 device. The recordings were manually scored by experienced sleep physiologists, according to the third International Classification of Sleep Disorders criteria [33]. Apnea was defined as a reduction in oro-nasal airflow by ≥90% for at least 10 s. Hypopnea was defined as a reduction in oro-nasal airflow by ≥30% for at least 10 s, that is associated with a ≥3% decrease in peripheral oxygen saturation. CPAP effective pressure autotitration in the sleep laboratory was determined using DreamStation Auto CPAP (Philips Respironics, Murrysville, PA, USA), REMstar Auto C-Flex CPAP (Philips Respironics, Murrysville, PA, USA), or a AirSense 10 Autoset CPAP (ResMed, San Diego, CA, USA). Follow-up cardiorespiratory polygraphy data were not collected due to the short follow-up of patients (8 weeks). Daytime sleepiness was assessed using the standard Epworth questionnaire at baseline and after 8-week CPAP therapy. The questionnaire was completed in the presence of a trained medical professional who offered guidance when necessary.

The exclusion criteria were prior CPAP therapy, central sleep apnea, use of supplemental oxygen, non-OSA primary sleep disorder, major surgery or acute medical conditions in the prior 30 days, prior cardiovascular events, psychological disturbances, alcohol dependence, or other chronic diseases except metabolic syndrome.

All patients signed a written informed consent for inclusion. The study was conducted in accordance with the Declaration of Helsinki [34], and the protocol was approved by the Ethics Committee of the Grigore T. Popa University of Medicine and Pharmacy in Iași (ethical approval code 1183/17.01.2018).

2.2. Study Design

After OSA diagnosis, the patients were admitted to the Cardiovascular Rehabilitation Clinic of the Rehabilitation Hospital in Iași, Romania. Subjects underwent standard clinical examination and biological panel, ambulatory blood pressure monitoring (ABPM), and Epworth questionnaire. All patients were informed of the need for daily CPAP use and the importance of a healthy lifestyle (diet and exercise); no change was made to their current drug regimen. OSA patients received standard CPAP therapy with DreamStation Auto CPAP (Philips Respironics, Murrysville, PA, USA), REMstar Auto C-Flex CPAP (Philips Respironics, Murrysville, PA, USA), or AirSense 10 AutoSet CPAP (ResMed, San Diego, CA, USA). OSA patients were reevaluated in the same clinic, using the same procedures, 8 weeks after initiating CPAP therapy. After assessing CPAP adherence (at the 8-week follow-up), we divided our initial study population into two subgroups: adherent and nonadherent patients. Adherence was defined as a device usage time ≥ 4 h/night, while nonadherence was defined as a CPAP usage time < 4 h/night [35].

In the a priori calculation of the sample size and according to previous results on the effects of 8-week CPAP therapy on the arterial stiffness [12], we estimated that at least eight subjects were required for each subgroup to detect a mean absolute maximal improvement difference in Aix of 6.4%, after treatment, at a significance level α of 5%, β cut-off of 20% and statistical power of 80%. A previous meta-analysis reported an average adherence rate to CPAP of 83% (with a variation from 40 to 100%) [18]. As such, we recruited 39 patients to obtain at least 13 patients for each group.

2.3. Measurements

2.3.1. Body Measurements

All measurements were performed three times. Height and weight were assessed without shoes and with light clothing in the morning. Body mass index (BMI) was calculated as weight (kg)/height (m^2). Waist circumference (WC) was measured at the end of a normal expiration, horizontally at the top of the right iliac crest, ensuring that the tape was snug, without compressing the patients' skin.

2.3.2. Smoking Status

Smoking status was classified as current smoker, former smoker, and never smoker, according to the National Health Interview Survey (NHIS) definition [36].

2.3.3. CPAP Adherence

CPAP adherence data (device usage, hours per night at the prescribed pressure) was recorded by the machine and downloaded using the appropriate software: Encore Pro 2 v.2.17 (Philips Respironics, Murrysville, PA, USA), EncoreBasic v.2.1 (Philips Respironics, Murrysville, PA, USA), or ResScan v.6.0 (ResMed, San Diego, CA, USA). Adherence was defined by the time of CPAP use ($\geq$4 h/night).

2.3.4. ABPM

The ABPM monitoring was performed with the DMS-300 ABP device (DM Software, Stateline, NV, USA) and was interpreted by an experienced cardiologist. The frequency of daytime (6:00–22:00) and nighttime (22:00–6:00) measurements was set at 30 and 60 min, respectively. The recording was considered satisfactory if it included at least 70% of the expected measurements. The first ABPM was performed before the initiation of CPAP. The second ABPM was performed after 8 weeks, with a full night of controlled CPAP use at home (data regarding accumulated CPAP use/56 days obtained from the device smart card).

2.3.5. Holter-ECG

The Holter-ECG monitoring was performed using the three-channel DMS-300 4A Cardioscan (DM Software Stateline, NV, USA) device. The seven electrodes were positioned according to the Standard B pattern, following the manufacturer's instructions [37]. The duration of the recording was 24 h. All recordings were manually interpreted by an experienced cardiologist. The first Holter-ECG was performed before the initiation of CPAP. The second Holter-ECG monitoring was performed after 8 weeks, with a full night of controlled CPAP use.

2.3.6. Assessment of Arterial Function

All patients underwent arterial stiffness assessment, before and after 8-week CPAP therapy, with the Arteriograph (TensioMed, Budapest, Hungary), using an appropriate cuff size, according to the patient's arm circumference [38]. The 2 month re-evaluation of arterial stiffness was performed after a night of controlled CPAP use. The examination was conducted by a single operator, from 9:00 to 10:00 in accordance with the manufacturer's instructions [38], in a quiet, temperature-controlled environment, after at least a 10 min rest period. The patient was not allowed to speak or move during the examination. Alcohol, caffeine, and smoking were not permitted 10 h prior to the examination. Central (aortic) systolic blood pressure (aoSBP), central (aortic) pulse pressure (aoPP), aortic augmentation index (aoAix), and aortic pulse wave velocity (aoPWV) were measured.

2.4. Statistical Analysis

The results were expressed as mean ± standard deviation or median (25th and 75th percentiles) for continuous variables and as percentages (%) for categorical variables. Statistical analysis was performed in SPSS v 20.0, using paired Student's t-test and the

Mann–Whitney U test for comparisons between groups for parametric and non-parametric variables, respectively. A linear mixed model using BMI as a covariate was performed for arterial stiffness parameters before and after CPAP. A potential relationship between variables was evaluated using the Pearson correlation coefficient. A p-value < 0.05 was considered the threshold for statistical significance.

3. Results
3.1. All Patients

Of the 154 patients referred to our sleep unit between January and December 2018, 55 met the inclusion criteria. Of the remaining subjects, 20 had OSA but no MS, and 16 patients were lost during follow-up (Figure 1).

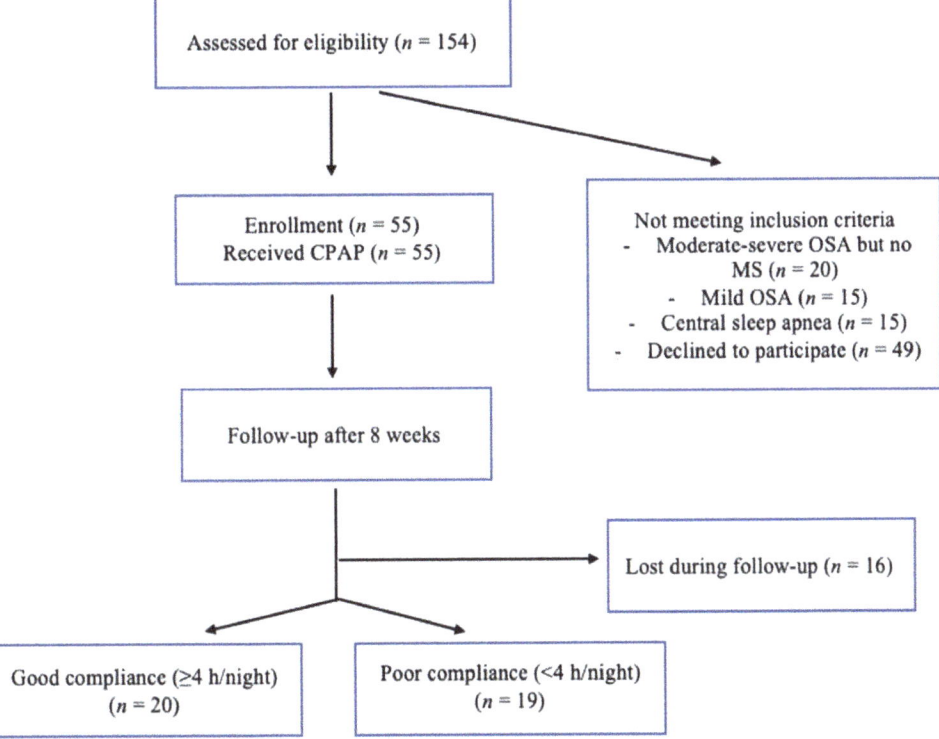

Figure 1. Flowchart diagram of patients examined in the sleep unit between January and December 2018; OSA: obstructive sleep apnea; MS: metabolic syndrome; CPAP: continuous positive airway therapy.

Our final study group included 39 patients (29 males and 10 females) with moderate–severe OSA and MS. The demographic, anthropometric, biochemical, and cardiorespiratory polygraphy characteristics are reported in Table 1. The average CPAP use in our entire study population (39 patients) was 4.0 ± 1.0 h/night. Average CPAP use was 2.3 ± 1.0 h/night and 6.1 ± 1.2 h/night in the non-adherent and adherent subgroups, respectively. The use of anti-hypertensive, anti-diabetic, and lipid-lowering medications were balanced across the two subgroups (Figure 2).

Table 1. Baseline demographic, anthropometric, biochemical, and cardiorespiratory polygraphy characteristics in the study population.

	All Patients (n = 39)	Adherent (n = 20)	Non-Adherent (n = 19)	p-Value [#]
Age (years)	57 ± 9	60 ± 7	55 ± 10	0.080
Smoking status				
Current smoker (%)	12.8%	5%	21.1%	0.133
Former smoker (%)	56.4%	55%	57.9%	0.857
Never smoker	30.8%	40%	21.1%	0.200
Weight (kg)	101 ± 17	97 ± 17	105 ± 16	0.143
BMI (kg/m^2)	33.8 ± 4.7	32.9 ± 4.8	34.7 ± 4.8	0.224
WC (cm)	114 ± 10	112 ± 10	116 ± 10	0.181
Blood tests				
Fasting blood glucose (mg/dL)	112.31 ± 19.84	111.77 ± 13.4	112.89 ± 25.31	0.863
HDL-cholesterol (mg/dL)	50.58 ± 12.87	52.80 ± 14.76	48.23 ± 10.41	0.274
TG (mg/dL)	167.44 ± 86.09	154.95 ± 98.88	180.60 ± 70.50	0.359
OSA parameters				
AHI (events/h)	39.7 ± 19.5	35.9 ± 15.9	45.4 ± 22.7	0.142
DI (events/h)	38.6 ± 18.4	35.6 ± 15.1	41.7 ± 21.4	0.312
Mean nocturnal O_2Sa (%)	91.8 ± 2.6	91.8 ± 2.5	91.8 ± 2.7	0.907
ESS (points)	6.2 ± 3.9	6.9 ± 3.9	5.4 ± 3.9	0.245
CPAP pressure (cmH$_2$0)	10.9 ± 2.3	11.5 ± 2.1	10.4 ± 2.5	0.159

Data are presented as mean ± SD. BMI: body mass index; WC: waist circumference; HDL: high-density lipoproteins; TG: triglycerides; OSA: obstructive sleep apnea; AHI: apnea–hypopnea index; DI: desaturation index; O_2Sa: oxygen saturation; ESS: Epworth sleepiness score; CPAP: continuous positive airway pressure; [#]: comparison between adherent and non-adherent subgroups.

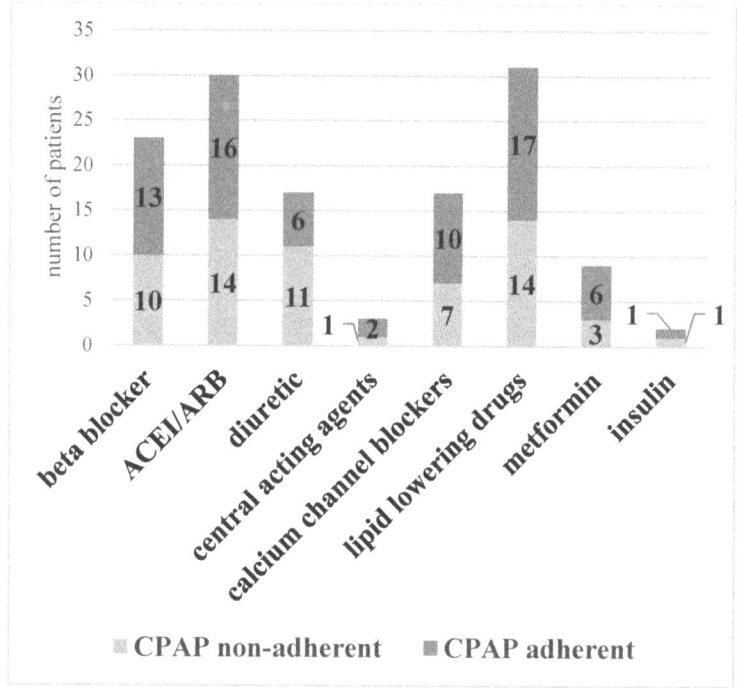

Figure 2. The use of anti-hypertensive, anti-diabetic, and lipid-lowering medications in the two subgroups, CPAP non-adherent and CPAP adherent. ACEI: angiotensin-converting enzyme inhibitors, ARB: angiotensin receptor blockers; CPAP: continuous positive airway pressure.

3.2. Comparison between Groups

After 8-week CPAP therapy, we observed a statistically significant decrease in almost all arterial stiffness parameters (aoSBP, aoAix, and aoPWV) only in the CPAP adherent subgroup (Table 2). Both subgroups exhibited minor, but statistically significant changes in weight, BMI, and WC; however, this was not the case with BP and HR values, where no significant changes were observed (Table 2).

Table 2. Impact of 8-week CPAP therapy on arterial stiffness parameters in our study group.

	All Patients (n = 39)			Adherent (n = 20)			Non-Adherent (n = 19)		
	Baseline	After 8-Week CPAP	p-Value	Baseline	After 8-Week CPAP	p-Value	Baseline	After 8-Week CPAP	p-Value
Age (years)	57 ± 9			60 ± 7			55 ± 10		
Weight (kg)	101 ± 17	98 ± 16	0.007	97 ± 17	95 ± 16	0.002	105 ± 16	102 ± 16	0.016
BMI (kg/m2)	33.7 ± 4.7	33.0 ± 4.6	0.0001	32.9 ± 4.8	32.3 ± 4.5	0.002	34.7 ± 4.8	33.8 ± 4.8	0.018
WC (cm)	114 ± 10	111 ± 11	<0.0001	112 ± 10	109 ± 10	0.000	116 ± 10	112 ± 12	0.002
ESS (points)	6.2 ± 3.9	3.1 ± 2.7	0.0001	6.9 ± 3.9	3.2 ± 2.5	0.0007	5.4 ± 3.9	3.1 ± 3.1	0.049
ABPM (mmHg)									
Mean SBP/24 h	129 ± 14	130 ± 13	0.597	129 ± 16	132 ± 9	0.372	129 ± 13	129 ± 15	0.965
Mean DBP/24 h	76 ± 8	75 ± 8	0.372	74 ± 7	75 ± 5	0.846	78 ± 8	75 ± 10	0.268
Mean daytime SBP	131 ± 16	133 ± 13	0.527	130 ± 19	134 ± 10	0.390	132 ± 13	132 ± 15	0.974
Mean daytime DBP	78 ± 9	77 ± 8	0.859	75 ± 10	77 ± 5	0.304	81 ± 8	78 ± 10	0.294
Mean nighttime SBP	122 ± 15	123 ± 14	0.877	125 ± 15	125 ± 11	0.936	120 ± 15	121 ± 17	0.796
Mean nighttime SBP	71 ± 10	68 ± 9	0.243	71 ± 8	69 ± 7	0.326	71 ± 12	68 ± 11	0.459
Holter ECG monitoring									
Mean HR/24 h (bpm)	71 ± 10	70 ± 9	0.641	70 ± 12	70 ± 10	0.526	70 ± 10	71 ± 8	0.175
Arterial stiffness									
aoSBP (mmHg)	122 ± 19	115 ± 13	0.029	125 ± 22	114 ± 15	0.009	118 ± 15	116 ± 13	0.696
aoPP (mmHg)	43.9 ± 11.9	41.9 ± 10.2	0.248	46.4 ± 13.4	42.4 ± 9.8	0.090	41.2 ± 9.9	41.6 ± 10.9	0.864
aoAix (%)	28.4 ± 15.2	24.7 ± 15.1	0.061	32.6 ± 16.2	24.3 ± 15.7	0.013	24.0 ± 13.1	25.2 ± 14.9	0.481
aoPWV (m/s)	9.3 ± 1.7	8.5 ± 1.4	0.004	9.2 ± 1.8	8.5 ± 1.3	0.036	9.3 ± 1.7	8.6 ± 1.6	0.057

Data are presented as mean ± SD. BMI: body mass index; WC: waist circumference; ESS: Epworth sleepiness score; SBP: systolic blood pressure; DBP: diastolic blood pressure; HR: heart rate; aoSBP: aortic systolic blood pressure; aoPP: central (aortic) pulse pressure; aoAix: aortic augmentation index; aoPWV: aortic pulse wave velocity.

After adjusting for BMI (linear mixed method), changes in aoPWV, aoAix and aoSBP remained significant in the adherent subgroup, but not among non-adherent patients, as follows: $p = 0.004$, 0.032 and 0.050 for aoPWV in all subjects, adherent and non-adherent patients, respectively; $p = 0.024$, 0.006 and 0.688 for aoSBP in all subjects, adherent and non-adherent patients, respectively; and $p = 0.058$, 0.011 and 0.468 for aoAix in all subjects, adherent and non-adherent patients, respectively. The change in aoPP was not significant in any of the analyzed subgroups after adjusting for BMI (linear mixed model).

The prevalence of patients with aoPWV > 10 m/s decreased from 35.89% (baseline) to 12.82% (after CPAP), $p < 0.00001$. A similar trend ($p < 0.00001$) was observed in the adherent and non-adherent subgroups (35% to 15% and 36.84% to 15%, respectively) (Figure 3).

3.3. Correlations between Arterial Stiffness and OSA Parameters

Mean nocturnal O_2Sa was significantly correlated with weight, BMI, and WC as well as exhibited a strong indirect correlation with aoPWV ($r = -0.507$, $p = 0.0009$) (Figure 4).

AHI was significantly correlated with the other OSA severity parameters, but not with age ($p = 0.10$) or arterial stiffness variables (Table 3).

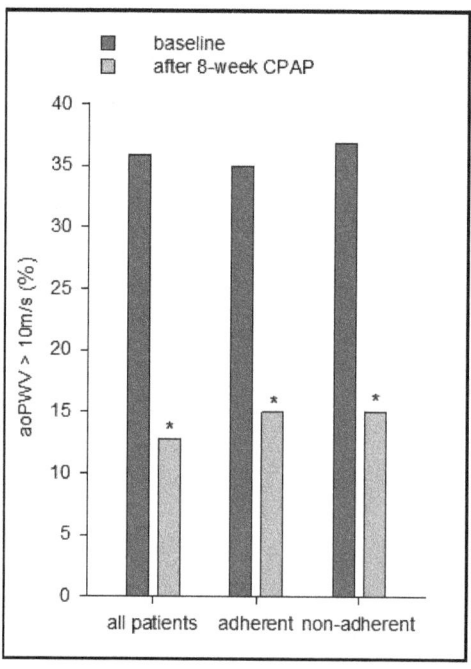

Figure 3. The prevalence of patients with aoPWV > 10 m/s at baseline and after 8-week CPAP therapy in the study population. aoPWV: aortic pulse wave velocity; CPAP: continuous positive airway pressure; *: $p < 0.00001$ vs. baseline.

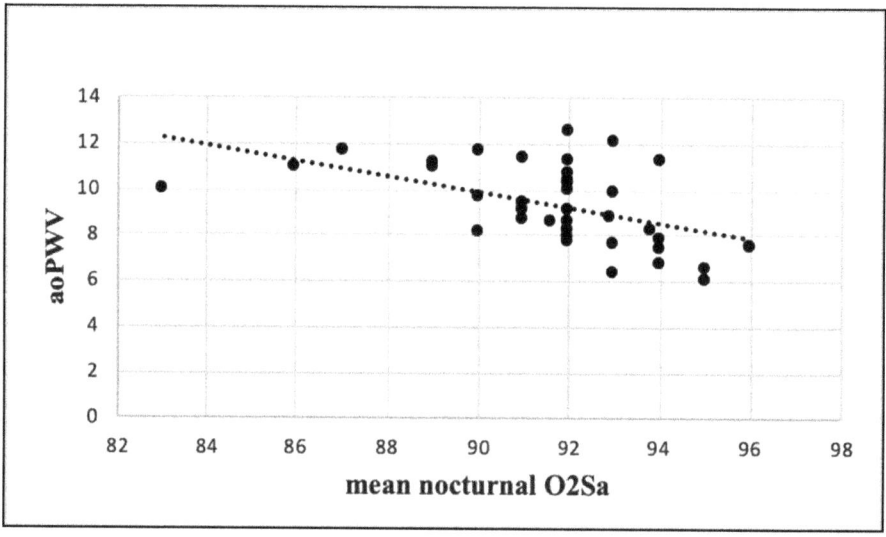

Figure 4. Correlation between aoPWV and mean nocturnal O2Sa. aoPWV: aortic pulse wave velocity; O_2Sa: oxygen saturation.

Table 3. Correlations between OSA parameters with demographic and arterial stiffness parameters ($n = 39$).

	AHI r	p-Value	Mean Nocturnal O_2Sa r	p-Value
AHI	-	-	−0.353	**0.027**
Mean nocturnal O_2Sa (%)	−0.353	**0.027**	—	-
Desaturation index (events/h)	0.964	**<0.0000001**	−0.390	**0.013**
Age	−0.009	0.956	−0.101	0.537
Weight	0.257	0.112	−0.402	**0.010**
BMI	0.294	0.069	−0.469	**0.002**
WC	0.310	0.054	−0.568	**0.0001**
ESS	−0.088	0.598	−0.248	0.133
aoSBP (mmHg)	0.026	0.872	0.015	0.923
aoPP (mmHg)	−0.075	0.646	0.082	0.616
aoAix (%)	−0.235	0.149	0.201	0.218
aoPWV (m/s)	0.264	0.103	−0.507	**0.0009**

AHI: apnea–hypopnea index; O_2Sa: oxygen saturation; BMI: body mass index; WC: waist circumference; ESS: Epworth sleepiness score; aoSBP: aortic systolic blood pressure; aoPP: aortic pulse pressure; aoAix: aortic augmentation index; aoPWV: aortic pulse wave velocity. Values in bold indicate statistically significant results.

4. Discussion

Our study showed that short-term CPAP therapy significantly improved the arterial stiffness parameters in patients with moderate–severe OSA and MS; however, the benefit is greatly influenced by CPAP adherence, remaining statistically significant only in patients who used the device for >4 h/night. CPAP adherence in our study (51.28%) was significantly lower than that in previous reports [18,39], but similar to that observed by Dorkova et al. [40] in patients with severe OSA and MS. The poor CPAP adherence could be explained by the relatively low average ESS score observed in our study group [41], as well as by the presence of MS per se [42].

Determination using SphygmoCor (AtCor Medical, Sydney, Australia) or Complior (Artech Medical, Pantin, France) is the gold-standard for arterial stiffness evaluation [5]. However, cfPWV measurement is associated with a risk of carotid plaque rupture in the elderly and requires exposure of the groin area [5], thus limiting its routine clinical use. On the other hand, the advantages of Arteriograph (TensioMed, Budapest, Hungary) include the higher reproducibility of parameters, due to the simple and time-effective methodology [5]. Although it has been suggested that the Arteriograph (TensioMed, Budapest, Hungary) actually measures axillo-brachial stiffness (a parameter closely correlated with aoPWV) [43], the results we obtained with the Arteriograph (TensioMed, Budapest, Hungary) are similar to those obtained by standard devices used for arterial stiffness assessment [5,7,8]. Furthermore, a previous RCT found no difference between PWV measurements using SphygmoCor (AtCor Medical, Sydney, Australia) and Arteriograph (TensioMed, Budapest, Hungary) [44]. AoPWV measured using Complior (Artech Medical, Pantin, France) is significantly higher than that obtained using SphygmoCor (AtCor Medical, Sydney, Australia) or Arteriograph (TensioMed, Budapest, Hungary), mostly due to the different techniques used to measure pulse wave travel distance [44]. In order to avoid unnecessary bias due to the jugulum-pubic symphysis range, we used the first measured value for both Arteriograph (TensioMed, Budapest, Hungary) evaluations.

The mean aoPWV in our study group was only 9.26 ± 1.73 m/s, and 35.89% of our patients had a baseline PWV value > 10 m/s. Short-term CPAP was associated with a decrease in the prevalence of patients with PWV > 10 m/s ($\Delta = -23.07\%$, $p < 0.00001$). OSA patients who associate hypertension or metabolic syndrome present the highest degree of arterial stiffening [11]. The initial threshold for PWV of 12 m/s proposed by the 2016 European guidelines on cardiovascular disease prevention [45] has been revised by the more recent 2018 guidelines for the management of arterial hypertension [4], in which a carotid-femoral PWV (cfPWV) > 10 m/s is considered a marker of asymptomatic hypertension-mediated organ damage (HMOD).

The arterial stiffness parameters were not significantly different between our moderate and severe OSA subgroups (data not shown). Similarly, Protogerou et al. [46] did not find statistically significant differences concerning PWV and Aix between patients suffering from moderate, severe, and very severe OSA in the presence of cardiovascular comorbidities. Most studies support an independent, dose-response association between OSA and elevated arterial stiffness parameters [11,17]. In accordance with two recent meta analyses [47,48], AHI was not correlated with the degree of arterial stiffening. However contrary to the results of Joyeux-Faure et al. [48], in our analysis aoPWV was strongly correlated with mean nocturnal O_2Sa, which was also associated with weight, BMI, and WC. Our results are in line with the "hypoxemic burden" theory in OSA patients, in which an integrated symptom–comorbidity approach aims to replace AHI as the central parameter in the OSA treatment algorithm [41].

Despite the lack of a significant correlation between arterial stiffness and AHI, we found that short-term CPAP therapy significantly improved AoPWV by 0.66 m/s in our CPAP adherent subgroup, which is in accordance with a recent meta-analysis that showed that CPAP decreases arterial stiffness by 0.65 m/s in hypertensive patients [19]. Buchner et al. [49] also observed significant improvements in both Aix and PWV values (SphygmoCor) after 6 months of CPAP; this was only among the 49 effectively treated OSA patients, thus emphasizing the importance of CPAP adherence. Contrary to our results, in the study by Buchner et al. [49], the decrease in central SBP after CPAP among OSA adherent patients was not statistically significant. Differences in anti-hypertensive regimens between our study groups could explain this inconsistency.

CPAP reduces PWV (Complior, Artech Medical, Pantin, France) in patients with severe OSA, even in the absence of associated cardiovascular disease [20]. Interestingly, the PWV changes were correlated with improvements in C reactive protein serum concentrations [20], isolating OSA as an independent risk factor for both atherosclerosis and systemic inflammation. On the other hand, Jones et al. [14], in a double-blind placebo-controlled trial, reported that 12-week CPAP therapy did not significantly influence Aix or PWV in a group of 43 OSA patients without associated cardiometabolic comorbidities. However, the study population of Jones et al. [14] had significantly lower average AHI and BMI values compared with our study group (31 events/h and 29.9 kg/m^2, respectively) and a baseline PWV of only 7.6 m/s (SphygmoCor, AtCor Medical, Sydney, Australia).

Medium-term CPAP use (6 months) was associated with a reduction in nighttime BP and arterial stiffness in patients with coexisting cardiovascular disease and OSA in a study by Picard et al. [50], but had no impact on arterial stiffness in patients with moderate–severe OSA and resistant HBP in another report by Cardoso et al. [51]. Kohler et al. [24] reported significant changes in Aix and mean arterial BP after only 4 weeks of therapeutic CPAP. One other study [25] evaluated CPAP-induced arterial stiffness changes in OSA patients with MS and reported significant improvements after 12 weeks of therapeutic CPAP [25].

Arterial stiffness is a composite measure of vascular health and an independent predictor of cardiovascular events [18]. Each 1 m/s increase in PWV is associated with a 15% increase in both cardiovascular and all-cause mortality [52]. As such, even a mild decrease in PWV can be clinically relevant, especially in patients with MS who are at increased cardiovascular risk. Recent studies have questioned whether arterial stiffness assessment using an oscillometric method (Mobil-O-Graph) can be used to predict cardiovascular outcome, since the measured PWV is highly dependent on patient's age and SBP [53,54]. Although similar limitations could be attributed to the Arteriograph (TensioMed, Budapest, Hungary) device, aoPWV and aoSBP improvement occurred in the absence of statistically significant BP or HR variations (the most important confounding factors for PWV [29]), and remained significant after BMI adjustment. The mild decrease in aoPWV can be explained by the rather low baseline aoPWV ("pathological" values of >10 m/s [4] in only 35% of patients; Figure 1), by the short follow-up duration (8 weeks) and by the low initial ESS score [41]. CPAP seems to be more effective in improving BP in symptomatic OSA patients (excessive sleepiness) with associated cardiovascular comorbidities, including MS

Although aoSBP improved in CPAP adherent patients (Δ = −11.4 mmHg), average 24 h BP remained unaffected, suggesting that excessive sleepiness could be a more important predictor for positive CPAP effect on BP than the presence of MS.

Interestingly, it was previously shown [26] that while PWV decreases over the first 6 months, it gradually increases during the following 18 months, without exceeding the baseline value. While this can be explained by the direct effect of aging and OSA on arterial stiffening, CPAP adherence and changes in chronic medication are important confounding factors and should be considered in the interpretation of these findings [23].

Despite being markedly dependent on cardiac characteristics and vascular tone (which are, in turn, altered in the presence of obesity in MS), Aix is sometimes used as a substitute parameter for arterial stiffness assessment [48]. A previous randomized trial reported a significant reduction in Aix after only one month of CPAP [24] and another study [12] reported that 8-week CPAP therapy improved morning (but not evening) Aix (Δ = 6.49%). Despite the identical therapy duration, the authors reported no improvement concerning PWV values, possibly due to preexisting irreversible OSA-related vascular damage [12]. Another explanation for the lack of significant PWV reduction is the relatively low prevalence of hypertension (63.9%). Furthermore, the study population of Paz y Mar et al. [12] included a high percentage of African Americans (45%) and females (47.3%) but had a significantly lower average AHI (19.3 events/h).

Smoking status is an important confounder in arterial stiffness assessment [55]. Smoking is not permitted 10 h prior to Arteriograph (TensioMed, Budapest, Hungary) measurement, which could bias BP and arterial stiffness parameters in heavy smokers. We limited this confounding factor by scheduling an early Arteriograph (TensioMed, Budapest, Hungary) measurement (9.00 a.m.–10.00 a.m.).

Whether CPAP impacts on anthropometric parameters is controversial [56,57]. Our study group exhibited mild weight loss after 8 weeks of CPAP. All subjects received standard advice regarding diet and exercise as part of a healthy lifestyle; therefore weight-loss should not be attributed to CPAP only. Adherence to lifestyle changes was not the purpose of this study and was not quantified. Similar to other studies of short or medium-term CPAP therapy on arterial stiffness [20,24,49,51], we performed only a baseline evaluation of OSA severity.

To the best of our knowledge, our study is the first to use the Arteriograph (TensioMed, Budapest, Hungary) device to analyze the effect of CPAP on arterial stiffness in OSA patients with MS. Although the use of oschillometry to evaluate arterial stiffness has been recently criticized, the gold-standard evaluation of cfPWV is difficult to implement in clinical practice, as it is time-consuming, operator-dependent and subject to significant errors regarding the anatomical estimation of arterial length [53]. The impact of positive airway therapy on PWV and Aix is influenced by treatment duration and patient characteristics, i.e., daytime sleepiness, smoking status, medication, cardiovascular comorbidities, apnea severity and OSA duration before diagnosis [55]. Anti-hypertensive drugs are effective in reducing arterial stiffness [58], with significant variations between classes and within the same class [59]. However, the impact of these drugs on arterial stiffness parameters is partly (or mostly) attributable to their ability to reduce SBP values [58], which remained unchanged in our study group. The use of lipid-lowering and anti-diabetic drugs was relatively balanced between the two study groups. Subgroup analysis regarding the effect of each class of medicine on arterial stiffness parameters measured with the Arteriograph (TensioMed, Budapest, Hungary) was irrelevant due to the small number of patients, but should be addressed in future research.

Our analysis shows that the beneficial effects of CPAP on arterial stiffness are apparent only in adherent patients and occur in the early stages of CPAP therapy, in the absence of significant changes in mean BP or HR values. The oscillometric evaluation of arterial stiffness can be easily performed in daily practice and can be used as a surrogate marker of CPAP adherence, which could motivate the patient to use the device accordingly. As

OSA and metabolic syndrome are cumulative cardiovascular risk factors, special attention should be given to patient education regarding optimal CPAP use.

5. Conclusions

Short-term (8 weeks) CPAP significantly reduced values for the aortic pulse wave velocity (aoPWV: $\Delta = -0.66$ m/s, $p = 0.03$), aortic augmentation index (aoAix: $\Delta = -8.25\%$, $p = 0.01$) and central systolic blood pressure ($\Delta = -11.4$ mmHg, $p = 0.009$) only in the CPAP adherent subgroup of OSA patients with MS. The Arteriograph (TensioMed, Budapest, Hungary) device is a noninvasive and time-effective way to assess arterial stiffness in patients with moderate–severe OSA and MS, yielding an in-depth analysis of individual cardiovascular risk.

Author Contributions: Conceptualization, I.M.Z. and F.M.; data curation, I.M.Z. and C.M.G.; formal analysis, C.M.G. and L.C.D.-C.; investigation, C.S., R.A.S., M.R., L.A., D.B., R.A. and S.R.C.; methodology, I.M.Z. and C.M.G.; project administration, I.M.Z. and F.M.; resources, D.B. and F.M.; software, C.M.G. and M.R.; supervision, F.M.; validation, L.C.D.-C.; visualization, I.M.Z., O.M., S.R.C. and L.C.D.-C.; writing—original draft, I.M.Z.; writing—review and editing, I.M.Z., C.S., R.A.S., O.M., C.M.G., S.R.C., L.C.D.-C. and F.M. All authors have read and agreed to the published version of the manuscript.

Funding: This research received no external funding.

Institutional Review Board Statement: The study was conducted according to the guidelines of the Declaration of Helsinki, and ap-proved by the Ethics Committee of the Grigore T. Popa University of Medicine and Pharmacy in Iași, Romania (protocol code 1183; approval date 17 January 2018).

Informed Consent Statement: Informed consent was obtained from all subjects involved in the study

Conflicts of Interest: M.R. and D.B. have received financial support for conference attendance from Linde Gas and Vital Aire.

References

1. Akkus, O.; Sahin, D.Y.; Bozkurt, A.; Nas, K.; Ozcan, K.S.; Illyés, M.; Molnár, F.; Demir, S.; Tüfenk, M.; Acarturk, E. Evaluation of arterial stiffness for predicting future cardiovascular events in patients with st segment elevation and non-st segment elevation myocardial infarction. *Sci. World J.* **2013**, *2013*, 1–6. [CrossRef]
2. Parati, G.; De Buyzere, M. Evaluating aortic stiffness through an arm cuff oscillometric device: Is validation against invasive measurements enough? *J. Hypertens.* **2010**, *28*, 2003–2006. [CrossRef] [PubMed]
3. Laurent, S.; Boutouyrie, P.; Asmar, R.; Gautier, I.; Laloux, B.; Guize, L.; Ducimetiere, P.; Benetos, A. Aortic stiffness is an independent predictor of all-cause and cardiovascular mortality in hypertensive patients. *Hypertension* **2001**, *37*, 1236–1241. [CrossRef] [PubMed]
4. Williams, B.; Mancia, G.; Spiering, W.; Rosei, E.A.; Azizi, M.; Burnier, M.; Clement, D.L.; Coca, A.; De Simone, G.; Dominiczak, A.; et al. 2018 ESC/ESH Guidelines for the management of arterial hypertension. *Eur. Heart J.* **2018**, *39*, 3021–3104. [CrossRef] [PubMed]
5. Boutouyrie, P.; Revera, M.; Parati, G. Obtaining arterial stiffness indices from simple arm cuff measurements: The holy grail? *J. Hypertens.* **2009**, *27*, 2159–2161. [CrossRef]
6. Baibata, E.D.; Cosor, O.C.; Mitu, F.; Iurciuc, M.; Mancas, S. Arterial stiffness and cardiovascular risk. *Rom. J. Cardiol.* **2016**, *26*, 450–454.
7. Jatoi, A.N.; Mahmud, A.; Bennett, K.; Feely, J. Assessment of arterial stiffness in hypertension: Comparison of oscillometric (Arteriograph), piezoelectronic (Complior) and tonometric (SphygmoCor) techniques*. *J. Hypertens.* **2009**, *27*, 2186–2191. [CrossRef]
8. Baulmann, J.; Schillings, U.; Rickert, S.; Uen, S.; Düsing, R.; Illyes, M.; Cziraki, A.; Nickenig, G.; Mengden, T. A new oscillometric method for assessment of arterial stiffness: Comparison with tonometric and piezo-electronic methods. *J. Hypertens.* **2008**, *26*, 523–528. [CrossRef]
9. Boutouyrie, P.; Tropeano, A.I.; Asmar, R.; Gautier, I.; Benetos, A.; Lacolley, P.; Laurent, S. Aortic stiffness is an independent predictor of primary coronary events in hypertensive patients: A longitudinal study. *Hypertension* **2002**, *39*, 10–15. [CrossRef]
10. Ring, M.; Eriksson, M.J.; Zierath, J.R.; Caidahl, K. Arterial stiffness estimation in healthy subjects: A validation of oscillometric (Arteriograph) and tonometric (SphygmoCor) techniques. *Hypertens. Res.* **2014**, *37*, 999–1007. [CrossRef]
11. Phillips, C.L.; Butlin, M.; Wong, K.K.; Avolio, A.P. Is obstructive sleep apnoea causally related to arterial stiffness? A critical review of the experimental evidence. *Sleep Med. Rev.* **2013**, *17*, 7–18. [CrossRef]

2. Mar, H.L.P.Y.; Hazen, S.L.; Tracy, R.P.; Strohl, K.P.; Auckley, D.; Bena, J.; Wang, L.; Walia, H.K.; Patel, S.; Mehra, R. Effect of Continuous Positive Airway Pressure on Cardiovascular Biomarkers. *Chest* **2016**, *150*, 80–90. [CrossRef] [PubMed]
3. Bercea, R.M.; Patacchioli, F.R.; Ghiciuc, C.M.; Cojocaru, E.; Mihaescu, T. Serum testosterone and depressive symptoms in severe OSA patients. *Andrologia* **2013**, *45*, 345–350. [CrossRef]
4. Jones, A.; Vennelle, M.; Connell, M.; McKillop, G.; Newby, D.E.; Douglas, N.J.; Riha, R.L. The effect of continuous positive airway pressure therapy on arterial stiffness and endothelial function in obstructive sleep apnea: A randomized controlled trial in patients without cardiovascular disease. *Sleep Med.* **2013**, *14*, 1260–1265. [CrossRef] [PubMed]
5. Ghiciuc, C.M.; Dima-Cozma, L.C.; Bercea, R.M.; Lupusoru, C.E.; Mihaescu, T.; Cozma, S.; Patacchioli, F.R. Imbalance in the diurnal salivary testosterone/cortisol ratio in men with severe obstructive sleep apnea: An observational study. *Braz. J. Otorhinolaryngol.* **2016**, *82*, 529–535. [CrossRef] [PubMed]
6. Ghiciuc, C.M.; Cozma, L.C.D.; Bercea, R.M.; Lupusoru, C.E.; Mihaescu, T.; Szalontay, A.; Gianfreda, A.; Patacchioli, F.R. Restoring the salivary cortisol awakening response through nasal continuous positive airway pressure therapy in obstructive sleep apnea. *Chronobiol. Int.* **2013**, *30*, 1024–1031. [CrossRef] [PubMed]
7. Doonan, R.J.; Scheffler, P.; Lalli, M.; Kimoff, R.J.; Petridou, E.; Daskalopoulos, E.M.; Daskalopoulou, S.S. Increased arterial stiffness in obstructive sleep apnea: A systematic review. *Hypertens. Res.* **2010**, *34*, 23–32. [CrossRef]
8. Vlachantoni, I.-T.; Dikaiakou, E.; Antonopoulos, C.N.; Stefanadis, C.; Daskalopoulou, S.S.; Petridou, E.T. Effects of continuous positive airway pressure (CPAP) treatment for obstructive sleep apnea in arterial stiffness: A meta-analysis. *Sleep Med. Rev.* **2013**, *17*, 19–28. [CrossRef]
9. Lin, X.; Chen, G.; Qi, J.; Chen, X.; Zhao, J.; Lin, Q. Effect of continuous positive airway pressure on arterial stiffness in patients with obstructive sleep apnea and hypertension: A meta-analysis. *Eur. Arch. Oto Rhino Laryngol.* **2016**, *273*, 4081–4088. [CrossRef]
10. Drager, L.F.; Bortolotto, L.A.; Figueiredo, A.C.; Krieger, E.M.; Lorenzi-Filho, G. Effects of Continuous Positive Airway Pressure on Early Signs of Atherosclerosis in Obstructive Sleep Apnea. *Am. J. Respir. Crit. Care Med.* **2007**, *176*, 706–712. [CrossRef]
11. Ning, Y.; Zhang, T.-S.; Wen, W.-W.; Li, K.; Yang, Y.-X.; Qin, Y.-W.; Zhang, H.-N.; Du, Y.-H.; Li, L.-Y.; Yang, S.; et al. Effects of continuous positive airway pressure on cardiovascular biomarkers in patients with obstructive sleep apnea: A meta-analysis of randomized controlled trials. *Sleep Breath.* **2018**, *23*, 77–86. [CrossRef]
12. Mineiro, M.A.; Da Silva, P.M.; Alves, M.; Papoila, A.L.; Gomes, M.J.M.; Cardoso, J. The role of sleepiness on arterial stiffness improvement after CPAP therapy in males with obstructive sleep apnea: A prospective cohort study. *BMC Pulm. Med.* **2017**, *17*, 1–8. [CrossRef] [PubMed]
13. Drager, L.F.; Lorenzi-Filho, G. Is CPAP preventing the long-term progression of arterial stiffness in patients with obstructive sleep apnea? *Hypertens. Res.* **2010**, *33*, 788–789. [CrossRef] [PubMed]
14. Kohler, M.; Pepperell, J.C.T.; Casadei, B.; Craig, S.; Crosthwaite, N.; Stradling, J.R.; Davies, R.J.O. CPAP and measures of cardiovascular risk in males with OSAS. *Eur. Respir. J.* **2008**, *32*, 1488–1496. [CrossRef] [PubMed]
15. Yandieva, A.; Ovsyannikov, K. Effect of CPAP-Treatment on the arterial stiffness and systemic inflammation in patients with metabolic syndrome and obstructive sleep apnea. *J. Clin. Exp. Cardiol.* **2017**, *8*, C1–C086.
16. Saito, T.; Saito, T.; Sugiyama, S.; Asai, K.; Yasutake, M.; Mizuno, K. Effects of long-term treatment for obstructive sleep apnea on pulse wave velocity. *Hypertens. Res.* **2010**, *33*, 844–849. [CrossRef] [PubMed]
17. Punjabi, N.M.; Caffo, B.S.; Goodwin, J.L.; Gottlieb, D.J.; Newman, A.B.; O'Connor, G.; Rapoport, D.; Redline, S.; Resnick, H.E.; Robbins, J.A.; et al. Sleep-Disordered Breathing and Mortality: A Prospective Cohort Study. *PLoS Med.* **2009**, *6*, e1000132. [CrossRef]
18. Cozma, S.; Dima-Cozma, L.; Ghiciuc, C.; Pasquali, V.; Saponaro, A.; Patacchioli, F. Salivary cortisol and α-amylase: Subclinical indicators of stress as cardiometabolic risk. *Braz. J. Med. Biol. Res.* **2017**, *50*, e5577. [CrossRef]
19. Topouchian, J.; Labat, C.; Gautier, S.; Bäck, M.; Achimastos, A.; Blacher, J.; Cwynar, M.; de la Sierra, A.; Pall, D.; Fantin, F.; et al. Effects of metabolic syndrome on arterial function in different age groups: The Advanced Approach to Arterial Stiffness Study. *J. Hypertens.* **2018**, *36*, 824–833. [CrossRef]
20. Effects of CPAP on Metabolic Syndrome in Patients with Obstructive Sleep Apnea: The TREATOSA-MS Randomized Controlled trial. Available online: https://www.abstractsonline.com/pp8/#!/8998/presentation/17720 (accessed on 24 June 2020).
21. Galerneau, L.-M.; Tamisier, R.; Benmerad, M.; Bonsignore, M.R.; Borel, J.-C.; Pepin, J.-L. Arterial stiffness in obese CPAP-treated obstructive sleep apnea (OSA): A seven years prospective longitudinal study. *Eur. Respir. J.* **2017**, *50*, PA4716. [CrossRef]
22. Grundy, S.M.; Cleeman, J.I.; Daniels, S.R.; Donato, K.A.; Eckel, R.H.; Franklin, B.A.; Gordon, D.J.; Krauss, R.M.; Savage, P.J.; Smith, S.C.; et al. Diagnosis and management of the metabolic syndrome: An American Heart Association/National Heart, Lung, and Blood Institute Scientific Statement. *Circulation* **2005**, *112*, 2735–2752. [CrossRef] [PubMed]
23. Sateia, M.J. International classification of sleep disorders-third edition. *Chest* **2014**, *146*, 1387–1394. [CrossRef]
24. World Medical Association. World Medical Association declaration of Helsinki: Ethical Principles for medical research involving human subjects. *JAMA* **2013**, *310*, 2191–2194. [CrossRef]
25. Engleman, H.M.; Wild, M.R. Improving CPAP use by patients with the sleep apnoea/hypopnoea syndrome (SAHS). *Sleep Med. Rev.* **2003**, *7*, 81–99. [CrossRef]
26. Ryan, H.; Trosclair, A.; Gfroerer, J. Adult current smoking: Differences in definitions and prevalence estimates—NHIS and NSDUH. *J. Environ. Public Health* **2012**, *2012*, 1–11. [CrossRef]

37. Operator's Manual for DMS 300-4A Holter ECG Recorder. Available online: http://www.holterdms.com/manuals/300-4A%20Manual.pdf (accessed on 17 April 2021).
38. Tensiomed. Innovative Method to Ease Arterial Stiffness Measurement. Available online: https://www.tensiomed.com (accessed on 17 April 2021).
39. Nsair, A.; Hupin, D.; Chomette, S.; Barthélémy, J.C.; Roche, F. Factors influencing adherence to auto-CPAP: An observational monocentric study comparing patients with and without cardiovascular diseases. *Front. Neurol.* **2019**, *10*, 801. [CrossRef]
40. Dorkova, Z.; Petrasova, D.; Molcanyiova, A.; Popovnakova, M.; Tkacova, R. Effects of Continuous positive airway pressure on cardiovascular risk profile in patients with severe obstructive sleep apnea and metabolic syndrome. *Chest* **2008**, *134*, 686–692. [CrossRef]
41. Randerath, W.J.; Herkenrath, S.; Treml, M.; Grote, L.; Hedner, J.; Bonsignore, M.R.; Pépin, J.L.; Ryan, S.; Schiza, S.; Verbraecken, J. et al. Evaluation of a multicomponent grading system for obstructive sleep apnoea: The Baveno classification. *ERJ Open Res* **2021**, *7*, 00928–02020. [CrossRef]
42. Alefishat, E.A.; Abu Farha, R.; Al-Debei, M.M. Self-Reported Adherence among Individuals at High Risk of Metabolic Syndrome: Effect of Knowledge and Attitude. *Med. Princ. Pract.* **2016**, *26*, 157–163. [CrossRef] [PubMed]
43. Trachet, B.; Reymond, P.; Kips, J.; Vermeersch, S.; Swillens, A.; Stergiopulos, N.; Segers, P. Validation of the Arteriograph working principle: Questions still remain. *J. Hypertens.* **2011**, *29*, 619. [CrossRef] [PubMed]
44. Rajzer, M.W.; Wojciechowska, W.; Klocek, M.; Palka, I.; Brzozowska-Kiszka, M.; Kawecka-Jaszcz, K. Comparison of aortic pulse wave velocity measured by three techniques: Complior, SphygmoCor and Arteriograph. *J. Hypertens.* **2008**, *26*, 2001–2007. [CrossRef]
45. Piepoli, M.F.; Hoes, A.W.; Agewall, S.; Albus, C.; Brotons, C.; Catapano, A.L.; Cooney, M.T.; Corrà, U.; Cosyns, B.; Deaton C.; et al. 2016 European Guidelines on cardiovascular disease prevention in clinical practice: The Sixth Joint Task Force of the European Society of Cardiology and Other Societies on Cardiovascular Disease Prevention in Clinical Practice (Constituted by Representatives of 10 Societies and by Invited Experts)Developed with the Special Contribution of the European Association for Cardiovascular Prevention & Rehabilitation (EACPR). *Eur. Heart J.* **2016**, *37*, 2315–2381. [CrossRef] [PubMed]
46. Protogerou, A.D.; Laaban, J.-P.; Czernichow, S.; Kostopoulos, C.; Lekakis, J.; E Safar, M.; Blacher, J. Structural and functional arterial properties in patients with obstructive sleep apnoea syndrome and cardiovascular comorbidities. *J. Hum. Hypertens.* **2007**, *22*, 415–422. [CrossRef] [PubMed]
47. Tamisier, R.; Borel, J.C.; Millasseau, S.; Galerneau, L.; Destors, M.; Perrin, M.; Pepin, J. Arterial stiffness in patients with obstructive sleep apnea syndrome: An individual meta-analysis of contributing factors. *J. Hypertens.* **2016**, *34*, e100. [CrossRef]
48. Joyeux-Faure, M.; Tamisier, R.; Borel, J.-C.; Millasseau, S.; Galerneau, L.-M.; Destors, M.; Bailly, S.; Pepin, J.L. Contribution of obstructive sleep apnoea to arterial stiffness: A meta-analysis using individual patient data. *Thorax* **2018**, *73*, 1146–1151. [CrossRef] [PubMed]
49. Buchner, N.J.; Quack, I.; Stegbauer, J.; Woznowski, M.; Kaufmann, A.; Rump, L.C. Treatment of obstructive sleep apnea reduces arterial stiffness. *Sleep Breath.* **2011**, *16*, 123–133. [CrossRef] [PubMed]
50. Picard, F.; Panagiotidou, P.; Weinig, L.; Steffen, M.; Tammen, A.-B.; Klein, R.M. Effect of CPAP therapy on nocturnal blood pressure fluctuations, nocturnal blood pressure, and arterial stiffness in patients with coexisting cardiovascular diseases and obstructive sleep apnea. *Sleep Breath.* **2020**, *25*, 151–161. [CrossRef] [PubMed]
51. Cardoso, C.R.L.; Roderjan, C.N.; Cavalcanti, A.H.; Cortez, A.F.; Muxfeldt, E.S.; Salles, G.F. Effects of continuous positive airway pressure treatment on aortic stiffness in patients with resistant hypertension and obstructive sleep apnea: A randomized controlled trial. *J. Sleep Res.* **2020**, *29*, e12990. [CrossRef] [PubMed]
52. Vlachopoulos, C.; Aznaouridis, K.; Stefanadis, C. Prediction of cardiovascular events and all-cause mortality with arterial stiffness: A systematic review and meta-analysis. *J. Am. Coll. Cardiol.* **2010**, *55*, 1318–1327. [CrossRef]
53. Schwartz, J.E.; Feig, P.U.; Izzo, J.L. Pulse wave velocities derived from cuff ambulatory pulse wave analysis. *Hypertension* **2019**, *74*, 111–116. [CrossRef]
54. Salvi, P.; Scalise, F.; Rovina, M.; Moretti, F.; Salvi, L.; Grillo, A.; Gao, L.; Baldi, C.; Faini, A.; Furlanis, G.; et al. Noninvasive estimation of aortic stiffness through different approaches. *Hypertension* **2019**, *74*, 117–129. [CrossRef]
55. Ryan, S. The effect of continuous positive airway pressure therapy on vascular function in obstructive sleep apnea: How much is enough? *Sleep Med.* **2013**, *14*, 1231–1232. [CrossRef] [PubMed]
56. Drager, L.F.; Brunoni, A.R.; Jenner, R.; Lorenzi-Filho, G.; Benseñor, I.M.; Lotufo, P. Effects of CPAP on body weight in patients with obstructive sleep apnoea: A meta-analysis of randomised trials. *Thorax* **2014**, *70*, 258–264. [CrossRef]
57. Tachikawa, R.; Ikeda, K.; Minami, T.; Matsumoto, T.; Hamada, S.; Murase, K.; Tanizawa, K.; Inouchi, M.; Oga, T.; Akamizu, T.; et al. Changes in energy metabolism after continuous positive airway pressure for obstructive sleep apnea. *Am. J. Respir. Crit. Care Med.* **2016**, *194*, 729–738. [CrossRef] [PubMed]
58. Liu, M.; Li, G.-L.; Li, Y.; Wang, J.-G. Effects of various antihypertensive drugs on arterial stiffness and wave reflections. *Pulse* **2013**, *1*, 97–107. [CrossRef] [PubMed]
59. Dudenbostel, T.; Glasser, S. Effects of antihypertensive drugs on arterial stiffness. *Cardiol. Rev.* **2012**, *20*, 259–263. [CrossRef]

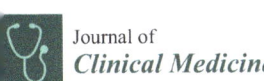

Association of IL-10 and CRP with Pulse Wave Velocity in Patients with Abdominal Aortic Aneurysm

Ida Åström Malm [1,*], Rachel De Basso [1], Peter Blomstrand [1,2] and Dick Wågsäter [3]

1. Department of Natural Sciences and Biomedicine, School of Health and Welfare, Jönköping University, SE-551 11 Jönköping, Sweden; rachel.de.basso@rjl.se (R.D.B.); peter.blomstrand@rjl.se (P.B.)
2. Department of Clinical Physiology, County Hospital Ryhov, SE-551 85 Jönköping, Sweden
3. Department of Medical Cell Biology, Uppsala University, SE-751 23 Uppsala, Sweden; dick.wagsater@mcb.uu.se
* Correspondence: ida.astrom-malm@ju.se

Abstract: Background: Markers of inflammation and arterial stiffness are predictors of cardiovascular morbidity and events, but their roles in the mechanisms and progression of abdominal aortic aneurysm (AAA) in males have not been fully investigated. This study explored possible associations between inflammatory marker levels and arterial stiffness in males with AAA. Methods: A total of 270 males (191 AAA and 79 controls) were included in the study. Arterial stiffness was assessed using non-invasive applanation tonometry to measure the regional pulse wave velocity between the carotid and femoral arteries and the carotid and radial arteries. Blood samples were obtained, and interleukin-10 (IL-10) and CRP levels were analysed. Results: Subjects with an AAA had higher levels of IL-10 (21.5 ± 14.0 ng/mL versus 16.6 ± 9.3 ng/mL) compared to controls ($p = 0.007$). In the AAA cohort, subjects with T2DM showed higher levels of IL-10 (26.4 ± 17.3 versus 20.4 ± 13.0, $p = 0.036$). We observed a positive correlation between PWVcf and CRP in the control group ($r = 0.332$) but not the AAA group. PWVcf and CRP were negatively correlated ($r = 0.571$) in the T2DM subjects treated with metformin in the AAA group. Conclusion: Arterial stiffness is related to the degree of inflammation reflected by CRP and IL-10 levels in males with an AAA. IL-10 is negatively correlated with arterial stiffness in these subjects. This finding suggests that IL-10 may decrease arterial stiffness in males with AAA. The negative correlation between CRP and PWVcf in males with T2DM treated with metformin may indicate that metformin influences the arterial wall to decrease stiffness in subjects with AAA.

Keywords: arterial stiffness; abdominal aortic aneurysm; diabetes mellitus type 2; inflammatory marker

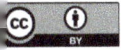

1. Introduction

Stiffening in large elastic arteries significantly contributes to cardiovascular disease (CVD) and is a well-known independent predictor of cardiovascular morbidity and mortality [1,2]. Inflammation has a considerable role in the development of arterial stiffness. Macrophages and monocytes generate pro-inflammatory and pro-oxidant cytokines in regions with inflammation. Local inflammation is a protective response of the vascular tissue to eliminate the cause of injury [3,4]. There is an association between arterial stiffness and inflammation measured as C-reactive protein (CRP) levels in healthy individuals [5] and middle-aged and elderly subjects [6], as well as patients with diabetes [7]. Several conditions characterized by increased systemic inflammation are associated with increased arterial stiffness [8–10]; for example, abdominal aortic aneurysm (AAA) is a form of CVD characterised by chronic inflammation [11]. Two studies have reported a correlation between increased inflammatory mediator levels and AAA [12,13], and some have found correlations between aneurysm size and inflammatory markers [12,14,15]. Males with AAA have increased arterial stiffness compered to controls [16], indicating that increased arterial stiffness may contribute to the overall higher cardiovascular risk seen in patients with AAA [16].

Immune system activation is related to diabetes incidence and prevalence, and a well known clinical relationship exists between diabetes, atherosclerosis, and CVD [17]. However, even though type 2 diabetes mellitus (T2DM) is a risk factor for CVD in general, the disease is uncommon in patients with AAA. Indeed, T2DM may protect against AAA through effects on pathophysiological mechanisms and antidiabetic drug treatment [18]. Metformin use in AAA patients is strongly associated with a slower AAA growth rate [19–21]. Kunath et al. (2021) demonstrated that metformin reduced vascular contraction and restored the anti-contractile function of perivascular adipose tissue in a mouse model of diabetes [22]. Metformin was also shown to decrease arterial stiffness in patients with non-alcoholic fatty liver disease [23] and polycystic ovary syndrome [24]. Thus, the anti-inflammatory effect of metformin may also influence arterial stiffness. Metformin treatment increases levels of interleukin (IL)-10, an anti-inflammatory cytokine involved in the atherosclerotic process that inhibits both macrophage activation and the expression of matrix metalloproteinases (MMPs), pro-inflammatory cytokines and cyclooxygenase-2 in lipid-loaded and activated macrophage foam cells [25]. Low IL-10 has been associated with an increased risk of future cardiovascular events in patients with acute coronary syndrome [26].

Inflammatory markers and arterial stiffness are predictors of cardiovascular events, however, the roles of these markers in the development and progression of arterial stiffness have not been fully investigated. The aim of the present study was to explore possible associations between inflammatory marker levels and metformin use and arterial stiffness in males with AAA.

2. Materials and Methods

2.1. Study Population

Participants were recruited from an ongoing ultrasound AAA screening program and a regional ultrasound surveillance program of known AAA in two neighbouring regions in southern Sweden. From 2011–2016, a total of 270 males (mean age 70 ± 4 years) were included in the study: 191 patients with AAA and 79 controls (Table 1). Subjects with the following conditions were excluded: cardiac arrhythmia, severe disability, advanced cancer and language barriers. Subjects with an AAA had a maximum infrarenal aortic diameter of at least 30 mm on their most recent clinical ultrasound examination. Patients with an AAA diameter >55 mm were referred for surgical intervention and excluded from the study. All subjects in the control group had an infrarenal aortic diameter within the reference range (<30 mm) at their screening examinations in the previous 5 years [16].

The regional ethical review board in Linköping, Sweden, approved the study (Dnr 2016/143-32), and all patients accepting gave written consent to participate in the study.

2.2. Study Protocol

The participants were instructed to abstain from alcohol for 12 h and from caffeinated beverages and tobacco for 4 h prior to their examination. Examinations were performed at the Department of Clinical Physiology at Linköping University Hospital and Ryhov County Hospital. At the time of the examination, a questionnaire regarding smoking status, CVD, and current medications was completed by the examiner based on participant responses. Arterial stiffness was measured with a SphygmoCor system (Model MM3, AtCor Medical, Sydney, Australia). Simultaneous electrocardiogram recording allowed pulse wave velocity (PWV) to be calculated. The pulse pressure waveforms were non-invasively recorded with a Millar pressure tonometer (Millar, Houston, TX, USA) at the carotid to the femoral PWV (central PWV) and the carotid to the radial artery PWV (peripheral PWV) [16].

Table 1. Characteristics of the study population.

	AAA n = 191	Controls n = 79	p Value
Age (year)	70.2 ± 3.0	68.6 ± 3.0	<0.001
Weight (kg)	87.9 ± 13.6	85.0 ± 12.1	0.336
Height (cm)	176.9 ± 6.1	177.6 ± 4.7	0.271
BMI (kg/m^2)	28.1 ± 4.3	27.2 ± 3.6	0.122
SBP (mmHg)	134 ± 1.4	131 ± 1.9	0.280
DBP (mmHg)	77 ± 0.7	75 ± 2	0.210
CRP (mg/L)	4.5 ± 6.8	3.0 ± 4.0	0.018
Self-reported smoking			
Current n (%)	116 (60.7)	26 (32.9)	<0.001
Former n (%)	42 (22.0)	6 (7.6)	<0.001
Non-smoker n (%)	17 (8.9)	39 (49.5)	<0.001
Self-reported medical treatment			
ACE inhibitors n (%)	91 (47.6)	24 (30.4)	0.008
β blockers n (%)	84 (44.0)	16 (20.3)	<0.001
Ca antagonists n (%)	51 (26.7)	9 (11.4)	0.005
Diuretics n (%)	39 (20.4)	5 (6.3)	0.004
Aspirin n (%)	117 (61.3)	15 (19.0)	<0.001
Statins n (%)	122 (63.9)	3 (3.8)	0.07
Self-reported disease			
HT n (%)	153 (80.1)	31 (39.2)	<0.001
HD n (%)	73 (38.2)	10 (12.7)	<0.001
T2DM n (%)	35 (18.3)	11 (13.9)	0.405
CVD n (%)	24 (12.6)	1 (1.3)	0.004
HL n (%)	119 (62.3)	17 (21.5)	<0.001

Values are presented as mean ± SD for continuous variables, or as numbers and percentage of participants for categorical variables. p values were calculated with t-tests or Mann–Whitney U tests. ACE, angiotensin-converting enzyme; BMI, body mass index; Ca, calcium; CRP, C-reactive protein; CVD, history of symptomatic cerebrovascular disease; DBP: diastolic blood pressure; HD, heart disease; HL, history of hyperlipidaemia; HT, hypertension or taking blood pressure-lowering drugs; SBP: systolic blood pressure; T2DM, type 2 diabetes mellitus.

2.3. Laboratory Analyses

After an overnight fast, morning blood samples were collected in prechilled plastic Vacutainer tubes (Terumo EDTA K-3, Tokyo, Japan). Plasma was prepared by centrifugation at 3000× g for 10 min at 4 °C. All samples were stored at −70 °C until analysis in the chemistry laboratories at Linköping University Hospital and Ryhov County Hospital, Jönköping. Both laboratories are ISO/IEC 17025-accredited by the Swedish Board for Accreditation and Conformity Assessment. CRP was analysed by an immunoturbidimetric method according to the manufacturer's recommendations with ADVIA 1800 (Siemens, Munich, Germany). An inflammatory biomarker panel was analysed with commercial Bio-Plex Pro™ Human Chemokine Panel, 40-Plex kits (Bio-Rad Laboratories, Inc., Hercules, CA, USA) according to the manufacturer's recommendations. The panel measures a variety of cytokines, chemokines (e.g., eotoxins, Gro, MIP-family), interleukins (e.g., IL-1b, IL-6), interferon gamma, and tumour necrosis factor alpha. An automatic magnetic washer (Magpix, Austin, TX, USA) was used during assay implementation. The 96-well microtiter plates were measured with the Luminex 200 system (Luminex Corp., Austin, TX, USA). A five-parameter logistic curve was generated for each analyte using the Masterplex computer software.

2.4. Statistics

Data were analysed using SPSS 27.0 for Windows (IBM Corp., Armonk, NY, USA). Continuous variables are expressed as mean ± standard deviation (SD), and categorical variables are expressed as number of participants and per cent. Comparisons between the AAA and control groups were performed using unpaired Student's t-tests, Fisher's exact tests, or non-parametric means tests (Mann–Whitney U tests). Pearson's bivariate correlation coefficients were calculated used to investigate the relationships between PWV and IL-10. Multivariate analysis was made in order to adjust for confounders. Differences were considered significant at $p \leq 0.05$.

3. Results

3.1. Demographic Data

Demographic data are presented in Table 1. We saw no differences between AAA and controls regarding height, weight, body mass index, or blood pressure. The AAA cohort was significantly older ($p < 0.01$) compared to the control group. The AAA group also included more current and former smokers ($p < 0.01$). The prevalence rates of T2DM and the reported occurrence of symptomatic cerebrovascular disease were similar between the two groups, while hyperlipidaemia, hypertension, and heart diseases were more frequent in the AAA cohort. A greater proportion of subjects in the AAA population were treated with b-blockers and aspirin ($p < 0.001$). No differences were found in the reported use of other anti-hypertension drugs, including diuretics, calcium channel blockers and statins.

3.2. Pulse Wave Parameters, IL-10, and CRP

The AAA cohort had a significantly higher mean level of IL-10 (21.5 ± 14.0 ng/mL) compared to controls (16.6 ± 9.3 ng/mL) ($p = 0.007$). When the AAA cohort was divided into no T2DM ($n = 156$) and T2DM ($n = 35$), the latter subgroup showed a significantly higher level of IL-10 ($p = 0.036$) (Table 2). Among the 35 subjects with T2DM in the AAA group, 12 were treated with metformin and 17 were not, but these subjects had similar IL-10 levels. Several other ILs and chemokines were analysed, but none were significantly correlated with arterial stiffness in the AAA or control group (data not shown) [27].

Table 2. PWV, IL-10, T2DM and AAA measurements.

	AAA without T2DM	AAA with T2DM	p-Value
	($n = 156$)	($n = 35$)	
PWVcf (m/s)	12.1 ± 2.8	13.2 ± 3.4	0.068
PWVcr (m/s)	9.5 ± 1.3	9.2 ± 1.2	0.259
IL-10 (ng/mL)	20.4 ± 13.0	26.4 ± 17.3	0.036
CRP (mg/L)	4.3 ± 6.3	5.2 ± 8.7	0.774
	AAA with T2DM and Metformin	AAA with T2DM without Metformin	p-Value
	($n = 12$)	($n = 17$)	
PWVcf (m/s)	12.8 ± 3.8	13.5 ± 3.2	0.565
PWVcr (m/s)	9.0 ± 1.4	9.3 ± 1.0	0.205
IL-10 (ng/mL)	29.9 ± 21.4	24.2 ± 14.3	0.468
CRP (mg/L)	6.5 ± 11.0	3.2 ± 2.9	0.875

Values are presented as mean $\pm$ SD. AAA, abdominal aortic aneurysm; CRP, C-reactive protein; IL-10, interleukin-10; PWVcf, carotid femoral pulse wave velocity; PWVcr, carotid-radial pulse wave velocity; T2DM, type 2 diabetes mellitus.

CRP levels were higher in subjects with AAA compared to controls, 4.5 ± 6.8 mg/L versus 3.0 ± 4.0 mg/L ($p = 0.018$, Table 1). Pearson's bivariate correlation analyses were performed between central pulse wave velocity (PWVcf) and periphery pulse PWV (PWVcr) and CRP and IL-10 in the AAA and control groups. A significant positive correlation between PWVcf and CRP was found in the controls ($r = 0.332$, $p < 0.01$) but not in the AAA group. This correlation remained in controls without T2DM ($r = 0.359$, $p < 0.01$) but disappeared in controls with T2DM. In the AAA group, we found a negative correlation between PWVcf and CRP ($r = 0.571$, $p = 0.05$), but only in the metformin-treated T2DM subgroup, not in subjects with T2DM without metformin. PWVcr was not correlated with CRP in the control or AAA group. A significant negative correlation was found between PWVcf and IL-10 in subjects with T2DM in the AAA cohort ($r = 0.424$). However, the significant correlation disappeared after adjusting age, smoking, and blood pressure. The correlation data are summarized in Tables 3 and 4. No difference was found in PWVcf or PWVcr when we compared AAA subjects with or without T2DM. PWV values were also comparable between AAA subjects with metformin treatment and those without (Table 2). In addition, there was no difference in the control group without AAA for PWV between subjects with or without T2DM.

Table 3. Correlations between PWV and CRP.

PWVcf (m/s)	R	PWVcr (m/s)	R
All AAA	−0.080		−0.083
AAA without T2DM	−0.061		−0.093
AAA with T2DM	−0.142		−0.055
AAA with T2DM and metformin	−0.571 **		−0.122
AAA with T2DM without metformin	−0.106		−0.122
All control	0.332 *		−0.173
Control with T2DM	0.094		−0.296
Control without T2DM	0.359 *		−0.182

Pearson's variate correlation, * $p < 0.01$, ** $p = 0.05$. AAA, abdominal aortic aneurysm; PWVcf, carotid femoral pulse wave velocity; PWVcr, carotid-radial pulse wave velocity; T2DM, type 2 diabetes mellitus.

Table 4. Correlations between PWV and IL-10.

PWVcf (m/s)	R	PWVcr (m/s)	R
All AAA	−0.206 *		−0.233 *
AAA without T2DM	−0.181 *		−0.232 *
AAA with T2DM	−0.424 *		−0.143
AAA with T2DM and metformin	−0.433		−0.059
AAA with T2DM without metformin	−0.408		−0.244
All control	0.008		0.001
Control with T2DM	−0.012		0.589
Control without T2DM	−0.016		−0.094

Pearson's bivariate correlation, * $p < 0.05$. AAA, abdominal aortic aneurysm; IL-10, interleukin 10; PWVcf, carotid femoral pulse wave velocity; PWVcr, carotid-radial pulse wave velocity; T2DM, type 2 diabetes mellitus.

4. Discussion

The main novel finding of our study is the negative correlation between aortic PWV and anti-inflammatory cytokine IL-10 levels in males with AAA. In addition, males with AAA and T2DM had further IL-10 increases compared to subjects with AAA but without T2DM. Interestingly, we found no correlation between aortic and brachial PWV and CRP in the AAA cohort, but these factors were associated with the control group. These data suggest that arterial stiffness is related to inflammation as measured as CRP and IL-10, but this relationship varies in males with and without AAA. This indicates that these inflammatory markers do not affect PWV in males with an AAA, but the results do not exclude the possibility that the vascular inflammation is affected. Further investigations are needed to assess local inflammation and vessel wall morphology.

PWVcf is the gold-standard measurement for arterial stiffness through its proven association with cardiovascular morbidity and mortality [28]. AAA leads to mechanical changes in the aortic wall, which may include a delayed propagation of the pressure wave [29]. It has been suggested that the presence of an aneurysm invalidate the reliability of PWV as a method for arterial stiffness [30]. The speed at which a pulse wave travels through arteries provides a measure of arterial stiffness through the Moens–Kortweg equation [31]. This calculation presumes isotropy within the measured arterial segment, which is not present in AAA, especially in advanced aneurysms. However, it is reasonable to suppose that the structural wall properties along the aorta in the AAA group are far more important for the regional pressure wave propagation speed than the altered geometry in the aneurysmal dilatation [32].

AAA pathogenesis is characterized by chronic inflammation and MMP-mediated aortic wall destruction [11]. Previous studies demonstrated that subjects with AAAs have higher CRP levels [33,34], which was confirmed in our study. CRP is an acute-phase protein that is rapidly produced and released in response to various cellular injuries, making it a useful prognostic marker for CVD [35]. CRP levels are also associated with aneurysm size [33], but this was not found in our study that only included males with small AAAs (<55 mm). CRP levels correlate with PWV-measured arterial stiffness in healthy individuals [5], in line with our results. Nakhai-Pour et al. suggested that elevated CRP may be a consequence of arterial stiffening [6], but we found no association between PWV and CRP in males with AAA. This is surprising because inflammation is an essential feature of AAA and plays an important role in the development of arterial stiffness. However, the AAA cohort was more frequently treated with antihypertensive drugs, which seems to have an impact on low-grade inflammation [36,37]. It is not surprising that a higher percentage in the AAA group were treated with statins, anti-platelet therapy and blood pressure-lowering agents. According to current guidelines should these drugs be considered in all patients with AAA [16,38]. CRP is a strong risk factor for clinical CVD, and arterial stiffness is a known predictor of cardiovascular morbidity and mortality. Interestingly, the relationship between these factors in males with AAA is different compared to other populations. CRP levels should be used with caution to predict CVD in males with AAA. In the subgroup of males with AAA and T2DM who were treated with metformin, we observed a negative correlation between CRP and PWVcf. This suggests that metformin decreases arterial stiffness in subjects with AAA and is in accordance with results in mice showing that metformin reduces vascular contraction [22].

We found higher levels of IL-10 in the AAA cohort compared to controls, and AAA subjects with T2DM had higher levels compared to those without T2DM. IL-10 is an anti-inflammatory cytokine involved in the atherosclerotic process. AAA is characterized by the destruction of elastin, increased collagen levels, and smooth muscle cell apoptosis [39]. Since local inflammation is a protective response of the vascular tissue to eliminate the cause of injury [3,4], the increased levels of IL-10 in subjects with AAA and/or T2DM are not surprising.

The diabetic drug metformin has anti-inflammatory effects [40], but we found no difference in IL-10 levels between T2DM subjects with or without metformin in the AAA cohort. Although metformin can decrease arterial stiffness in several diseases [23,24], these effects are not found in T2DM patients [41]. We found a negative correlation between arterial stiffness and IL-10 levels in AAA subjects with T2DM. However, no difference was found in this correlation between T2DM subjects treated with or without metformin.

The AAA group was not only affected by AAA, but they were also more affected by other CVD. This may not be surprising; AAA shares a number of risk factors in common with other CVD. It was more current and former smokers in the AAA and one of the most well-known risk factors for AAA as well as for CVD is smoking [41].

Limitations

Our results should be considered in the context of several potential limitations. This was a cross-sectional study, so direct cause-and-effect associations can be derived. The size of the T2DM cohort was small, and even fewer patients were treated with metformin. Moreover, the durations of T2DM and metformin treatment were not assessed. Finally, only males with small AAAs were included in the study. However, the prevalence of AAA is higher in males than females, females are less than one fourth as likely as males to have an AAA.

5. Conclusions

Arterial stiffness in males with AAA is related to the level of inflammation as measured by CRP and IL-10 in a different way than in male subjects without AAA. Males with AAA had higher IL-10 levels, which were negatively correlated with arterial stiffness, suggesting that IL-10 may decrease arterial stiffness in males with AAA. We found no relationship between CRP and arterial stiffness in males with AAA, even though they had higher CRP levels and increased arterial stiffness compared to controls. The negative correlation between CRP and PWVcf in males with T2DM who were treated with metformin could indicate that metformin influences the arterial wall and decreases arterial stiffness in subjects with AAA.

Author Contributions: Conceptualization, R.D.B.; methodology, R.D.B., I.Å.M. and D.W.; validation, I.Å.M. and D.W.; formal analysis, I.Å.M. and D.W.; investigation, I.Å.M.; resources, P.B. and R.D.B.; data curation, I.Å.M.; writing—original draft preparation, I.Å.M.; writing—review and editing, I.Å.M., R.D.B., P.B. and D.W.; supervision, R.D.B., P.B. and D.W.; project administration, R.D.B.; funding acquisition, R.D.B. and P.B. All authors have read and agreed to the published version of the manuscript.

Funding: This study was supported by grants from The Swedish Research Council (#12661); Swedish Heart and Lung Foundation (#20130650); Futurum–the Academy for Healthcare, County Council, Jönköping, Sweden (#259701); and King Gustav V and Queen Victoria's Foundation and Medical Research Council of Southeast Sweden (FORSS) (#34931). None of the grant providers influenced the results of the current study. The funders had no role in study design, data collection and analysis, decision to publish, or preparation of the manuscript.

Institutional Review Board Statement: The study was conducted in accordance with the Declaration of Helsinki, and approved by the regional ethical review board in Linköping, Sweden, (Dnr 108 2016/143-32).

Informed Consent Statement: Informed written consent was obtained from all subjects involved in the study.

Data Availability Statement: The data supporting reported results can be found at Department of Natural Sciences and Biomedicine, School of Health and Welfare, Jönköping University, Jönköping, Sweden.

Conflicts of Interest: The authors declare no conflict of interest. The funders had no role in the design of the study; in the collection, analyses, or interpretation of data; in the writing of the manuscript, or in the decision to publish the results.

References

1. Laurent, S.; Boutouyrie, P.; Asmar, R.; Gautier, I.; Laloux, B.; Guize, L.; Ducimetiere, P.; Benetos, A. Aortic Stiffness Is an Independent Predictor of All-Cause and Cardiovascular Mortality in Hypertensive Patients. *Hypertension* **2001**, *37*, 1236–1241. [CrossRef] [PubMed]
2. Boutouyrie, P.; Tropeano, A.I.; Asmar, R.; Gautier, I.; Benetos, A.; Lacolley, P.; Laurent, S. Aortic stiffness is an independent predictor of primary coronary events in hypertensive patients: A longitudinal study. *Hypertension* **2002**, *39*, 10–15. [CrossRef] [PubMed]
3. Cecelja, M.; Chowienczyk, P. Arterial stiffening: Causes and consequences. *Artery Res.* **2012**, *7*, 22–27. [CrossRef]
4. Pearson, T.A.; Mensah, G.A.; Alexander, R.W.; Anderson, J.L.; Cannon, R.O., III; Criqui, M.; Fadl, Y.Y.; Fortmann, S.P.; Hong, Y.; Myers, G.L.; et al. Markers of Inflammation and Cardiovascular Disease. *Circulation* **2003**, *107*, 499–511. [CrossRef]
5. Yasmin, N.; McEniery, C.M.; Wallace, S.; Mackenzie, I.S.; Cockcroft, J.R.; Wilkinson, I.B. C-Reactive Protein Is Associated with Arterial Stiffness in Apparently Healthy Individuals. *Arterioscler. Thromb. Vasc. Biol.* **2004**, *24*, 969–974. [CrossRef]
6. Nakhai-Pour, H.R.; E Grobbee, D.; Bots, M.L.; Muller, M.; Van Der Schouw, Y.T. C-reactive protein and aortic stiffness and wave reflection in middle-aged and elderly men from the community. *J. Hum. Hypertens.* **2007**, *21*, 949–955. [CrossRef]
7. Llaurado, G.; Ceperuelo-Mallafre, V.; Vilardell, C.; Simo, R.; Freixenet, N.; Vendrell, J.; Gonzalez-Clemente, J.M. Arterial Stiffness Is Increased in Patients With Type 1 Diabetes Without Cardiovascular Disease: A potential role of low-grade inflammation. *Diabetes Care* **2012**, *35*, 1083–1089. [CrossRef]
8. Dregan, A. Arterial stiffness association with chronic inflammatory disorders in the UK Biobank study. *Heart* **2018**, *104*, 1257–1262. [CrossRef]
9. Sacre, K.; Escoubet, B.; Pasquet, B.; Chauveheid, M.-P.; Zennaro, M.-C.; Tubach, F.; Papo, T. Increased Arterial Stiffness in Systemic Lupus Erythematosus (SLE) Patients at Low Risk for Cardiovascular Disease: A Cross-Sectional Controlled Study. *PLoS ONE* **2014**, *9*, e94511. [CrossRef]
10. Anyfanti, P.; Triantafyllou, A.; Gkaliagkousi, E.; Koletsos, N.; Aslanidis, S.; Douma, S. Association of non-invasive hemodynamics with arterial stiffness in rheumatoid arthritis. *Scand. Cardiovasc. J.* **2018**, *52*, 171–176. [CrossRef]
11. Jagadesham, V.P.; Scott, D.J.A.; Carding, S.R. Abdominal aortic aneurysms: An autoimmune disease? *Trends Mol. Med.* **2008**, *14*, 522–529. [CrossRef] [PubMed]

12. Lindberg, S.; Zarrouk, M.; Holst, J.; Gottsäter, A. Inflammatory markers associated with abdominal aortic aneurysm. *Eur. Cytokine Netw.* 2016, *27*, 75–80. [CrossRef]
13. Parry, D.J.; Al-Barjas, H.S.; Chappell, L.; Rashid, S.T.; Ariens, R.; Scott, D.J.A. Markers of inflammation in men with small abdominal aortic aneurysm. *J. Vasc. Surg.* 2010, *52*, 145–151. [CrossRef]
14. Flondell-Sité, D.; Lindblad, B.; Kölbel, T.; Gottsäter, A. Cytokines and systemic biomarkers are related to the size of abdominal aortic aneurysms. *Cytokine* 2009, *46*, 211–215. [CrossRef]
15. Sánchez-Infantes, D.; Nus, M.; Navas-Madroñal, M.; Fité, J.; Pérez, B.; Barros-Membrilla, A.; Soto, B.; Martínez-González, J.; Camacho, M.; Rodriguez, C.; et al. Oxidative Stress and Inflammatory Markers in Abdominal Aortic Aneurysm. *Antioxidants* 2021, *10*, 602. [CrossRef]
16. Åström Malm, I.; De Basso, R.; Blomstrand, P.; Bjarnegård, N. Increased arterial stiffness in males with abdominal aortic aneurysm. *Clin. Physiol. Funct. Imaging* 2021, *41*, 68–75. [CrossRef] [PubMed]
17. Tsalamandris, S.; Antonopoulos, A.S.; Oikonomou, E.; Papamikroulis, G.-A.; Vogiatzi, G.; Papaioannou, S.; Deftereos, S.; Tousoulis, D. The Role of Inflammation in Diabetes: Current Concepts and Future Perspectives. *Eur. Cardiol. Rev.* 2019, *14*, 50–59. [CrossRef] [PubMed]
18. Raffort, J.; Lareyre, F.; Clement, M.; Hassen-Khodja, R.; Chinetti, G.; Mallat, Z. Diabetes and aortic aneurysm: Current state of the art. *Cardiovasc. Res.* 2018, *114*, 1702–1713. [CrossRef]
19. Unosson, J.; Wågsäter, D.; Bjarnegård, N.; de Basso, R.; Welander, M.; Mani, K.; Gottsäter, A.; Wanhainen, A. Metformin Prescription Associated with Reduced Abdominal Aortic Aneurysm Growth Rate and Reduced Chemokine Expression in a Swedish Cohort. *Ann. Vasc. Surg.* 2021, *70*, 425–433. [CrossRef]
20. Fujimura, N.; Xiong, J.; Kettler, E.; Xuan, H.; Glover, K.J.; Mell, M.W.; Xu, B.; Dalman, R.L. Metformin treatment status and abdominal aortic aneurysm disease progression. *J. Vasc. Surg.* 2016, *64*, 46–54.e8. [CrossRef]
21. Golledge, J.; Moxon, J.; Pinchbeck, J.; Anderson, G.; Rowbotham, S.; Jenkins, J.; Bourke, M.; Bourke, B.; Dear, A.; Buckenham T.; et al. Association between metformin prescription and growth rates of abdominal aortic aneurysms. *Br. J. Surg.* 2017, *104*, 1486–1493. [CrossRef] [PubMed]
22. Kunath, A.; Unosson, J.; Friederich-Persson, M.; Bjarnegård, N.; Becirovic-Agic, M.; Björck, M.; Mani, K.; Wanhainen, A.; Wågsäter, D. Inhibition of angiotensin-induced aortic aneurysm by metformin in apolipoprotein E–deficient mice. *JVS Vasc. Sci.* 2021, *2*, 33–42. [CrossRef] [PubMed]
23. Shargorodsky, M.; Omelchenko, E.; Matas, Z.; Boaz, M.; Gavish, D. Relation between augmentation index and adiponectin during one-year metformin treatment for nonalcoholic steatohepatosis: Effects beyond glucose lowering? *Cardiovasc. Diabetol.* 2012, *11*, 61. [CrossRef]
24. Agarwal, N.; Rice, S.P.L.; Bolusani, H.; Luzio, S.; Dunseath, G.; Ludgate, M.; Rees, A. Metformin Reduces Arterial Stiffness and Improves Endothelial Function in Young Women with Polycystic Ovary Syndrome: A Randomized, Placebo-Controlled, Crossover Trial. *J. Clin. Endocrinol. Metab.* 2010, *95*, 722–730. [CrossRef] [PubMed]
25. Tedgui, A.; Mallat, Z. Cytokines in Atherosclerosis: Pathogenic and Regulatory Pathways. *Physiol. Rev.* 2006, *86*, 515–581 [CrossRef] [PubMed]
26. Liu, J.; Jia, Y.; Li, X.; Xu, R.; Zhu, C.; Guo, Y.; Wu, N.; Li, J. Serum interleukin-10 levels and adverse events in patients with acute coronary syndrome: A systematic review and meta-analysis. *Chin. Med. J.* 2014, *127*, 150–156. [PubMed]
27. Laurent, S.; Cockcroft, J.; Van Bortel, L.; Boutouyrie, P.; Giannattasio, C.; Hayoz, D.; Pannier, B.; Vlachopoulos, C.; Wilkinson, I.; Struijker-Boudier, H.; et al. Expert consensus document on arterial stiffness: Methodological issues and clinical applications. *Eur. Heart J.* 2006, *27*, 2588–2605. [CrossRef]
28. Fujikura, K.; Luo, J.; Gamarnik, V.; Pernot, M.; Fukumoto, R.; Tilson, M.D., 3rd; Konofagou, E.E. A novel noninvasive technique for pulse-wave imaging and characterization of clinically-significant vascular mechanical properties in vivo. *Ultrason. Imaging* 2007, *29*, 137–154. [CrossRef]
29. Lee, S.J.; Park, S.H. Arterial ageing. *Korean Circ. J.* 2013, *43*, 73–79. [CrossRef]
30. Callaghan, F.J.; Geddes, L.A.; Babbs, C.F.; Bourland, J.D. Relationship between pulse-wave velocity and arterial elasticity. *Med. Biol. Eng. Comput.* 1986, *24*, 248–254. [CrossRef]
31. Cameron, S.J.; Russell, H.M.; Owens, A.P., 3rd. Antithrombotic therapy in abdominal aortic aneurysm: Beneficial or detrimental? *Blood* 2018, *132*, 2619–2628. [CrossRef] [PubMed]
32. Vainas, T.; Lubbers, T.; Stassen, F.R.; Herngreen, S.B.; Van Dieijen-Visser, M.P.; Bruggeman, C.A.; Kitslaar, P.J.; Schurink, G.W.H Serum C-Reactive Protein Level Is Associated With Abdominal Aortic Aneurysm Size and May Be Produced by Aneurysmal Tissue. *Circulation* 2003, *107*, 1103–1105. [CrossRef] [PubMed]
33. Shangwei, Z.; Yingqi, W.; Jiang, X.; Zhongyin, W.; Juan, J.; Dafang, C.; Yonghua, H.; Wei, G. Serum High-Sensitive C-Reactive Protein Level and CRP Genetic Polymorphisms Are Associated with Abdominal Aortic Aneurysm. *Ann. Vasc. Surg.* 2017, *45*, 186–192. [CrossRef]
34. Verma, A.; Lavie, C.J.; Milani, R.V. C-Reactive Protein: How Has JUPITER Impacted Clinical Practice? *Ochsner J.* 2009, *9*, 204–210. [PubMed]
35. Fulop, T.; Rule, A.D.; Schmidt, D.W.; Wiste, H.J.; Bailey, K.R.; Kullo, I.J.; Schwartz, G.L.; Mosley, T.H.; Boerwinkle, E.; Turner, S.T. C-reactive protein among community-dwelling hypertensives on single-agent antihypertensive treatment. *J. Am. Soc. Hypertens.* 2009, *3*, 260–266. [CrossRef] [PubMed]

26. Hage, F. C-reactive protein and Hypertension. *J. Hum. Hypertens.* **2013**, *28*, 410–415. [CrossRef]
27. JCS Joint Working Group. Guidelines for diagnosis and treatment of aortic aneurysm and aortic dissection (JCS 2011): Digest version. *Circ. J.* **2013**, *77*, 789–828. [CrossRef]
28. Rabkin, S.W. The Role Matrix Metalloproteinases in the Production of Aortic Aneurysm. *Prog. Mol. Biol. Transl. Sci.* **2017**, *147*, 239–265.
29. Cameron, A.R.; Morrison, V.; Levin, D.; Mohan, M.; Forteath, C.; Beall, C.; McNeilly, A.; Balfour, D.J.; Savinko, T.; Wong, A.K.; et al. Anti-Inflammatory Effects of Metformin Irrespective of Diabetes Status. *Circ. Res.* **2016**, *119*, 652–665. [CrossRef]
30. Driessen, J.H.M.; de Vries, F.; van Onzenoort, H.A.W.; Schram, M.T.; van der Kallen, C.; Reesink, K.D.; Simoneg, S.; Coen, D.A.S.; Nicolaasg, S.; Kroon, A.A.; et al. Metformin use in type 2 diabetic patients is not associated with lower arterial stiffness: The Maastricht Study. *J. Hypertens.* **2019**, *37*, 365–371. [CrossRef]
31. Piepoli, M.F.; Hoes, A.W.; Agewall, S.; Albus, C.; Brotons, C.; Catapano, A.L.; Cooney, M.; Corrà, U.; Cosyns, B.; Deaton, C.; et al. 2016 European Guidelines on cardiovascular disease prevention in clinical practice: The Sixth Joint Task Force of the European Society of Cardiology and Other Societies on Cardiovascular Disease Prevention in Clinical Practice (constituted by representatives of 10 societies and by invited experts) Developed with the special contribution of the European Association for Cardiovascular Prevention & Rehabilitation (EACPR). *Atherosclerosis* **2016**, *252*, 207–274. [PubMed]

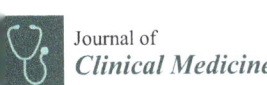

Association of Increased Vascular Stiffness with Cardiovascular Death and Heart Failure Episodes Following Intervention on Symptomatic Degenerative Aortic Stenosis

Jakub Baran [1,2], Anna Kablak-Ziembicka [1,3], Pawel Kleczynski [1,2], Ottavio Alfieri [4], Łukasz Niewiara [2,5], Rafał Badacz [1,2], Piotr Pieniazek [2,6], Jacek Legutko [1,2], Krzysztof Zmudka [1,2], Tadeusz Przewlocki [2,6] and Jakub Podolec [1,2,*]

[1] Department of Interventional Cardiology, Institute of Cardiology, Jagiellonian University Medical College, Prądnicka 80 Str., 31-202 Krakow, Poland; jakub_baran@yahoo.pl (J.B.); kablakziembicka@op.pl (A.K.-Z.); kleczu@interia.pl (P.K.); rbadacz@gmail.com (R.B.); jacek.legutko@uj.edu.pl (J.L.); zmudka@icloud.com (K.Z.)
[2] The John Paul II Hospital, Prądnicka 80 Str., 31-202 Krakow, Poland; lniewiara@gmail.com (Ł.N.); kardio@kki.krakow.pl (P.P.); tadeuszprzewlocki@op.pl (T.P.)
[3] Noninvasive Cardiovascular Laboratory, The John Paul II Hospital, Prądnicka 80 Str., 31-202 Krakow, Poland
[4] San Raffaele University Hospital and Alfieri Heart Foundation, 20132 Milan, Italy; alfieri.ottavio@hsr.it
[5] Department of Emergency Medicine, Faculty of Health Sciences, Jagiellonian University Medical College, 31-126 Krakow, Poland
[6] Department of Cardiac and Vascular Diseases, Institute of Cardiology, Jagiellonian University Medical College, the John Paul II Hospital, Prądnicka 80 Str., 31-202 Krakow, Poland
* Correspondence: jakub.podolec@uj.edu.pl; Tel.: +48-12-614-3501

Abstract: Background. The resistive (RI) and pulsatile (PI) indices are markers of vascular stiffness (VS) which are associated with outcomes in patients with cardiovascular disease. We aimed to assess whether VS might predict incidence of cardiovascular death (CVD) and heart failure (HF) episodes following intervention on degenerative aortic valve stenosis (DAS). Methods. The distribution of increased VS (RI $\geq$ 0.7 and PI $\geq$ 1.3) from supra-aortic arteries was assessed in patients with symptomatic DAS who underwent aortic valve replacement (AVR, n = 127) or transcatheter aortic valve implantation (TAVI, n = 119). During a 3-year follow-up period (FU), incidences of composite endpoint (CVD and HF) were recorded. Results. Increased VS was found in 100% of TAVI patients with adverse event vs. 88.9% event-free TAVI patients (p = 0.116), and in 93.3% of AVR patients with event vs. 70.5% event-free (p = 0.061). Kaplan–Mayer free-survival curves at 1-year and 3-year FU were 90.5% vs. 97.1 % and 78% vs. 97.1% for patients with increased vs. lower VS. (p = 0.014). In univariate Cox analysis, elevated VS (HR 7.97, p = 0.04) and age (HR 1.05, p = 0.024) were associated with risk of adverse outcomes; however, both failed in Cox multivariable analysis. Conclusions. Vascular stiffness is associated with outcome after DAS intervention. However, it cannot be used as an independent outcome predictor.

Keywords: vascular stiffness; cardiovascular death; degenerative aortic stenosis; heat failure episodes; pulsatile index; resistive index; aortic valve replacement; transcatheter aortic valve implantation

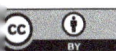

1. Introduction

Resistive (RI) and pulsatile index (PI) are parameters corresponding to vascular stiffness (VS) which have been investigated in various clinical conditions, including renovascular and coronary atherosclerotic disease, hypertension, diabetes, and heart failure [1,2]. Vascular stiffness is a potential predictor of all-cause mortality, including cardiovascular mortality [3].

According to epidemiological data, even in young patients with increased VS, there is an increased risk of cardiovascular events, which carries with it a higher mortality rate [4]. Development and progression of degenerative aortic valve stenosis (DAS) is driven by similar factors to those of VS, including aging, atherosclerosis, inflammation, fibrosis, calcification processes, and genetic susceptibility [5–7]. In addition, the data behind genetic predispositions in patients with ischemic heart disease have proven to favor its significant importance in progression of VS [7].

However, it is still unclear whether RI and PI might predict the incidence of cardiovascular death (CVD) and heart failure (HF) episodes following transcatheter (TAVI) or surgical (AVR) intervention on DAS [8].

Therefore, in the present study, we aimed to assess whether VS is associated with outcomes in post-intervention DAS patients.

2. Materials and Methods

2.1. Study Population

The study group comprised 246 consecutive patients with severe symptomatic DAS (aortic valve area, AVA < 1.0 cm^2) referred for surgical or interventional treatment. From this group, 119 patients underwent transcatheter aortic valve implantation (TAVI), while 127 patients underwent surgical aortic valve replacement (AVR). Afterwards, patients were followed up for 36 months for the composite endpoint: CVD and HF episodes requiring hospital readmission.

Subjects were eligible if they (1) had preserved left ventricular ejection fraction (LVEF), (2) had never been diagnosed with stroke or transient ischemic attack (TIA), and (3) were $\geq$40 years of age. The exclusion criteria for both study groups included significant stenosis of any carotid or vertebral artery (exceeding 50% lumen reduction), persistent atrial fibrillation or other severe arrhythmia, significant concomitant valvular diseases, ongoing or recent myocardial infarction (<3 months), hemodynamic instability (NYHA class IV or acute heart failure), aortic dissection, and lack of informed consent.

Prevalence of cardiovascular risk factors including age, sex, hypertension, diabetes and dyslipidemia was evaluated in compliance with guidelines of the European Society of Cardiology [9,10].

Carotid and vertebral arterial compliance parameters (RI and PI) of vascular stiffness indices and echocardiographic parameters of DAS were assessed. All measurements were done before final Heart Team qualification and performed by sonographers blinded to the subjects' characteristics.

The study protocol was consistent with the requirements of the Helsinki Declaration and approved by the local Institutional Ethics Committee. All subjects gave their informed consent for participation in the study.

2.2. Echocardiographic Study

All patients underwent a complete echocardiographic study in compliance with guidelines of the European Association of Cardiovascular Imaging [11]. Peak velocity and mean gradient across the aortic valve, AVA, and LVEF were assessed in all subjects.

2.3. Arterial Compliance Assessment

High-resolution B-Mode, color Doppler, and pulse Doppler ultrasonography of both carotid and vertebral arteries were performed with an ultrasound machine (TOSHIBA APLIO 450) equipped with a linear-array 5–10 MHz transducer on a patient lying in the supine position with head tilted slightly backward. Examinations were performed by experienced sonographers who were blinded to the subject's characteristics. Data comprised bilateral recording of peak systolic (PSV) and end diastolic velocities (EDV) measured within 1.0 to 1.5 cm of the proximal segment of the internal carotid artery and proximal V2 segment of the vertebral artery.

The averaged values of RI and PI from all assessed segments were calculated for each patient in accordance with the following equations: Resistive Index (RI) = [PSV − EDV/PSV], and Pulsatile Index (PI) = PSV − EDV/[(PSV + 2 × EDV)/3].

Frequencies of high RI (equal to 0.7 or higher) and high PI (equal to 1.3 or higher) from carotid and vertebral arteries were assessed [12,13].

2.4. Follow-Up Period

During an observation period of up to 36 months, the incidences of CVD and HF episodes were recorded. Cardiovascular disease was defined as fatal ischemic stroke, fatal myocardial infarction, fatal acute heart failure episode, or other CVD (i.e., any sudden or unexpected death unless proven as non-cardiovascular on autopsy). Heart failure episodes were defined as hospitalization for newly diagnosed or exacerbated congestive heart failure requiring administration of intravenous diuretics and/or vasoactive drugs (dopamine, dobutamine, epinephrine, or norepinephrine).

The final follow-up (FU) visit was conducted via telephone with the patient or an appointed family member. For all patients, data regarding patient vital status were obtained from the national health registry at the closing database.

2.5. Statistical Analysis

Data are presented as mean ± standard deviation or median (interquartile range) for continuous variables and as proportions for categorical variables. Differences between mean values were verified using the Student's t test and analysis of variance (ANOVA) test, while frequencies were compared using the chi squared test for independence, as appropriate. Normal distribution of the studied variables was determined using the Shapiro–Wilk test.

We assessed incidence of CVD and HF events in groups classified by high versus low PI and RI using the univariate Cox model, followed by the multivariable age-adjusted Cox models, with $PI \geq 1.3$ and $RI \geq 0.7$ as references [12,13]. We included age, sex, diabetes mellitus, hypertension, hyperlipidemia, previous myocardial infarction (MI), previous percutaneous coronary intervention (PCI), previous coronary artery bypass graft (CABG), chronic obstructive pulmonary disease (COPD), lower extremity artery disease (LEAD), LVEF, and pre-interventional AVA as factors which are potentially associated with the composite endpoint.

Results of the multivariate Cox proportional hazards analysis were expressed as hazard ratio (HR) and 95% confidence interval (CI). A two-sided value of $p < 0.05$ was considered statistically significant. The Kaplan-Mayer survival curves were constructed for groups with high vs. low VS. Statistical analyses were performed with Statistica version 13.3 software (TIBCO Software, Palo Alto, CA, USA) and with R Statistic Language 3.6.3 (R-Core Team, Vienna, Austria) [14].

3. Results

Out of 249 initially screened patients with severe DAS, 246 were eligible for follow-up evaluation. Three patients died from perioperative complications: 2 in the AVR and 1 in the TAVI groups.

Successful AVR was performed in 127 patients having a mean age of 69.3 ± 7.2 years (range: 53–86), including 75 (59.1%) females. Successful TAVI was performed in 119 patients having a mean age of 80.5 ± 5.8 years (range: 58–88), including 85 (71.4%) females.

The distribution of cardiovascular risk factors, including hyperlipidemia ($p = 0.346$), type 2 diabetes mellitus ($p = 0.748$), arterial hypertension ($p = 0.292$), history of previous MI ($p = 0.833$), and previous coronary interventions were similar between the AVR and the TAVI groups. Of note, patients referred for TAVI were older ($p < 0.001$) and more often were female ($p = 0.042$).

Patients with DAS referred for TAVI more frequently presented with symptoms corresponding to class 3 according to the New York Heart Association functional class (NYHA) when compared to AVR group (64.7% vs. 20.5%; $p < 0.001$).

All echocardiographic DAS parameters, as well as LVEF, were similar in both groups. Detailed study group characteristics are presented in Table 1.

Table 1. Study group clinical data.

	AVR Group N = 127	TAVI Group N = 119	p-Value
Demographic data			
Age, years, (SD)	69.3 (7.2)	80.5 (5.8)	<0.001
Female, n (%)	75 (59.1)	85 (71.4)	0.042
Hypertension, n (%)	118 (92.9)	106 (89.1)	0.292
Diabetes, n (%)	43 (33.9)	38 (31.9)	0.748
Dyslipidemia, n (%)	124 (97.6)	118 (99.2)	0.346
Previous MI, n (%)	27 (21.3)	24 (20.2)	0.833
COPD, n (%)	9 (7.1)	14 (11.8)	0.208
Previous PCI, n (%)	31 (24.4)	34 (28.6)	0.459
Previous CABG, n (%)	7 (5.5)	9 (7.6)	0.514
LEAD, n (%)	24 (18.9)	19 (16.0)	0.545
NYHA III vs. I + II, n (%)	26 (20.5)	77 (64.7)	<0.001
Echocardiographic data			
Aortic valve area (cm^2) ± SD	0.80 ± 0.2	0.70 ± 0.2	0.197
Peak aortic velocity (m/s) ± SD	4.76 ± 0.62	4.81 ± 0.68	0.193
Mean aortic gradient (mmHg) ± SD	52.6 ± 15.7	55.3 ± 19.2	0.596
Left ventricular ejection fraction (LVEF) (%) ± SD	61.8 ± 5.8	60.7 ± 7.0	0.368
Vascular stiffness parameters			
Resistive Index, median (Q1;Q3)	0.724 (0.685;0.784)	0.727 (0.714;0.756)	0.501
Pulsatile Index, median (Q1;Q3)	1.394 (1.272;1.650)	1.418 (1.364;1.527)	0.513
Resistive Index ≥ 0.7, n (%)	93 (78.2)	109 (91.6)	<0.001
Pulsatile Index ≥ 1.3, n (%)	93 (78.2)	109 (91.6)	<0.001

Abbreviations: AVR, aortic valve replacement; CABG, coronary artery bypass graft; COPD, chronic obstructive pulmonary disease; LEAD, lower extremities artery disease; MI, myocardial infarction; PCI, percutaneous coronary intervention; TAVI, transcatheter aortic valve implantation.

Increased RI ≥ 0.7 and PI ≥ 1.3 were found in 91.6% of DAS patients in the TAVI group vs. 78.2% in the AVR group ($p < 0.001$) (Table 1).

After each valvular intervention, during a mean FU period of 29.3 ± 10.4 months, the composite endpoint occurred in 29 of 119 (24.4%) TAVI patients, including CVD in 21 (17.7%) and non-fatal HF episodes in 8 (6.7%) patients. In AVR patients, the composite endpoint occurred in 15 of 127 (11.8%) patients, including CVD in 7 (5.5%) and non-fatal HF episodes in 8 (6.3%) patients. A detailed comparison of patients with adverse events in TAVI and AVR groups is presented in Table 2.

Among patients with the composite endpoint compared to event-free patients, increased VS parameters (RI ≥ 0.7 and PI ≥ 1.3) were found in 29/29 (100%) vs. 80/90 (88.9%) patients in the TAVI group ($p = 0.116$), and in 14/15 (93.3%) vs. 79/112 (70.5%) in the AVR group ($p = 0.061$). In the entire study group (AVR plus TAVI), patients with increased VS more frequently suffered from a cardiovascular event when compared to patients with lower VS values ($p = 0.011$).

However, there was a large overlap of median and interquartile RI and PI values between event vs. event-free groups (Figure 1).

In the entire study group, Kaplan-Mayer free-survival curves at 1-year and 3-year FU were 90.5% vs. 97.1% and 78% vs. 97.1% for patients with increased VS compared to patients with lower RI and PI values ($p = 0.014$). Additionally, when TAVI and AVR groups were analyzed separately, patients with increased VS had lower free-survival curves when compared to patients with normal RI and PI values; however, this did not reach the level of statistical significance (Figure 2).

Table 2. Comparison of patients with composite endpoint and event-free patients in AVR and TAVI groups.

	AVR Group without Composite Endpoint N = 112	AVR Group with Composite Endpoint N = 15	p-Value	TAVI Group without Composite Endpoint N = 90	TAVI Group with Composite Endpoint N = 29	p-Value
Demographic data						
Age, years, (SD)	69.3 ± 7.2	68.9 ± 7.1	0.952	80.0 ± 5.9	82.3 ± 5.4	0.032
Female, n (%)	65 (58.0)	10 (66.7)	0.523	61 (67.8)	24 (82.8)	0.120
Hypertension, n (%)	103 (92.0)	15 (100)	0.598	78 (86.7)	21 (72.4)	0.349
Diabetes, n (%)	37 (33.0)	6 (40.0)	0.592	28 (31.1)	9 (31.0)	0.994
Dyslipidemia, n (%)	109 (97.3)	15 (100)	1.000	89 (98.9)	28 (96.6)	0.395
Previous MI, n (%)	8 (7.1)	1 (6.7)	0.946	12 (13.3)	2 (6.9)	0.349
COPD, n (%)	27 (24.1)	0 (0)	0.04	18 (20.0)	6 (20.7)	0.934
Previous PCI, n (%)	28 (25.0)	3 (20.0)	0.672	21 (23.3)	12 (41.4)	0.059
Previous CABG, n (%)	6 (5.3)	1 (6.7)	0.835	5 (5.6)	4 (13.8)	0.145
LEAD, n (%)	19 (17.0)	5 (33.3)	0.128	12 (13.3)	7 (24.1)	0.167
NYHA III vs. I + II, n(%)	21 (18.8)	5 (33.3)	0.189	59 (65.6)	18 (62.1)	0.733
Echocardiographic data						
Aortic valve area (cm^2) ± SD	0.80 (0.20)	0.80 (0.27)	0.431	0.69 (0.19)	0.71 (0.22)	0.027
Peak aortic velocity (m/s) ± SD	4.79 (0.61)	4.54 (0.63)	0.296	4.79 (0.64)	4.84 (0.79)	0.064
Mean aortic gradient (mmHg) ± SD	53.0 (15.3)	49.5 (18.6)	0.284	54.7 (16.9)	58.1 (23.3)	0.091
LVEF (%) ± SD	61.7 (5.7)	62.8 (6.9)	0.341	60.7 (6.8)	60.9 (7.9)	0.460
Vascular stiffness parameters						
Resistive Index, median (Q1;Q3)	0.728 (0.678;0.797)	0.722 (0.705;0.755)	0.952	0.737 (0.715;0.758)	0.718 (0.712;0.737)	0.764
Pulsatile Index, median (Q1;Q3)	1.417 (1.242;1.713)	1.390 (1.335;1.526)	0.897	1.454 (1.368;1.538)	1.388 (1.361;1.451)	0.569
Resistive Index ≥ 0.7, n (%)	79 (70.5)	14 (93.3)	0.061	80 (88.9)	29 (100)	0.116
Pulsatile Index ≥ 1.3, n (%)	79 (70.5)	14 (93.3)	0.061	80 (88.9)	29 (100)	0.116

Abbreviations: AVR, aortic valve replacement; CABG, coronary artery bypass graft; COPD, chronic obstructive pulmonary disease; LEAD, lower extremities artery disease; MI, myocardial infarction; PCI, percutaneous coronary intervention; TAVI, transcatheter aortic valve implantation; VS, vascular stiffness.

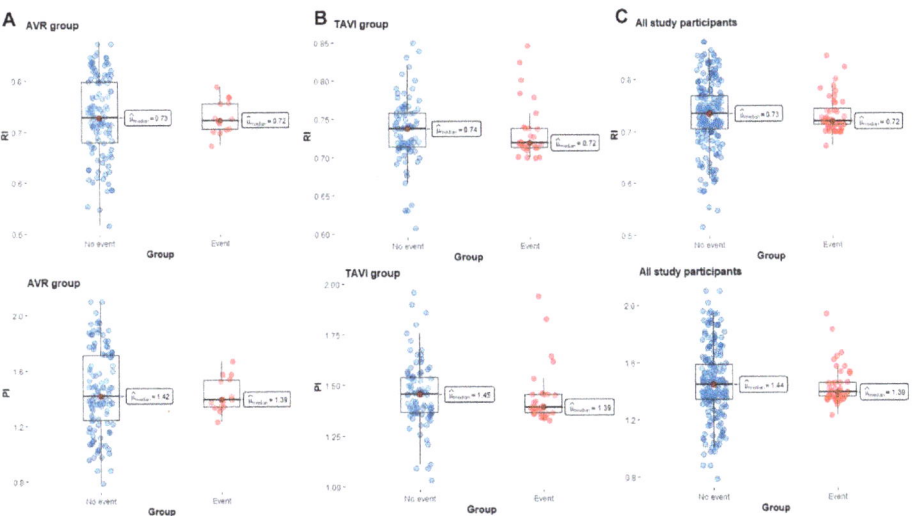

Figure 1. Median and interquartile range for mean RI and PI in patients with the composite endpoint and in patients without the endpoint. Panel (**A**), AVR group; Panel (**B**), TAVI group; Panel (**C**), all study participants (AVR and TAVI patients). Abbreviations: PI, pulsatile index; RI, resistive index.

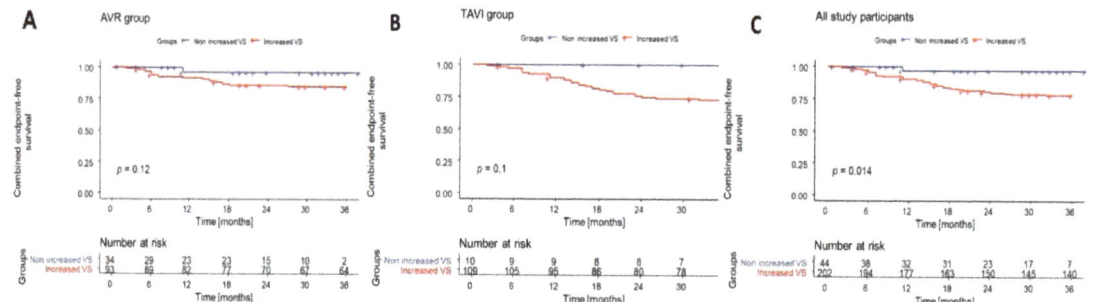

Figure 2. Kaplan-Meier survival curves showing time-to-event curves for 3-year cumulative survival to cardiovascular death and heart failure episodes dependent on increased vascular stiffness (defined as RI ≥ 0.7 and PI ≥ 1.3) compared to non-increased vascular stiffness. Panel (**A**), AVR group; Panel (**B**), TAVI group; Panel (**C**), all study participants (AVR and TAVI patients). Abbreviations: VS vascular stiffness.

In univariate Cox analysis, factors potentially associated with increased risk of adverse outcomes included elevated VS (HR 7.97, 95% CI 1.10 to 57.9; p = 0.04), age (HR 1.05, 95% CI 1.01 to 1.09; p = 0.024), female gender (HR 1.90, 95% CI 0.94 to 3.85, p = 0.074), LEAD (HR 1.76, 95% CI 0.91 to 3.42; p = 0.094), and NYHA class III (HR 1.73, 95% CI 0.96 to 3.13; p = 0.069) (Table 3).

Table 3. Univariate and multivariate Cox proportional hazard analysis presenting risk of cardio vascular death and heart failure episodes for increased VS (RI ≥ 0.7 and PI ≥ 1.3 in all study group participants.

Variable	Univariate Cox Proportional Hazard Analysis			Multivariate Cox Proportional Hazard Analysis		
	Hazard Ratio	95% Confidence Interval	p-Value	Hazard Ratio	95% Confidence Interval	p-Value
Age	1.05	1.01–1.09	0.024	1.02	0.97–1.06	0.420
Female gender	1.90	0.94–3.85	0.074	1.60	0.79–3.28	0.194
Hypertension	2.31	0.56–9.56	0.246			
Diabetes	1.10	0.59–2.04	0.774			
Dyslipidemia	0.50	0.07–3.61	0.488			
Previous MI	0.54	0.23–1.27	0.156			
COPD	0.69	0.21–2.23	0.534			
Previous PCI	1.41	0.75–2.62	0.284			
Previous CABG	1.94	0.76–4.92	0.163			
LEAD	1.76	0.91–3.42	0.094	2.22	1.12–4.39	0.023
Aortic valve area	0.90	0.20–3.99	0.893			
LVEF	1.00	0.96–1.05	0.943			
NYHA III vs. I + II	1.73	0.96–3.13	0.069	1.56	0.81–3.01	0.183
Increased VS (RI ≥ 0.7 and PI ≥ 1.3)	7.97	1.10–57.9	0.04	7.12	0.97–52.5	0.054

Abbreviations: CABG, coronary artery bypass graft; COPD, chronic obstructive pulmonary disease; LEAD, lower extremities artery disease; MI, myocardial infarction; LVEF, left ventricular ejection fraction; PCI, percutaneous coronary intervention; VS, vascular stiffness.

In multivariate Cox proportional hazard analysis, only LEAD (HR 2.22, 95% CI 1.12 to 4.39; p = 0.023) showed associations with risk of an adverse event, while increased VS failed to show an independent value (HR 7.12, 95% CI 0.97 to 52.5; p = 0.054) (Table 3).

4. Discussion

Our results support the hypothesis that high VS may be associated with risk of CVD and HF episodes in patients who underwent intervention for DAS, and that this risk can be elevated long after the intervention. Our findings are in line with studies by Makkar et al. and Mistiaen et al., who observed fatal cardiovascular events in patients with DAS and preserved LVEF, despite treatment of the valve [15,16].

Interestingly, the prognostic value of HF in patients with a preserved EF (HFpEF) in the TAVI population was presented by Seoudy et al. [17]. Importantly, the postulated multifactorial mechanisms of the HFpEF also may contribute to VS development and progression [18], while microvascular dysfunction underlies pathophysiological mechanisms of both VS and HF episodes despite a preserved systolic left ventricle contractility, constituting the main pathophysiological mechanism of recurrent HF episodes [19].

In the present study, preoperative values of RI $\geq$ 0.7 and PI $\geq$ 1.3, corresponding to increased VS, were associated with a 7.97-fold risk increase (p = 0.040) in univariate Cox proportional hazard analysis and a 7.12-fold risk increase (p = 0.054) in the occurrence of the composite endpoint in multivariate analysis. Similarly, Saeed et al. showed that event-free survival was significantly lower in patients with PWV $\geq$ 10 m/s when compared to those with lower PWV (p = 0.015); however, they observed an impact of PWV on all-cause mortality only in univariate Cox analysis (HR 1.80, 95% CI 1.14 to 2.83; p = 0.012) and not in multivariate analysis (HR 0.91, 95% CI 0.48 to 1.74, p = 0.778) [20].

In patients who underwent AVR for symptomatic DAS, increased left ventricular filling pressures were associated with cardiovascular mortality after AVR [21].

Similarly, in TAVI patients, VS is proposed as an important risk factor for adverse outcomes [22,23].

Tanaka et al. assessed the impact of pre-procedural brachial-ankle pulse wave velocity (PWV) on 1-year post-TAVI adverse outcomes in a group of 161 patients with severe DAS [22]. In the group with increased PWV, the incidence of all-cause death and re-hospitalization related to HF episodes was 3.42-fold greater (95% CI 1.62 to 7.85; p = 0.002) when compared to that of patients with lower PWV values [22]. Broyd et al. indicated an optimum cut-off for PWV higher than 11 m/s to be the only predictor of 1-year mortality following TAVI in 186 patients (OR 3.57, 95% CI 1.36–9.42, p = 0.01) associated with survival (log-rank p = 0.04) [23]. In line with these studies, our results indicate an important role for VS in the prediction of event-free survival at 1-year and 3-year FU, which were 90.5% vs. 97.1% and 78% vs. 97.1% for patients with increased VS when compared to patients with lower RI and PI values (p = 0.014).

Some researchers have investigated further, comparing VS parameters after DAS intervention. Musa et al. compared the impact of TAVI and AVR on VS as measured with PWV. They found that there was a further significant increase in PWV parameters following AVR at the 6-month FU, while in the TAVI arm, the postprocedural PWV increase did not reach the level of statistical significance [24]. However, in a TAVI population, Terentes-Printzios et al. showed that the arterial system exhibited increased stiffness in response to acute relief of the obstruction following intervention, which was retained in the long term [25]. Of note, in this high-risk subset of patients, such as patients referred for TAVI, the intervention on the valve has a beneficial effect on supra-aortic artery flow parameters during the orthostatic stress test, resulting from the alleviated obstruction to cerebral in-flow [26]. On the other hand, Cantürk et al. did not observe a significant change in PWV values following AVR [27].

In our study, we did not find a relationship between pre-interventional VS values and the NYHA class symptoms to the support findings of Kidher et al., which showed that PWV was an independent predictor of NYHA class pre-operatively (OR 8.3, 95% CI 2.27 to 33.33) and post-operatively (OR 14.44, 95% CI 1.49 to 139.31) [28]. Of interest, the baseline NYHA class (OR 1.02, 95% CI 1.005 to 1.041, p = 0.041) may be an independent predictor of improvement in PWV following AVR [28].

Our study shows the limitations of using VS parameters in daily clinical practice. The main disadvantage in result interpretation is the large overlap in median RI and PI values between groups with adverse events when compared to those without (Figure 1). A potential explanation for this finding is the presence of multifactorial associations between VS, traditional, and non-traditional cardiovascular risk factors [13,29].

Therefore, more data are required from studies in a larger scaled population to determine the role of VS in predicting outcome following aortic valve interventions. Recently published data from the OCEAN Japanese multicenter registry including 2588 patients who underwent TAVI demonstrated that male sex, body mass index, Clinical Frailty Scale, atrial fibrillation, peripheral artery disease, prior cardiac surgery, serum albumin level, renal function, and presence of pulmonary disease were independent predictors of 1-year mortality following TAVI [30]. However, in the registry of Yamamoto et al., arterial compliance was not investigated at all. Similarly, our present study showed LEAD to be an independent risk factor for CVD and HF episodes following aortic valve intervention. In summary, the Heart Team is at the center of the decision-making process in patients with DAS [31–33]. The gathered experience indicates that a multidimensional and multidisciplinary pre-procedural work-up in patients with severe DAS, including a thorough assessment of coexisting disorders, results in an optimal treatment strategy and can be associated with a superior prognosis when compared to conservative medical management [31–33].

Accordingly, future studies are required to elucidate whether routine VS assessment should be incorporated as an additional parameter in this risk stratification model.

Seoudy et al. showed the clinical importance of a potential role in routine assessment of patients with HFpEF using the novel diagnostics algorithm (HFA-PEFF score) among the DAS population [17], where the same VS advancement score could be beneficial for better patient monitoring and treatment.

5. Conclusions

Our data demonstrates that VS is common in patients with severe DAS. We have demonstrated that increased VS can be a predictor of post-procedure outcome. In patients with PI $\geq$ 1.3 or RI $\geq$ 0.7, there is an increased risk of cardiovascular death and heart failure episodes despite intervention on the aortic valve (AVR or TAVI). However, huge the large overlap of RI and PI values between patients with or without adverse events during follow-up may limit the clinical value of routine vascular stiffness assessment.

Author Contributions: Conceptualization, J.B., P.K., A.K.-Z. and J.P.; data curation, J.B., Ł.N., R.B., P.P., J.L. and K.Z.; formal analysis, Ł.N., J.P. and P.P.; funding acquisition, A.K.-Z. and J.P.; investigation, P.K., Ł.N., R.B., P.P. and A.K.-Z.; methodology, J.B., Ł.N., R.B., T.P. and A.K.-Z.; project administration, K.Z.; resources, J.B. and T.P.; software, J.B. and Ł.N.; supervision, A.K.-Z.; validation, O.A., J.L. and K.Z.; visualization, J.B., Ł.N. and R.B.; writing—original draft, J.B., P.K. and J.P.; writing—review and editing, O.A., J.L., K.Z., T.P. and A.K.-Z. All authors have read and agreed to the published version of the manuscript.

Funding: This research was funded by grants from the Jagiellonian University (grant numbers: N41/DBS/000038 and N41/DBS/000437).

Institutional Review Board Statement: The study was conducted in accordance with the Declaration of Helsinki and approved by the Institutional Ethics Committee of the Jagiellonian University (KBET/118/B/2014 and KBET/1072.6120.148.2018).

Informed Consent Statement: Informed consent was obtained from all subjects involved in the study.

Data Availability Statement: The data presented in this study are available on request from the corresponding author. The data are not publicly available due to privacy.

Conflicts of Interest: The authors declare no conflict of interest.

References

1. Kabłak-Ziembicka, A.; Rosławiecka, A.; Badacz, R.; Sokołowski, A.; Rzeźnik, D.; Trystuła, M.; Musiałek, P.; Przewłocki, T. Simple clinical scores to predict blood pressure and renal function response to renal artery stenting for atherosclerotic renal artery stenosis. *Pol. Arch. Intern. Med.* **2020**, *130*, 953–959. [CrossRef] [PubMed]
2. Wielicka, M.; Neubauer-Geryk, J.; Kozera, G.; Bieniaszewski, L. Clinical application of pulsatility index. *Med. Res. J.* **2020**, *52*, 201–210. [CrossRef]
3. Sutton-Tyrrell, K.; Najjar, S.S.; Boudreau, R.M.; Venkitachalam, L.; Kupelian, V.; Simonsick, E.M.; Havlik, R.; Lakatta, E.G.; Spurgeon, H.; Kritchevsky, S.; et al. Health ABC Study. Elevated aortic pulse wave velocity, a marker of arterial stiffness, predicts cardiovascular events in well-functioning older adults. *Circulation* **2005**, *111*, 3384–3390. [CrossRef] [PubMed]
4. Nilsson, P.M.; Boutouyrie, P.; Cunha, P.; Kotsis, V.; Narkiewicz, K.; Parati, G.; Rietzschel, E.; Scuteri, A.; Laurent, S. Early vascular ageing in translation: From laboratory investigations to clinical applications in cardiovascular prevention. *J. Hypertens.* **2013**, *31*, 1517–1526. [CrossRef] [PubMed]
5. Yan, A.T.; Koh, M.; Chan, K.K.; Guo, H.; Alter, D.A.; Austin, P.C.; Tu, J.V.; Wijeysundera, H.C.; Ko, D.T. Association Between Cardiovascular Risk Factors and Aortic Stenosis: The CANHEART Aortic Stenosis Study. *J. Am. Coll. Cardiol.* **2017**, *69*, 1523–1532. [CrossRef]
6. Podolec, J.; Baran, J.; Siedlinski, M.; Urbanczyk, M.; Krupinski, M.; Bartus, K.; Niewiara, L.; Podolec, M.; Guzik, T.; Tomkiewicz-Pajak, L.; et al. Serum rantes, transforming growth factor-β1 and interleukin-6 levels correlate with cardiac muscle fibrosis in patients with aortic valve stenosis. *J. Physiol. Pharmacol.* **2018**, *69*, 615–623. [CrossRef]
7. Severino, P.; D'Amato, A.; Prosperi, S.; Magnocavallo, M.; Mariani, M.V.; Netti, L.; Birtolo, L.I.; De Orchi, P.; Chimenti, C.; Maestrini, V.; et al. Potential Role of eNOS Genetic Variants in Ischemic Heart Disease Susceptibility and Clinical Presentation. *J. Cardiovasc. Dev. Dis.* **2021**, *8*, 116. [CrossRef]
8. Gardikioti, V.; Terentes-Printzios, D.; Iliopoulos, D.; Aznaouridis, K.; Sigala, E.; Tsioufis, K.; Vlachopoulos, C. Arterial biomarkers in the evaluation, management, and prognosis of aortic stenosis. *Atherosclerosis* **2021**, *332*, 1–15. [CrossRef]
9. Mach, F.; Baigent, C.; Catapano, A.L.; Koskinas, K.C.; Casula, M.; Badimon, L.; Chapman, M.J.; De Backer, G.G.; Delgado, V.; Ference, B.A.; et al. 2019 ESC/EAS Guidelines for the management of dyslipidaemias: Lipid modification to reduce cardiovascular risk. *Eur. Heart J.* **2020**, *41*, 111–188. [CrossRef]
10. Williams, B.; Mancia, G.; Spiering, W.; Agabiti Rosei, E.; Azizi, M.; Burnier, M.; Clement, D.L.; Coca, A.; de Simone, G.; Dominiczak, A.; et al. 2018 ESC/ESH Guidelines for the management of arterial hypertension: The Task Force for the management of arterial hypertension of the European Society of Cardiology and the European Society of Hypertension: The Task Force for the management of arterial hypertension of the European Society of Cardiology and the European Society of Hypertension. *J. Hypertens.* **2018**, *36*, 1953–2041. [CrossRef]
11. Baumgartner, H.; Hung, J.; Bermejo, J.; Chambers, J.B.; Edvardsen, T.; Goldstein, S.; Lancellotti, P.; LeFevre, M.; Miller, F., Jr.; Otto, C.M. Recommendations on the echocardiographic assessment of aortic valve stenosis: A focused update from the European Association of Cardiovascular Imaging and the American Society of Echocardiography. *J. Am. Soc. Echocardiogr.* **2017**, *30*, 372–392. [CrossRef] [PubMed]
12. Frauchiger, B.; Schmid, H.P.; Roedel, C.; Moosmann, P.; Staub, D. Comparison of carotid arterial resistive indices with intima-media thickness as sonographic markers of atherosclerosis. *Stroke* **2001**, *32*, 836–841. [CrossRef] [PubMed]
13. Baran, J.; Kleczyński, P.; Niewiara, Ł.; Podolec, J.; Badacz, R.; Gackowski, A.; Pieniążek, P.; Legutko, J.; Żmudka, K.; Przewłocki, T.; et al. Importance of Increased Arterial Resistance in Risk Prediction in Patients with Cardiovascular Risk Factors and Degenerative Aortic Stenosis. *J. Clin. Med.* **2021**, *10*, 2109. [CrossRef] [PubMed]
14. Robin, X.; Turck, N.; Hainard, A.; Tiberti, N.; Lisacek, F.; Sanchez, J.C.; Müller, M. pROC: An open-source package for R and S+ to analyze and compare ROC curves. *BMC Bioinf.* **2011**, *12*, 77. [CrossRef]
15. Makkar, R.R.; Thourani, V.H.; Mack, M.J.; Kodali, S.K.; Kapadia, S.; Webb, J.G.; Yoon, S.H.; Trento, A.; Svensson, L.G.; Herrmann, H.C. PARTNER 2 Investigators. Five-Year Outcomes of Transcatheter or Surgical Aortic-Valve Replacement. *N. Engl. J. Med.* **2020**, *382*, 799–809. [CrossRef]
16. Mistiaen, W.P.; Van Cauwelaert, P.; Muylaert, P.; Wuyts, F.; Bortier, H. Risk factors for congestive heart failure after aortic valve replacement with a Carpentier-Edwards pericardial prosthesis in the elderly. *J. Heart Valve Dis.* **2005**, *14*, 774–779.
17. Seoudy, H.; von Eberstein, M.; Frank, J.; Thomann, M.; Puehler, T.; Lutter, G.; Lutz, M.; Bramlage, P.; Frey, N.; Saad, M.; et al. HFA-PEFF score: Prognosis in patients with preserved ejection fraction after transcatheter aortic valve implantation. *ESC Heart Fail.* **2022**, *9*, 1071–1079. [CrossRef]
18. Severino, P.; D'Amato, A.; Prosperi, S.; Fanisio, F.; Birtolo, L.I.; Costi, B.; Netti, L.; Chimenti, C.; Lavalle, C.; Maestrini, V.; et al. Myocardial Tissue Characterization in Heart Failure with Preserved Ejection Fraction: From Histopathology and Cardiac Magnetic Resonance Findings to Therapeutic Targets. *Int. J. Mol. Sci.* **2021**, *22*, 7650. [CrossRef]
19. Kontogeorgos, S.; Thunström, E.; Pivodic, A.; Dahlström, U.; Fu, M. Prognosis and outcome determinants after heart failure diagnosis in patients who underwent aortic valvular intervention. *ESC Heart Fail.* **2021**, *8*, 3237–3247. [CrossRef]
20. Saeed, S.; Saeed, N.; Grigoryan, K.; Chowienczyk, P.; Chambers, J.B.; Rajani, R. Determinants and clinical significance of aortic stiffness in patients with moderate or severe aortic stenosis. *Int. J. Cardiol.* **2020**, *315*, 99–104. [CrossRef]

21. Thaden, J.J.; Balakrishnan, M.; Sanchez, J.; Adigun, R.; Nkomo, V.T.; Eleid, M.; Dahl, J.; Scott, C.; Pislaru, S.; Oh, J.K.; et al. Left ventricular filling pressure and survival following aortic valve replacement for severe aortic stenosis. *Heart* **2020**, *106*, 830–837. [CrossRef] [PubMed]
22. Tanaka, T.; Asami, M.; Yahagi, K.; Ninomiya, K.; Okuno, T.; Horiuchi, Y.; Komiyama, K.; Tanaka, J.; Yokozuka, M.; Miura, S.; et al. Prognostic impact of arterial stiffness following transcatheter aortic valve replacement. *J. Cardiol.* **2021**, *78*, 37–43. [CrossRef] [PubMed]
23. Broyd, C.J.; Patel, K.; Pugliese, F.; Chehab, O.; Mathur, A.; Baumbach, A.; Ozkor, M.; Kennon, S.; Mullen, M. Pulse wave velocity can be accurately measured during transcatheter aortic valve implantation and used for post-procedure risk stratification. *J. Hypertens.* **2019**, *37*, 1845–1852. [CrossRef]
24. Musa, T.A.; Uddin, A.; Fairbairn, T.A.; Dobson, L.E.; Sourbron, S.P.; Steadman, C.D.; Motwani, M.; Kidambi, A.; Ripley, D.P.; Swoboda, P.P.; et al. Assessment of aortic stiffness by cardiovascular magnetic resonance following the treatment of severe aortic stenosis by TAVI and surgical AVR. *J. Cardiovasc. Magn. Reson.* **2016**, *18*, 37. [CrossRef] [PubMed]
25. Terentes-Printzios, D.; Gardikioti, V.; Aznaouridis, K.; Latsios, G.; Drakopoulou, M.; Siasos, G.; Oikonomou, E.; Tsigkou, V.; Xanthopoulou, M.; Vavuranakis, M.; et al. The impact of transcatheter aortic valve implantation on arterial stiffness and wave reflections. *Int. J. Cardiol.* **2021**, *323*, 213–219. [CrossRef]
26. Kleczyński, P.; Petkow Dimitrow, P.; Dziewierz, A.; Surdacki, A.; Dudek, D. Transcatheter aortic valve implantation improves carotid and vertebral arterial blood flow in patients with severe aortic stenosis: Practical role of orthostatic stress test. *Clin. Cardiol.* **2017**, *40*, 492–497. [CrossRef]
27. Cantürk, E.; Çakal, B.; Karaca, O.; Omaygenç, O.; Salihi, S.; Özyüksel, A.; Akçevin, A. Changes in Aortic Pulse Wave Velocity and the Predictors of Improvement in Arterial Stiffness Following Aortic Valve Replacement. *Ann. Thorac. Cardiovasc. Surg.* **2017**, *23*, 248–255. [CrossRef]
28. Kidher, E.; Harling, L.; Ashrafian, H.; Naase, H.; Francis, D.P.; Evans, P.; Athanasiou, T. Aortic stiffness as a marker of cardiac function and myocardial strain in patients undergoing aortic valve replacement. *J. Cardiothorac. Surg.* **2014**, *91*, 2. [CrossRef]
29. Baran, J.; Podolec, J.; Tomala, M.; Nawrotek, B.; Niewiara, Ł.; Gackowski, A.; Przewłocki, T.; Żmudka, K.; Kabłak-Ziembicka, A. Increased risk profile in the treatment of patients with symptomatic degenerative aortic valve stenosis over the last 10 years. *Adv. Interv. Cardiol.* **2018**, *14*, 276–284. [CrossRef]
30. Yamamoto, M.; Otsuka, T.; Shimura, T.; Yamaguchi, R.; Adachi, Y.; Kagase, A.; Tokuda, T.; Yashima, F.; Watanabe, Y.; Tada, N.; et al. Clinical risk model for predicting 1-year mortality after transcatheter aortic valve replacement. *Cath. Cardiovasc. Interv.* **2021**, *97*, E544–E551. [CrossRef]
31. Jonik, S.; Marchel, M.; Pędzich-Placha, E.; Huczek, Z.; Kochman, J.; Ścisło, P.; Czub, P.; Wilimski, R.; Hendzel, P.; Opolski, G.; et al. Heart Team for Optimal Management of Patients with Severe Aortic Stenosis-Long-Term Outcomes and Quality of Life from Tertiary Cardiovascular Care Center. *J. Clin. Med.* **2021**, *10*, 5408. [CrossRef] [PubMed]
32. Pighi, M.; Giovannini, D.; Scarsini, R.; Piazza, N. Diagnostic Work-Up of the Aortic Patient: An Integrated Approach toward the Best Therapeutic Option. *J. Clin. Med.* **2021**, *10*, 5120. [CrossRef] [PubMed]
33. Ciardetti, N.; Ciatti, F.; Nardi, G.; Di Muro, F.M.; Demola, P.; Sottili, E.; Stolcova, M.; Ristalli, F.; Mattesini, A.; Meucci, F.; et al. Advancements in Transcatheter Aortic Valve Implantation: A Focused Update. *Medicina* **2021**, *57*, 711. [CrossRef] [PubMed]

Energy Drinks and Their Acute Effects on Arterial Stiffness in Healthy Children and Teenagers: A Randomized Trial

Pengzhu Li, Guido Mandilaras, André Jakob, Robert Dalla-Pozza, Nikolaus Alexander Haas and Felix Sebastian Oberhoffer *

Division of Pediatric Cardiology and Intensive Care, University Hospital, LMU Munich, 81377 Munich, Germany; pengzhu.li.extern@med.uni-muenchen.de (P.L.); guido.mandilaras@med.uni-muenchen.de (G.M.); andre.jakob@med.uni-muenchen.de (A.J.); robert.dallapozza@med.uni-muenchen.de (R.D.-P.); nikolaus.haas@med.uni-muenchen.de (N.A.H.)
* Correspondence: felix.oberhoffer@med.uni-muenchen.de

Abstract: Adolescents are the main consumer group of energy drinks (ED). Studies suggest that acute ED consumption is associated with increased peripheral blood pressure. Little is known of the ED-induced effects on arterial stiffness. Therefore, this study aimed to investigate the acute effects of ED consumption on arterial stiffness in healthy children and teenagers by conducting a prospective, randomized, single-blind, placebo-controlled, crossover clinical trial. Study participants (n = 27, mean age = 14.53 years) consumed a body-weight-adjusted amount of an ED or a placebo on two consecutive days. Arterial stiffness was evaluated sonographically by two-dimensional speckle tracking of the common carotid artery (CCA) at baseline and up to four hours after beverage consumption. The ED intake led to a significantly decreased peak circumferential strain of the CCA (11.78 ± 2.70% vs. 12.29 ± 2.68%, $p = 0.043$) compared with the placebo. The results of this study indicate that the acute ED consumption might be associated with increased arterial stiffness in healthy children and teenagers. Minors, particularly those with increased cardiovascular morbidity, should be discouraged from ED consumption.

Keywords: energy drinks; arterial stiffness; pediatrics; prevention

1. Introduction

Energy drinks (EDs) are soft drinks that contain high amounts of sugar, caffeine, and other stimulant compounds such as guarana, taurine, or ginseng [1]. EDs were introduced in the 1960s and have become one of the fastest-growing beverages in the soft drink industry after widespread advertising in the 1990s [2]. EDs are particularly popular among teenagers and young adults. According to a review conducted by Seifert et al., 30% to 50% of adolescents and young adults consume EDs [3]. The main function of EDs is marketed as providing fatigue relief, physical performance enhancement, and concentration improvement [4]. However, heavy ED consumption is associated with a series of cardiovascular side effects, including arterial hypertension and arrhythmia in young adults [5–7]. Multiple studies demonstrated that heavy ED consumption is linked with increased blood pressure in young adults [5,8,9]. In addition, a recent publication by our department revealed that acute ED consumption significantly raised systolic and diastolic blood pressure in a pediatric cohort [10].

Arterial stiffness refers to the wall rigidity of the large arterial vessels, including the aorta, the carotid arteries, and the cervical arteries [11]. Healthy large arteries have a strong cushioning function. Arterial stiffening caused by aging and multiple cardiovascular risk factors (e.g., smoking, dyslipidemia, diabetes, excess weight) impairs this cushioning function [12]. The stiffness-induced increase in pulse pressure (PP) was shown to be an independent predictor of cardiovascular risk [13].

The current gold standard for the assessment of arterial stiffness is considered to be carotid-femoral pulse wave velocity (cfPWV) measurement [14]. Other techniques, such as performing an ultrasound of the great arteries, have been recently applied to evaluate arterial stiffness: two-dimensional speckle tracking (2DST) is an advanced, non-invasive imaging technique, which has been widely used to analyze left ventricular function [15]. Recently, 2DST has been applied to assess arterial stiffness by tracking the ultrasonic speckles of the arterial wall during systole and diastole. Through the calculation of the vessel's deformation (strain), arterial stiffness can be visualized [16,17].

Current studies support the hypothesis that caffeine increases arterial stiffness and thus has an impact on the cardiovascular system [18]. To the best of our knowledge, the acute effects of caffeine-containing ED consumption on arterial stiffness have not been investigated yet.

The aim of this study was to evaluate the acute effects of caffeine-containing ED consumption on arterial stiffness in healthy children and teenagers.

2. Materials and Methods

2.1. Ethical Statement

This study was conducted according to the guidelines of the Declaration of Helsinki and approved by the Ethics Committee of the Ludwig Maximilians University Munich (Munich, Germany) (protocol code: 20-0993, date of approval: 12 January 2021). We obtained prior written informed consent from all study participants. For minor study participants we additionally obtained prior written informed consent from parents or legal guardians.

2.2. Study Population

In total, 27 healthy children and teenagers aged 10–18 years were prospectively enrolled for this study. Study participants were examined for eligibility through personal interviews, clinical examination, conventional echocardiography, 24-h Holter ECG, and 24-h blood pressure monitoring before inclusion. The exclusion criteria were as follows: the presence of chronic diseases such as congenital heart disease, arterial hypertension, presence of severe dysrhythmia, family history of sudden cardiac death, allergies to beverage ingredients, regular use of medication with effects on cardiovascular function, regular use of drugs including smoking and alcohol consumption, and pregnancy.

In study participants <18 years, weight classification was assessed according to the body mass index (BMI, kg/m^2) percentiles (P.) established by Kromeyer-Hauschild et al. [19]. In study participants ≥18 years, normal weight was defined as BMI < 25 kg/m^2, overweight as BMI ≥ 25 kg/m^2 but < 30 kg/m^2, and obesity as BMI ≥ 30 kg/m^2.

The caffeine consumption behavior of study participants was assessed in accordance with Shah et al.: rare caffeine consumers if <1 caffeinated beverage per month, occasional caffeine consumers if 1 to 3 caffeinated beverages per month, frequent caffeine consumers if 1 to 6 caffeinated beverages per week, and daily caffeine consumers if ≥1 caffeinated beverage per day [5]. In addition, study participants' ED consumption behavior was investigated as described above.

2.3. Study Design

This study was a prospective, randomized, single-blind (study participants), placebo-controlled, crossover clinical trial conducted by the Division of Pediatric Cardiology and Intensive Care, University Hospital, LMU Munich (Munich, Germany), from April 2021 to October 2021. The study was registered in the German Clinical Trials Register (https://www.drks.de/drks_web/DRKS00027580 (accessed on 27 February 2022)).

Detailed information on the study design was described in a recent publication by our department [20]. In short, eligible study participants were randomized into two groups (Group I: day 1: ED, day 2: placebo; Group II: day 1: placebo, day 2: ED) and received either an ED or a placebo drink on two consecutive days. The administered ED amount was adjusted according to the maximal daily caffeine consumption for healthy children and teenagers (3 mg caffeine per kilogram of body weight per day) as recommended by the European Food Safety Authority [21]. The amount of the administered placebo drink was matched with the ED and did not contain typical ED ingredients such as caffeine, guarana, or taurine. ED and placebo had a similar sugar content and taste. The beverages were administered in an identical and masked drinking bottle at room temperature on both study days.

Participants were required not to consume any sources of caffeine or drugs 48 h before and 24 h after study participation. An overnight fast (apart from water) was requested before every study day. Study participants were asked not to consume any food or liquids during each examination duration. Lastly, after complete data collection, to assess blinding quality, study participants were asked to guess on which study day the ED beverage was administered.

2.4. Two-Dimensional Speckle Tracking of the Common Carotid Artery

An iE33 xMatrix and an Epiq 7G ultrasound machine (Philips, Amsterdam, The Netherlands) were used for examination. Both common carotid arteries (CCA) were recorded in short-axis view just below carotid bifurcation with a 3–8 MHz sector array transducer. During the entire examination period, study participants were in supine position, and the neck was extended to a 45° angle and turned to the opposite side of examination. Three consecutive loops were acquired under constant three-lead ECG tracking. Recorded clips were then transferred to a separate workstation (QLAB cardiovascular ultrasound quantification software, version 11.1, Philips, Amsterdam, The Netherlands). Peak circumferential strain (CS, %) and peak strain rate (SR, s^{-1}) of both CCAs were measured semi-automatically through the software's function "SAX-A". The vascular region of interest was manually adjusted. Speckles of the vessel wall were then two-dimensionally tracked, as visualized in Figure 1. A masked investigator analyzed the recorded loops three consecutive times, and an average was then calculated. Arterial distensibility (mmHg^{-1} × 10^{-3}) was defined as

Arterial distensibility = (2 × Peak Circumferential Strain)/(Systolic Blood Pressure − Diastolic Blood Pressure)

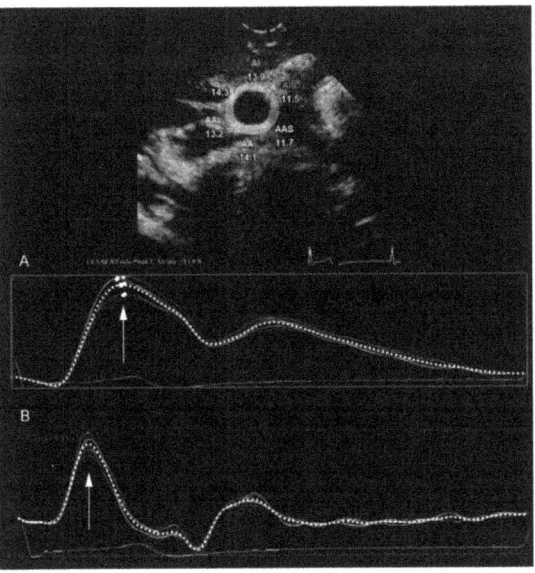

Figure 1. Two-dimensional speckle tracking of the common carotid artery. The arrow indicates (**A**) peak circumferential strain (CS, %) and (**B**) peak strain rate (SR, s^{-1}).

Data on ambulatory blood pressure, which were used for the calculation of arterial distensibility, were given in a recent publication by our department [10]. CS, SR, and arterial distensibility of the right and left CCA were averaged.

2.5. Endpoints Measurement

The endpoints were CS, SR, and arterial distensibility. For each study day, the endpoints were assessed at baseline as well as 30, 60, 120, and 240 min after beverage consumption.

2.6. Statistical Analysis

As this study was a pediatric pilot study, pediatric reference values for ED-induced changes in arterial stiffness did not exist and could not be considered in a power analysis. To test for normal distribution of continuous variables, histograms, QQ-plots, and the Shapiro–Wilk test were applied. Mean and standard deviation were used for all continuous variables. Ordinal and nominal variables are presented as percentages and counts. Sqrt or Ln data transformation was used if data were not normally distributed. A paired t-test was applied to compare baseline parameters between the ED and the placebo group. A two-way repeated-measures analysis of variance (ANOVA) was performed to evaluate the main effects of "beverage", "time", and interaction of "beverage and time" on CS, SR, and arterial distensibility. The Bonferroni-adjusted pairwise test was used for post hoc testing. Data analyses were performed independently by a masked statistician using SPSS (IBM SPSS Statistics for Windows, version 26.0. IBM Corp., Armonk, NY, USA). A p-value < 0.05 was considered statistically significant.

3. Results

3.1. Patient Characteristics

A total of 27 healthy children and teenagers were included in the analysis. The characteristics of participants are shown in Table 1. None of the subjects had chronic health conditions or was receiving medication. The parameters of arterial stiffness were not significantly different between the two groups at baseline (Table 2). Thirteen of the twenty-seven study participants (48.15%) correctly guessed the day of ED administration, indicating an appropriate blinding quality.

Table 1. Study Participants' Characteristics (n = 27).

Characteristics	Total
Age, years (mean ± SD)	14.53 ± 2.40
Sex, n (%)	
Male	14 (51.85)
Female	13 (48.15)
Weight Classification, n (%)	
Normal weight	23 (85.19)
Overweight	4 (14.81)
Obese	0 (0)
Caffeine Consumption Behavior, n (%) [a]	
Rare	17 (62.96)
Occasional	3 (11.11)
Frequent	5 (18.52)
Daily	2 (7.41)
Energy Drink Consumption Behavior, n (%) [b]	
Never	12 (44.44)
Rare	11 (40.74)
Occasional	1 (3.70)
Frequent	3 (11.11)
Daily	0 (0)

[a] Rare caffeine consumer if <1 caffeine-containing drink per month, occasional caffeine consumer if 1 to 3 caffeine-containing drinks per month, frequent caffeine consumer if 1 to 6 caffeine-containing drinks per week, and daily caffeine consumer if ≥1 caffeine-containing drink per day [5]. [b] Rare energy drink (ED) consumer if <1 ED per month, occasional ED consumer if 1 to 3 EDs per month, frequent ED consumer if 1 to 6 EDs per week, and daily ED consumer if ≥1 ED per day.

Table 2. Parameters of Arterial Stiffness at Baseline ($n = 27$).

Parameters	Energy Drink	Placebo	p-Value
CCA CS (%)	12.37 ± 3.01	12.29 ± 2.76	0.89
CCA SR (s^{-1})	3.23 ± 0.73	3.24 ± 0.73	0.94
Arterial Distensibility (mmHg^{-1} × 10^{-3})	538.68 ± 135.25	519.94 ± 117.22	0.49

CCA, common carotid artery; CS, peak circumferential strain; SR, peak strain rate. Mean ± standard deviation were used for normally distributed parameters.

3.2. Acute Effects of Energy Drinks on CS, SR, and Arterial Distensibility

The Shapiro–Wilk test revealed a non-normal distribution for the CS at time points baseline, 120 min, and 240 min within the ED group. It revealed a non-normal distribution for the SR at time point 30 min within the placebo group and at time points baseline and 120 min within the ED group. For arterial distensibility, a non-normal distribution was assessed at time points baseline, 60 min, and 120 min within the placebo group and at time points 30 min and 120 min within the ED group. To achieve a normal distribution, the original CS and SR data were transferred into Sqrt-form, and the original arterial distensibility data were transferred into Ln-form. According to Mauchly's sphericity hypothesis test for the interaction term "beverage and time", the variance and covariance matrices of the dependent variables were equal ($p > 0.05$).

The interaction between the variables "beverage and time" had no statistically significant effect on the CS, the SR, and arterial distensibility ($p > 0.05$). Hence, the main effect of "beverage consumption" was chosen.

A two-way repeated-measures ANOVA demonstrated that the CS was significantly lower after ED consumption compared with placebo intake (Table 3, Figure 2). In addition, the SR tended to be lower after ED consumption but did not reach statistical significance (Table 3). Regarding arterial distensibility, no significant differences were assessed between both groups (Table 3).

Table 3. CS, SR and, Arterial Distensibility after Energy Drink and Placebo Consumption ($n = 27$).

Parameters	Energy Drink	Placebo	p-Value
CCA CS (%)	11.78 ± 2.70	12.29 ± 2.68	0.043 *
CCA SR (s^{-1})	3.20 ± 0.73	3.34 ± 0.74	0.087
Arterial Distensibility (mmHg^{-1} × 10^{-3})	504.69 ± 145.50	521.92 ± 134.99	0.313

CCA, common carotid artery; CS, peak circumferential strain; SR, peak strain rate. * $p < 0.05$.

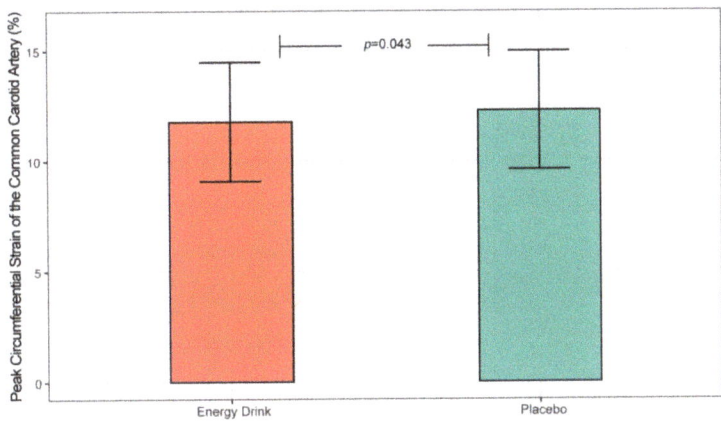

Figure 2. Peak Circumferential Strain (CS, %) of the Common Carotid Artery after Energy Drink and Placebo Consumption.

4. Discussion

To the best of our knowledge, this is the first study investigating the acute effects of ED consumption on arterial stiffness in healthy children and teenagers. In total, 27 children with a mean age of 14.53 years were included for strain imaging of the CCA. After ED consumption, a significant decrease in the CS was observed. In addition, the SR tended to be lower after ED intake. Therefore, the results of this study suggest an acute elevation of arterial stiffness in a cohort of healthy children and teenagers after ED consumption.

4.1. Pathophysiological Considerations and Clinical Implications

The ED-induced effects on arterial stiffness can mainly be attributed to the high content of caffeine and guarana in EDs. Caffeine is thought to increase peripheral vascular resistance through sympathetic stimulation and consequently effect arterial stiffness [18,22]. Interestingly, a recent publication by our department reported a significant increase in peripheral systolic and diastolic blood pressure in the same pediatric cohort after ED consumption [10]. The results of this study suggest that the increased peripheral vascular resistance may result in an elevation of arterial stiffness visualized by a significant decrease in CS after ED consumption.

For this study, the administered amount of caffeine corresponded to the maximal daily dose (3 mg caffeine per kilogram of body weight per day) recommended for healthy children and teenagers by the European Food Safety Authority [21]. Presumably, the cardiovascular system might respond even more severely to higher amounts of caffeinated EDs. Besides caffeine and guarana, other substances such as taurine, glucuronolactone, and vitamins are commonly added to EDs. It has been suggested that taurine may lower blood pressure and have a positive effect on arterial stiffness [23–26]. The potential impact of glucuronolactone and vitamins on the cardiovascular system, however, requires further research.

Increased arterial stiffness is associated with elevated cardiovascular risk: the literature suggests that increased arterial stiffness is linked with altered coronary perfusion, elevated left ventricular afterload, left ventricular dysfunction, and left ventricular hypertrophy [12,27]. Therefore, further studies investigating the acute and chronic effects of ED consumption on left ventricular function and morphology are required. Moreover, pediatric studies indicate that increased arterial stiffness leads to structural vascular changes early in life [28]. Besides caffeine, EDs are high in sugar and calories. In particular, chronic ED consumption can increase the risk for glucose metabolism disorders, excess weight, and arterial hypertension. All of these cardiovascular risk factors were shown to be involved in the process of arterial stiffening [11,29,30]. As EDs negatively affect the cardiovascular system, minors, particularly those with already present cardiovascular risk factors (e.g., arterial hypertension, diabetes, excess weight, congenital heart disease), should be discouraged from ED consumption. In the future, studies are needed that evaluate the cardiovascular morbidity, including arterial stiffness, of chronic ED consumers.

4.2. Limitations

The limitations of the study design were reported in previous publications of our department [10,20]. The sample size of this study can be considered relatively low, as only 27 study participants were included. As 2DST of the CCA is a relatively new method to evaluate arterial stiffness, pediatric reference values do not exist and could not be elaborated in the current study. In addition, solely healthy children and teenagers were included in the present study. Minors with pre-existing health conditions (e.g., arterial hypertension, congenital heart disease) might react more profoundly to ED ingestion. Further, the relatively small sample size did not allow for an analysis of the influence of sex and habitual caffeine consumption on the parameters studied. Moreover, the ED amount was matched with body weight instead of lean body mass. Lastly, only the acute ED-induced effects on arterial stiffness were investigated, and only one specific ED product was utilized for this study. Hence, further studies are required that take the abovementioned limitations into consideration.

5. Conclusions

The acute ED consumption is associated with a significant increase in arterial stiffness in healthy children and teenagers. Minors, particularly those with pre-existing health conditions such as arterial hypertension, diabetes, overweight, or congenital heart disease, should be discouraged from ED consumption. Further studies are required that evaluate the chronic effects of ED consumption on cardiovascular morbidity in children and teenagers.

Author Contributions: Conceptualization, R.D.-P., N.A.H. and F.S.O.; methodology, G.M., R.D.-P., N.A.H. and F.S.O.; software, G.M., R.D.-P, N.A.H. and F.S.O.; validation, G.M., R.D.-P., N.A.H. and F.S.O.; formal analysis, P.L. and F.S.O.; investigation, P.L., G.M. and F.S.O.; resources, A.J., R.D.-P., N.A.H. and F.S.O.; data curation, P.L., G.M. and F.S.O.; writing—original draft preparation, P.L., G.M. and F.S.O.; writing—review and editing, all authors; visualization, P.L., G.M., R.D.-P., N.A.H. and F.S.O.; supervision, G.M., A.J., R.D.-P., N.A.H. and F.S.O.; project administration, G.M. and F.S.O. All authors have read and agreed to the published version of the manuscript.

Funding: This study (project title: EDUCATE Study: Energy Drinks—Unexplored Cardiovascular Alterations in TEens and TwEens) was supported by the German Heart Foundation/German Foundation of Heart Research.

Institutional Review Board Statement: The study was conducted according to the guidelines of the Declaration of Helsinki and approved by the Ethics Committee of the Ludwig Maximilians University Munich (Munich, Germany) (protocol code: 20-0993, date of approval: 12 January 2021).

Informed Consent Statement: Prior written informed consent was obtained from all study participants. For minor study participants prior written informed consent from parents or legal guardians was additionally obtained.

Data Availability Statement: The data presented in this study are available upon reasonable request from the corresponding author.

Acknowledgments: We would like to thank Megan Crouse for editorial assistance.

Conflicts of Interest: The authors declare no conflict of interest.

References

1. Hampton, T. Energy Drinks Pose Worrisome Risks to Adolescents' Cardiovascular Health. *Circulation* **2016**, *134*, 1052–1053. [CrossRef] [PubMed]
2. Grasser, E.K.; Miles-Chan, J.L.; Charrière, N.; Loonam, C.R.; Dulloo, A.G.; Montani, J.P. Energy Drinks and Their Impact on the Cardiovascular System: Potential Mechanisms. *Adv. Nutr.* **2016**, *7*, 950–960. [CrossRef] [PubMed]
3. Seifert, S.M.; Schaechter, J.L.; Hershorin, E.R.; Lipshultz, S.E. Health effects of energy drinks on children, adolescents, and young adults. *Pediatrics* **2011**, *127*, 511–528. [CrossRef] [PubMed]
4. Sanchis-Gomar, F.; Pareja-Galeano, H.; Cervellin, G.; Lippi, G.; Earnest, C.P. Energy drink overconsumption in adolescents: Implications for arrhythmias and other cardiovascular events. *Can. J. Cardiol.* **2015**, *31*, 572–575. [CrossRef] [PubMed]
5. Shah, S.A.; Szeto, A.H.; Farewell, R.; Shek, A.; Fan, D.; Quach, K.N.; Bhattacharyya, M.; Elmiari, J.; Chan, W.; O'Dell, K.; et al. Impact of High Volume Energy Drink Consumption on Electrocardiographic and Blood Pressure Parameters: A Randomized Trial. *J. Am. Heart Assoc.* **2019**, *8*, e011318. [CrossRef] [PubMed]
6. Hussain, A.; Jiji, A.K.; Barke, P.; Biswas, S.; Tabrez, S.S.M. Cardiovascular Pathologies Associated with Excessive Energy Drink Consumption: A Review. *Crit. Rev. Eukaryot. Gene Exp.* **2018**, *28*, 107–113. [CrossRef] [PubMed]
7. Ehlers, A.; Marakis, G.; Lampen, A.; Hirsch-Ernst, K.I. Risk assessment of energy drinks with focus on cardiovascular parameters and energy drink consumption in Europe. *Food Chem. Toxicol.* **2019**, *130*, 109–121. [CrossRef]
8. Fletcher, E.A.; Lacey, C.S.; Aaron, M.; Kolasa, M.; Occiano, A.; Shah, S.A. Randomized Controlled Trial of High-Volume Energy Drink Versus Caffeine Consumption on ECG and Hemodynamic Parameters. *J. Am. Heart Assoc.* **2017**, *6*, e004448. [CrossRef]
9. Nowak, D.; Gośliński, M.; Nowatkowska, K. The Effect of Acute Consumption of Energy Drinks on Blood Pressure, Heart Rate and Blood Glucose in the Group of Young Adults. *Int. J. Environ. Res. Public Health* **2018**, *15*, 544. [CrossRef]
10. Oberhoffer, F.S.; Li, P.; Jacob, A.; Dalla-Pozza, R.; Haas, N.A.; Mandilaras, G. Energy Drinks: Effects on Blood Pressure and Heart Rate in Children and Teenagers. A Randomized Trial. *Front. Cardiovasc. Med.* **2022**, *9*, 512. [CrossRef]
11. Boutouyrie, P.; Chowienczyk, P.; Humphrey, J.D.; Mitchell, G.F. Arterial Stiffness and Cardiovascular Risk in Hypertension. *Circ. Res.* **2021**, *128*, 864–886. [CrossRef]

12. Chirinos, J.A.; Segers, P.; Hughes, T.; Townsend, R. Large-Artery Stiffness in Health and Disease: JACC State-of-the-Art Review. *J. Am. Coll. Cardiol.* **2019**, *74*, 1237–1263. [CrossRef] [PubMed]
13. Safar, M.E. Arterial stiffness as a risk factor for clinical hypertension. *Nat. Rev. Cardiol.* **2018**, *15*, 97–105. [CrossRef] [PubMed]
14. Laurent, S.; Cockcroft, J.; Van Bortel, L.; Boutouyrie, P.; Giannattasio, C.; Hayoz, D.; Pannier, B.; Vlachopoulos, C.; Wilkinson, I.; Struijker-Boudier, H.; et al. Expert consensus document on arterial stiffness: Methodological issues and clinical applications. *Eur. Heart J.* **2006**, *27*, 2588–2605. [CrossRef] [PubMed]
15. Krämer, J.; Niemann, M.; Liu, D.; Hu, K.; Machann, W.; Beer, M.; Wanner, C.; Ertl, G.; Weidemann, F. Two-dimensional speckle tracking as a non-invasive tool for identification of myocardial fibrosis in Fabry disease. *Eur. Heart J.* **2013**, *34*, 1587–1596. [CrossRef] [PubMed]
16. Oberhoffer, F.S.; Abdul-Khaliq, H.; Jung, A.M.; Rohrer, T.R.; Abd El Rahman, M. Two-dimensional speckle tracking of the abdominal aorta: A novel approach to evaluate arterial stiffness in patients with Turner syndrome. *Cardiovasc. Diagn. Ther.* **2019**, *9*, S228–S237. [CrossRef]
17. Oishi, Y.; Miyoshi, H.; Iuchi, A.; Nagase, N.; Ara, N.; Oki, T. Vascular aging of common carotid artery and abdominal aorta in clinically normal individuals and preclinical patients with cardiovascular risk factors: Diagnostic value of two-dimensional speckle-tracking echocardiography. *Heart Vessels* **2013**, *28*, 222–228. [CrossRef]
18. Papaioannou, T.G.; Karatzi, K.; Karatzis, E.; Papamichael, C.; Lekakis, J.P. Acute effects of caffeine on arterial stiffness, wave reflections, and central aortic pressures. *Am. J. Hypertens.* **2005**, *18*, 129–136. [CrossRef]
19. Kromeyer-Hauschild, K.; Wabitsch, M.; Kunze, D.; Geller, F.; Geiß, H.C.; Hesse, V.; von Hippel, A.; Jaeger, U.; Johnsen, D.; Korte, W.; et al. Perzentile für den Body-mass-Index für das Kindes- und Jugendalter unter Heranziehung verschiedener deutscher Stichproben. *Monatsschr. Kinderheilkd.* **2001**, *149*, 807–818. [CrossRef]
20. Mandilaras, G.; Li, P.; Dalla-Pozza, R.; Haas, N.A.; Oberhoffer, F.S. Energy Drinks and Their Acute Effects on Heart Rhythm and Electrocardiographic Time Intervals in Healthy Children and Teenagers: A Randomized Trial. *Cells* **2022**, *11*, 498. [CrossRef]
21. EFSA Panel on Dietetic Products, Nutrition and Allergies. Scientific Opinion on the safety of caffeine. *EFSA J.* **2015**, *13*, 4102.
22. Mahmud, A.; Feely, J. Acute Effect of Caffeine on Arterial Stiffness and Aortic Pressure Waveform. *Hypertension* **2001**, *38*, 227–231. [CrossRef] [PubMed]
23. Guan, L.; Miao, P. The effects of taurine supplementation on obesity, blood pressure and lipid profile: A meta-analysis of randomized controlled trials. *Eur. J. Pharmacol.* **2020**, *885*, 173533. [CrossRef] [PubMed]
24. Sun, Q.; Wang, B.; Li, Y.; Sun, F.; Li, P.; Xia, W.; Zhou, X.; Li, Q.; Wang, X.; Chen, J.; et al. Taurine Supplementation Lowers Blood Pressure and Improves Vascular Function in Prehypertension: Randomized, Double-Blind, Placebo-Controlled Study. *Hypertension* **2016**, *67*, 541–549. [CrossRef] [PubMed]
25. Ra, S.-G.; Choi, Y.; Akazawa, N.; Ohmori, H.; Maeda, S. Taurine supplementation attenuates delayed increase in exercise-induced arterial stiffness. *Appl. Physiol. Nutr. Metab.* **2016**, *41*, 618–623. [CrossRef] [PubMed]
26. Satoh, H.; Kang, J. Modulation by taurine of human arterial stiffness and wave reflection. *Adv. Exp. Med. Biol.* **2009**, *643*, 47–55. [CrossRef] [PubMed]
27. Zanoli, L.; Lentini, P.; Briet, M.; Castellino, P.; House, A.A.; London, G.M.; Malatino, L.; McCullough, P.A.; Mikhailidis, D.P.; Boutouyrie, P. Arterial Stiffness in the Heart Disease of CKD. *J. Am. Soc. Nephrol.* **2019**, *30*, 918–928. [CrossRef]
28. Ahmadizar, F.; Voortman, T. Arterial stiffness in childhood: A predictor for later cardiovascular disease? *Eur. J. Prev. Cardiol.* **2018**, *25*, 100–102. [CrossRef]
29. Wu, S.; Xu, L.; Wu, M.; Chen, S.; Wang, Y.; Tian, Y. Association between triglyceride-glucose index and risk of arterial stiffness: A cohort study. *Cardiovasc. Diabetol.* **2021**, *20*, 146. [CrossRef]
30. Cote, A.T.; Harris, K.C.; Panagiotopoulos, C.; Sandor, G.G.; Devlin, A.M. Childhood obesity and cardiovascular dysfunction. *J. Am. Coll. Cardiol.* **2013**, *62*, 1309–1319. [CrossRef]

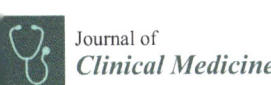

Article

Non-Invasive Assessment of Arterial Stiffness: Pulse Wave Velocity, Pulse Wave Analysis and Carotid Cross-Sectional Distensibility: Comparison between Methods

Paolo Salvi [1,*,†], Filippo Valbusa [2,†], Anna Kearney-Schwartz [3], Carlos Labat [4], Andrea Grillo [5], Gianfranco Parati [1,6] and Athanase Benetos [3,4]

1. Cardiology Unit, Istituto Auxologico Italiano, IRCCS, 20100 Milan, Italy; gianfranco.parati@unimib.it
2. Department of Internal Medicine, IRCCS Sacro Cuore-Don Calabria Hospital, 37024 Negrar, Italy; filippo.valbusa77@gmail.com
3. CHRU-Nancy, Pôle "Maladies du Vieillissement, Gérontologie et Soins Palliatifs", Université de Lorraine, 54000 Nancy, France; a.kearney-schwartz@chru-nancy.fr (A.K.-S.); a.benetos@chru-nancy.fr (A.B.)
4. INSERM, DCAC u1116, Université de Lorraine, 54000 Nancy, France; carlos.labat@inserm.fr
5. Medicina Clinica, Azienda Sanitaria Universitaria Giuliano Isontina, 34148 Trieste, Italy; andr.grillo@gmail.com
6. Department of Medicine and Surgery, University of Milano-Bicocca, 20100 Milan, Italy
* Correspondence: paolo.salvi@unimib.it; Tel.: +39-026-1911-2949; Fax: +39-026-1911-2956
† These authors contributed equally to this work.

Abstract: Background: The stiffening of large elastic arteries is currently estimated in research and clinical practice by propagative and non-propagative models, as well as parameters derived from aortic pulse waveform analysis. Methods: Common carotid compliance and distensibility were measured by simultaneously recording the diameter and pressure changes during the cardiac cycle. The aortic and upper arm arterial distensibility was estimated by measuring carotid–femoral and carotid–radial pulse wave velocity (PWV), respectively. The augmentation index and blood pressure amplification were derived from the analysis of central pulse waveforms, recorded by applanation tonometry directly from the common carotid artery. Results: 75 volunteers were enrolled in this study (50 females, average age 53.5 years). A significant inverse correlation was found between carotid distensibility and carotid–femoral PWV (r = −0.75; $p < 0.001$), augmentation index (r = −0.63; $p < 0.001$) and central pulse pressure (r = −0.59; $p < 0.001$). A strong correlation was found also between the total slope of the diameter/pressure rate carotid curves and aortic distensibility, quantified from the inverse of the square of carotid–femoral PWV (r = 0.67). No correlation was found between carotid distensibility and carotid–radial PWV. Conclusions: This study showed a close correlation between carotid–femoral PWV, evaluating aortic stiffness by using the propagative method, and local carotid cross-sectional distensibility.

Keywords: aorta; arterial distensibility; arterial stiffness; augmentation index; blood pressure amplification; cardiovascular prevention; elastic modulus; pulse wave analysis; pulse wave velocity

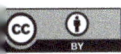

1. Introduction

Several studies have shown that the assessment of arterial function and structure provides prognostic information incremental to conventional cardiovascular risk stratification [1–4]. Arterial stiffness is strongly related to cardiovascular risk factors and cardiovascular morbidity and mortality [5], particularly in individuals with end-stage renal disease [6–9], in hypertensive patients [1,10,11], in diabetic patients [12], in very old individuals [13,14], and in coronary patients [2,3,15–17].

Different models were proposed to estimate the mechanical properties of the large arteries [18]: (i) propagative models, (ii) non-propagative models, and (iii) central pulse wave analysis.

In propagative models, arterial distensibility is defined from the propagation velocity of the pulse wave. The pulse wave runs through the arterial vessels at a speed that depends on the elasticity of the wall itself: the less elastic the wall, the greater the propagation velocity. In non-propagative models, the cross-sectional mechanical properties of the arteries can be assessed non-invasively on the basis of the volume/pressure relationship of an arterial segment [19,20]. Vascular distensibility is defined by the change in diameter in relation to the blood pressure (BP) change. It is possible to define the degree of vascular distensibility by simultaneously measuring the variation in BP and vascular diameter.

Parameters derived from the analysis of the pulse pressure (PP) waveform have been suggested as markers of arterial stiffness, such as augmentation index (AIx) [21] and BP amplification phenomenon [22]. AIx estimates the increase in systolic BP caused by an early return of reflected waves to the aorta and is defined by the difference between the second and first systolic peaks, expressed as a percentage of the central PP [22–24]. BP amplification is calculated from the increase of PP from the central aorta toward the periphery and is mainly attributed to systolic BP increase [22,23,25–27].

The purpose of the present study was to evaluate the relationship between variables derived from the above models: pulse wave analysis (AIx, PP amplification), propagative models (carotid–femoral and carotid–radial pulse wave velocity), and non-propagative models (carotid cross-sectional compliance and distensibility). Our study also aimed at determining, for each of them, the specific influence of age, sex, anthropometric parameters, and BP levels.

2. Materials and Methods

Participants in this study were volunteers (age range between 20 and 90 years) recruited among the medical and paramedical staff, day hospital patients or outpatients from the Geriatric Department of the University Hospital of Nancy (France), with an equal distribution in three age subgroups (20–45, 46–70, and 71–90 years). The absence of major systemic diseases was confirmed by physical and laboratory routine examinations. All the individuals recruited were given a clear explanation of the aims of the trial, and all were asked to give their consent to the study procedures. The protocol of this study was approved in Nancy, France, by the "Comité de Protection des Personnes" of Nancy CPP Est III 15 December 2006. After recording the weight and height of all recruited individuals, a rest period in supine position for 15′ for acclimatization was scheduled before data collection. Body mass index (BMI) was calculated as weight divided by height squared (kg/m^2). A validated oscillometric sphygmomanometer Omron 705IT (Omron Co., Kyoto, Japan) [28] was used for brachial BP measurement. After BP measurement, a Duplex sonography (Esaote) was performed on both carotid arteries to exclude vascular stenosis. The presence of atherosclerotic plaques, defined as a focal intima-media thickness >1.5 mm, was an additional study exclusion criterion.

2.1. Carotid Distensibility and Compliance

Common carotid compliance and distensibility were measured by simultaneously recording the carotid diameter and pressure change during the cardiac cycle [29]. The diameter variation curve was recorded by the Wall Track System (Pie Medical, Maastricht, The Netherlands) [30]. This system measures the variation of the carotid diameter during the cardiac cycle, using a radio frequency analysis implemented in the Esaote ultrasound system (Genoa, Italy) [31,32]. For this study, the Wall Track System was programmed to simultaneously record the vascular diameter variation curve and the electrocardiogram (ECG) tracing for a duration of 4 s, with a 200 Hz sampling rate (one signal acquired every 5 ms). A validated PulsePen (DiaTecne s.r.l., San Donato Milanese, Italy) [33–35] transcutaneous arterial tonometer was used to record the carotid BP wave. The PulsePen simultaneously records the pressure curve and the ECG tracing for a period of 10 cardiac cycles, with a 1 kHz sampling rate.

The synchronization of the two waves (diameter and pressure) is allowed by superimposing the ECG readings recorded at the same time as the two curves via a specifically software DiaPres (DiaTecne s.r.l., San Donato Milanese, Italy). This method was previously described in detail [29]. The change in diameter/change in pressure rate and the slope of the curve concerning this rate were estimated from the entire cardiac cycle (Figure 1), from the proto-mesosystolic phase (a–b phase in Figure 1), and from the diastolic phase (c–a′ phase in Figure 1).

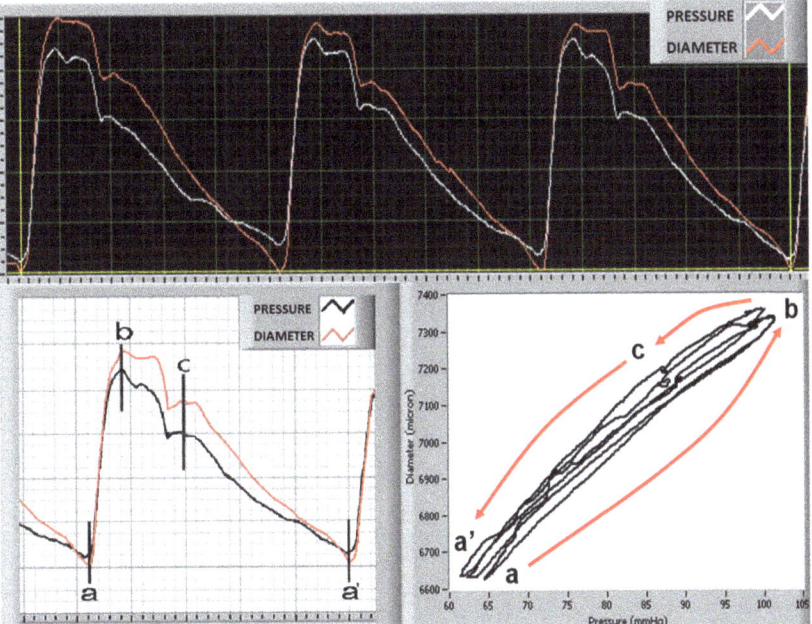

Figure 1. Upper panel: original tracings of carotid diameter (red line) and simultaneously acquired blood pressure (white line) wave. Lower panel: on the left arterial pressure wave (black line) and curves of cross-sectional diameter changes (red line); a–b interval indicates the proto-mesosystolic phase, and c–a′ is the late diastole phase (lower panel). Cross-sectional diameter/pressure curves are shown in the right lower panel.

Common carotid arterial cross-sectional compliance was calculated according to the following formula [19,36,37]:

$$Compliance = \frac{D_{max} - D_{min}}{PP}$$

where D_{max} and D_{min} are the maximal and minimal calculated carotid diameters obtained during a cardiac cycle, and PP is the carotid PP measured by arterial tonometer.

Arterial cross-sectional distensibility is the compliance value normalized for the carotid cross-sectional diameter:

$$Distensibility = \frac{D_{max} - D_{min}}{PP \times D_{min}}$$

Compliance and distensibility define, respectively, absolute and relative diameter change for every 1 mmHg increase in BP.

Common carotid elastic modulus was determined by the following formula:

$$Elastic\ Modulus = \frac{PP}{S_{AD}}$$

where S_{AD} is the strain of the common carotid diameter, defined as follows:

$$S_{AD} = \frac{(D_{max} - D_{min})}{D_{min}}$$

Carotid diameter measurements were obtained by assuming circular geometry of the common carotid artery. Elastic modulus is the pressure change required for theoretical 100% stretch from resting diameter. It is, thus, the inverse of distensibility.

The stiffness index was calculated according to the following formula:

$$Stiffness\ Index = \frac{ln(SBP/DBP)}{S_{AD}}$$

where SBP and DBP are carotid systolic and diastolic BP.

Two recordings were performed in quick succession. From the analysis of these diameter and pressure curves, we calculated the mean value of the arterial wall properties parameters required by our study protocol.

2.2. Pulse Wave Velocity (PWV)

The carotid, femoral, and radial pressure waves were recorded with the PulsePen tonometer to measure the carotid–femoral pulse wave velocity (cf-PWV) and the carotid–radial pulse wave velocity (cr-PWV). PWV, measured in m/s, is defined by the relationship between the distance travelled by the pressure wave and the delay in registering the distal wave (femoral artery for cf-PWV, and radial artery for cr-PWV) compared with the carotid wave [38]. The distance travelled was assessed by subtracting carotid to suprasternal notch distance from suprasternal notch to peripheral (femoral or radial) distance. We used the mathematical model proposed by Bramwell and Hill [39] to relate the arterial wall distensibility with the inverse of the square of pulse wave velocity.

2.3. Pulse Wave Analysis and Central Blood Pressure Measurement

Central BP values and central pulse pressure waveforms were recorded directly from the common carotid artery, using a validated applanation tonometer [40–42] (PulsePen device). This device was described in detail elsewhere [33,34]. As previously demonstrated, the pressure waves recorded non-invasively by the PulsePen tonometer at the site of the common carotid artery are almost equal to the pressure waveforms obtained invasively by means of an intra-arterial catheter in the same arterial segment [33]. Moreover, several studies have demonstrated that central BP values and pulse wave parameters recorded in the common carotid artery are reliable surrogates of the corresponding parameters recorded in the aorta by invasive methods [19,23,33]. Central BP values were obtained from carotid BP curve analysis and brachial BP measurements, using an appropriate validated algorithm [19,33]. The amplification phenomenon (from aorta to brachial artery) was expressed as (i) PP amplification rate, i.e., the percentage of increase of PP in the brachial artery (PP_B) relative to central PP (PP_C), according to the formula PPA = 100·(PP_B − PP_C)/PP_C; and (ii) systolic BP amplification, i.e., the difference between brachial systolic BP and aortic systolic BP, expressed in mmHg. We defined AIx as the difference between the second and first systolic peaks of carotid pressure waveform and expressed as a percentage of central PP.

2.4. Statistical Analysis

All statistical analyses were performed with NCSS version 9 Statistical Software (NCSS, LLC, Kaysville, UT, USA). Values are presented as means ± standard deviation. The relationship between hemodynamic parameters was tested with Spearman's correlation coefficient in univariate analysis. A simple regression test was performed for the analysis of bivariate linear correlations. A $p < 0.05$ was considered as the level of statistical significance. As a measure of BP for multiple regression analysis, we used only mean arterial pressure, because systolic BP and PP are influenced by arterial stiffness. Multivariate stepwise regression analyses were performed, including age, sex, weight, height, mean arterial pressure, and heart rate as independent variables, while arterial-stiffness-related variables were taken as dependent variables. In multivariate models, the *p*-to-enter was set at 0.10, and the *p*-to-stay to 0.05.

2.5. Preliminary Study: Standardization of the Method for Measuring Vascular Distensibility

We performed a preliminary study to overcome the difficulties in analyzing the diameter and pressure curves simultaneously in the same carotid artery before beginning a comparative study between the various methods. We explored whether the simultaneous acquisition of the diameter and pressure curves on the same carotid artery could be adequately replaced by the simultaneous acquisition of the same two curves on the two carotid arteries by deriving the pressure curve from the right carotid artery and the diameter curve from the left carotid artery. In fact, using both carotid arteries would make the test considerably simpler to perform.

Thus, in the first 10 healthy volunteers included in our study (3 males and 7 females, mean age of 30.0 ± 4.7 years), the diameter and pressure curves were first recorded simultaneously on the same carotid artery (right carotid artery), placing the tonometer in a distal position in relation to the ultrasound probe. Subsequently, the systolic–diastolic variations in diameter and pressure were simultaneously recorded on the two common carotid arteries, 2–3 cm proximal to the carotid bifurcation, by placing the ultrasound probe on the left common carotid, and the tonometer on the right common carotid. The results obtained from a single carotid artery and those obtained from both left and right carotid arteries were then compared. A data analysis was performed according to the recommendations of Bland and Altman [43]. The relative (positive or negative) differences between each pair of measurements were plotted against their mean to evaluate the relationship between the mean value of the considered parameter and the difference in the estimates provided by these two approaches. The level of agreement between the two series of measurements was estimated by their mean difference and the standard deviation of these differences [43]. The coefficient of variation was defined as the standard deviation of the differences between the methods divided by the mean of the absolute difference values.

The study highlighted the high reliability of the data obtained by positioning the two probes on the two carotid arteries. The mean difference between the values obtained by using the two approaches was always very close to zero, and the differences between the two series of data that appeared were homogeneously distributed across each parameter value distribution and were, in any case, always less than 10% of the mean values. As an example, for a mean value of arterial distensibility of 3.77 ± 0.71, the mean of the differences ± twice the standard deviation was 0.06 ± 0.33. The coefficient of variation values were lower than 5% for the parameters of vascular distensibility (coefficient of variation 4.5%) and vascular compliance (coefficient of variation 4.4%). Based on these initial results, we then decided to use recordings performed on both carotid arteries in our study. This choice was supported also by the fact that the test performed on both carotid arteries is considerably simpler to carry out, and the signal is easier to obtain, and its reliability is supported by another study [44]. Moreover, using both arteries avoids the possibility of technical interferences with the measurement, due to, for example, the slight compression of the carotid artery by the tonometer, which might affect ultrasound diameter assessment; or the interference between the gel used for the ultrasound recordings and the receiving end of the tonometric probe.

3. Results

A total of 75 volunteers were enrolled in the study (66% females, average age 53.5 years). Seven individuals (9.3%) were smokers, and none had a history of alcohol consumption, although three reported occasional drinking. Table 1 summarizes the clinical, hemodynamic, and anthropometric parameters.

Table 1. Clinical, anthropometric, and hemodynamic parameters.

Parameter	Pooled	Age Groups (years)			Trend
		20–45	46–70	>70	p
Subjects	75	25	25	25	
Gender, M/F	25/50	9/16	8/17	8/17	
BMI, kg/m^2	24.4 ± 3.4	23.3 ± 3.6	24.9 ± 3.4	24.9 ± 3.3	n.s.
Height, cm	166.9 ± 9.3	170.3 ± 8.8	166.9 ± 9.0	163.0 ± 9.0	0.03
Weight, kg	68.0 ± 12.2	67.6 ± 10.4	69.7 ± 13.5	66.6 ± 12.8	n.s.
Brachial Systolic BP, mmHg	126.4 ± 20.0	112.6 ± 11.2	124.2 ± 13.5	142.2 ± 21.4	<0.0001
Central Systolic BP, mmHg	114.3 ± 18.4	101.0 ± 11.2	113.0 ± 12.1	128.8 ± 19.2	<0.0001
Brachial PP, mmHg	55.7 ± 17.0	47.1 ± 7.9	49.6 ± 11.5	70.4 ± 18.7	<0.0001
Central PP, mmHg	43.6 ± 15.5	35.4 ± 8.0	38.3 ± 10.6	57.0 ± 16.6	<0.0001
Mean BP, mmHg	89.2 ± 11.7	81.3 ± 7.1	91.2 ± 8.6	95.3 ± 13.8	<0.0001
Diastolic BP, mmHg	70.± 10.1	65.6 ± 5.8	74.6 ± 8.0	71.8 ± 13.2	0.005
LVET, ms	296.1 ± 28.9	294.8 ± 22.0	303.4 ± 24.7	290.1 ± 37.3	n.s.
Diastolic Time, ms	592.0 ± 116.6	594.0 ± 101.0	575.2 ± 131.2	606.9 ± 118.2	n.s.
Heart Rate, bpm	69.1 ± 10.3	68.6 ± 8.7	70.1 ± 11.9	68.4 ± 10.4	n.s.
Amplification, mmHg	12.1 ± 4.3	11.6 ± 2.6	11.2 ± 4.7	13.4 ± 5.0	n.s.
PP Amplification, %	30.1 ± 11.5	34.6 ± 10.6	31.1 ± 12.9	24.8 ± 8.8	0.008
AIx, %	12.8 ± 20.7	−8.5 ± 11.7	20.1 ± 16.7	26.7 ± 13.1	<0.0001
cf-PWV, m/s	9.90 ± 4.81	6.35 ± 0.99	8.03 ± 2.38	15.33 ± 4.13	<0.0001
cr-PWV, m/s	8.41 ± 1.58	7.76 ± 1.75	8.82 ± 1.51	8.72 ± 1.24	0.04
Carotid cross-sectional Compliance, μm/mmHg	9.79 ± 4.89	15.28 ± 3.36	8.57 ± 2.22	5.54 ± 2.41	<0.0001
Distensibility, mmHg^{-1}	1.50 ± 0.86	2.49 ± 0.55	1.27 ± 0.37	0.74 ± 0.38	<0.0001
Elastic Modulus, mmHg	977 ± 663	427 ± 127	864 ± 276	1641 ± 691	<0.0001
Stiffness Index	4.26 ± 2.49	2.17 ± 0.61	3.77 ± 1.07	6.84 ± 2.40	<0.0001
Carotid Global Slope	9.4 ± 4.7	14.7 ± 3.3	8.2 ± 2.1	5.3 ± 2.2	<0.0001
Carotid Systolic Slope	9.7 ± 4.9	15.1 ± 3.6	8.7 ± 2.3	5.3 ± 1.9	<0.0001
Carotid Diastolic Slope	11.9 ± 5.9	18.4 ± 4.1	10.4 ± 3.3	6.9 ± 2.9	<0.0001

Data are shown for the whole cohort (first column), and by dividing the cohort in tertiles of age. Last column shows the statistical significance of the parameter variation trend as a function of age. Data are expressed as means ± standard deviations. AIx, augmentation index; BMI, body mass index; BP, blood pressure; cf-PWV, carotid–femoral pulse wave velocity; cr-PWV, carotid–radial pulse wave velocity; LVET, left ventricular ejection time; M/F, males/females; n.s., not significant; PP, pulse pressure.

The BP parameters, PP amplification, PWV and carotid cross-sectional distensibility appeared to be significantly correlated with age. The relationships of cf-PWV and cr-PWV with age were quite different. In the young age group, the cf-PWV values were lower than the cr-PWV values (in first tertile, cf-PWV was 6.350 ± 0.99 m/s, and cr-PWV was 7.76 ± 1.75 m/s). With aging, the cr-PWV increased much less than the cf-PWV (in third tertile, cf-PWV was 15.33 ± 4.13 m/s, and cr-PWV was 8.72 ± 1.24 m/s). Figure 2 clearly shows that the cf-PWV values in third tertile were more than two times greater than in the first tertile and increased quickly in the elderly. Thus, the relationship between age and PWV is more appropriately expressed by a quadratic non-linear model than by the conventional linear model approach.

Figure 3 shows the changes in carotid artery compliance curves with age. In this figure, only the first and third tertiles of age are shown: all curves of the youngest individuals are positioned in the upper and left part of the figure (small BP changes determine large changes in vascular diameter); on the contrary, curves related to the oldest people are positioned in the lower and right part of the figure (large pressure changes determine small changes in diameter).

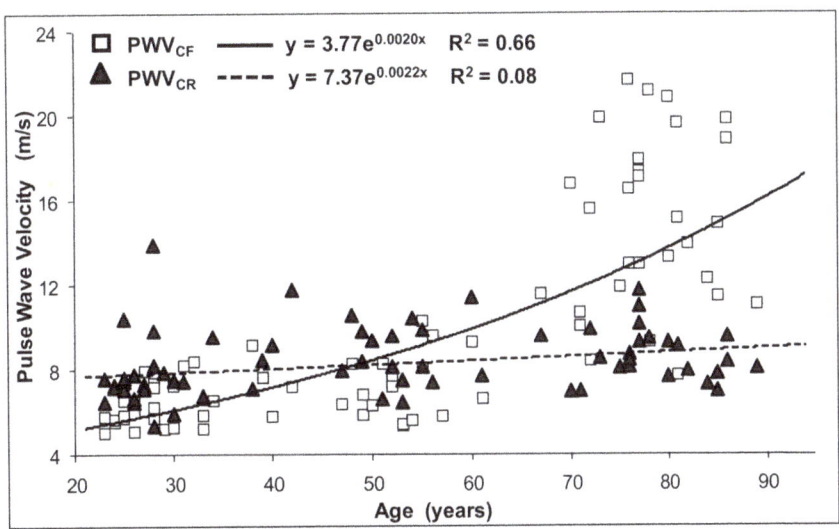

Figure 2. Relationship between age and carotid–femoral pulse wave velocity PWV_{CF} (continuous line, open squares) and carotid–radial pulse wave velocity PWV_{CR} (dotted line, closed triangles).

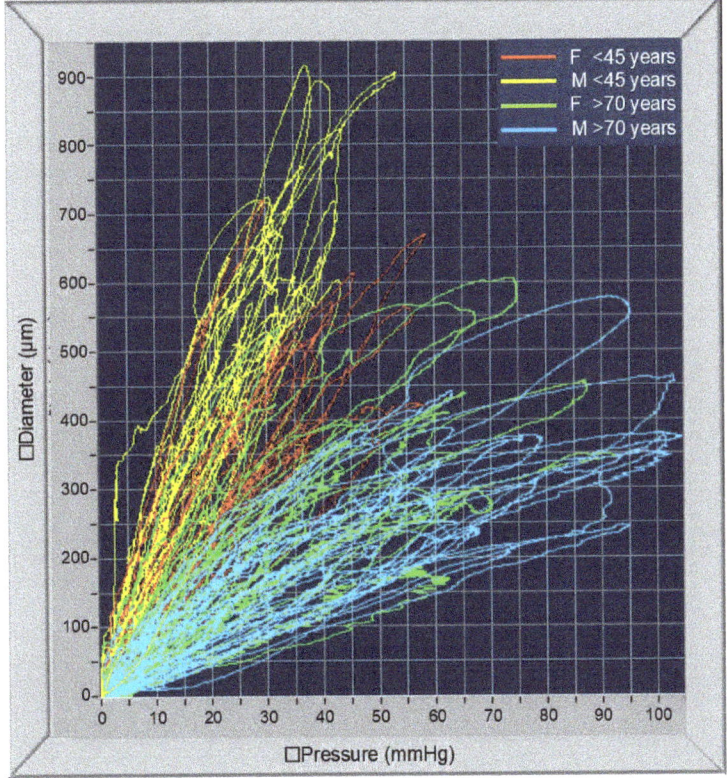

Figure 3. Carotid cross-section pressure curves in individuals aged 20–45 years (red lines, females; yellow lines, males) and over 70 years old (green lines, females; blue lines, males).

The global (systolic and diastolic) slopes of the diameter/pressure rate curves related to the different tertiles of age are shown in Figure 4. All slope values in the first tertile are higher than the mean value of the second, and all values of the third tertile are lower than mean values of the second tertile.

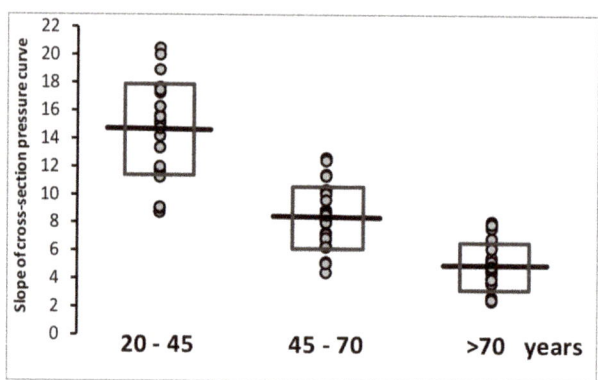

Figure 4. Slope of the cross-section diameter–pressure curves are separately shown for the different age tertiles. Mean values and standard deviation (open rectangles) are shown.

Table 2 shows the results of the bivariate analysis between PP amplification, AIx, cf-PWV, cr-PWV, and carotid artery distensibility and age, sex, anthropometric parameters, BP values, and heart rate. Height was directly correlated with carotid distensibility ($p < 0.02$) and inversely correlated with AIx ($p < 0.001$); BMI showed a significant inverse correlation with carotid distensibility ($p < 0.001$), cf-PWV ($p < 0.001$) and cr-PWV ($p < 0.04$). All the studied parameters showed a significant strong correlation with central and peripheral systolic BP and PP ($p < 0.001$), with the exception of cr-PWV, which instead appeared to be correlated with diastolic and mean BP. Heart rate was significantly correlated with PP amplification ($p < 0.004$) and inversely correlated with AIx ($p < 0.03$).

Table 2. Bivariate analysis (Spearman's correlation coefficient) between the main parameters for estimating arterial stiffness and clinical and anthropometric parameters.

Parameter	PPA		AIx		cf-PWV		CCS Distensibility	
	r	p	r	p	r	p	r	p
Sex	0.05	n.s.	0.33	0.005	−0.13	n.s.	0.02	n.s.
Age	−0.47	<0.001	0.76	<0.001	0.79	<0.001	−0.84	<0.001
BMI	−0.18	n.s.	0.15	n.s.	0.38	0.001	−0.40	<0.001
Height	0.19	n.s.	−0.53	<0.001	−0.14	n.s.	0.28	0.02
Weight	−0.03	n.s.	−0.26	0.03	0.17	n.s.	−0.09	n.s.
bSBP	−0.35	0.002	0.49	<0.001	0.59	<0.001	−0.67	<0.001
cSBP	−0.47	<0.001	0.52	<0.001	0.58	<0.001	−0.66	<0.001
bPP	−0.48	<0.001	0.41	<0.001	0.54	<0.001	−0.59	<0.001
cPP	−0.67	<0.001	0.46	<0.001	0.53	<0.001	−0.59	<0.001
MAP	−0.13	n.s.	0.40	<0.001	0.50	<0.001	−0.57	<0.001
DBP	0.10	n.s.	0.24	0.04	0.29	0.01	−0.35	0.002
LVET	−0.25	0.03	0.31	0.007	−0.24	0.04	0.16	n.s.
DT	−0.35	0.002	0.22	0.05	0.02	n.s.	0.08	n.s.
HR	0.33	0.004	−0.26	0.03	0.05	n.s.	−0.11	n.s.

AIx, augmentation index; BMI, body mass index; bPP, brachial pulse pressure; bSBP, brachial systolic blood pressure; CCS, carotid cross-sectional; cf-PWV, carotid–femoral pulse wave velocity; cPP, carotid pulse pressure; cSBP, carotid systolic blood pressure; DBP, diastolic blood pressure; DT, diastolic time; HR, heart rate; LVET, left ventricular ejection time; MAP, mean arterial pressure; n.s., not significant; PPA, pulse pressure amplification.

Table 3 shows the results of bivariate analysis between local carotid artery hemodynamic parameters and measurements derived from the central pulse wave analysis and by propagative models (cf-PWV). A strong inverse correlation was found between carotid distensibility and cf-PWV (r = −0.75; $p < 0.001$), AIx (r = −0.63; $p < 0.001$), and central PP (r = −0.59; $p < 0.001$). A significant, but weaker, correlation was found also between carotid distensibility and PP amplification (r = 0.34; $p < 0.003$) and cr-PWV (inverse correlation, r = −0.39; $p < 0.001$). Finally, an inverse relationship was found between carotid distensibility and amplification of systolic BP, expressed as the difference between brachial and carotid systolic BP (r = −0.24; $p < 0.04$).

Table 3. Bivariate analysis (Spearman's correlation coefficient) between carotid cross-sectional distensibility measurements and main hemodynamic parameters, derived from central pulse wave analysis, and carotid–femoral PWV.

Carotid Cross-Sectional Measurements	Peripheral PP		Central PP		PP Amplification		AIx		cf-PWV	
	r	p	r	p	r	p	r	p	r	p
Distensibility	−0.67	<0.001	−0.59	<0.001	0.34	0.003	−0.63	<0.001	−0.75	<0.001
Compliance	−0.65	<0.001	−0.59	<0.001	0.34	0.003	−0.65	<0.001	−0.72	<0.001
Elastic Modulus	0.67	<0.001	0.59	<0.001	−0.34	0.003	0.63	<0.001	0.75	<0.001
Stiffness Index	0.54	<0.001	0.51	<0.001	−0.33	0.004	0.61	<0.001	0.74	<0.001
Total slope	−0.65	<0.001	−0.59	<0.001	0.36	0.002	−0.65	<0.001	−0.71	<0.001
Systolic slope	−0.66	<0.001	−0.59	<0.001	0.32	0.005	−0.62	<0.001	−0.75	<0.001
Diastolic slope	−0.61	<0.001	−0.53	<0.001	0.25	0.03	−0.61	<0.001	−0.68	<0.001

AIx, augmentation index; cf-PWV, carotid–femoral pulse wave velocity; PP, pulse pressure.

The relationship between slope of the diameter/pressure rate curves across the entire cardiac cycle and aortic distensibility, quantified as the inverse of $(cf-PWV)^2$, is shown in Figure 5. AIx was strongly correlated with cf-PWV (r = 0.53; $p < 0.001$) and weakly related to cr-PWV (r = 0.29; $p < 0.02$).

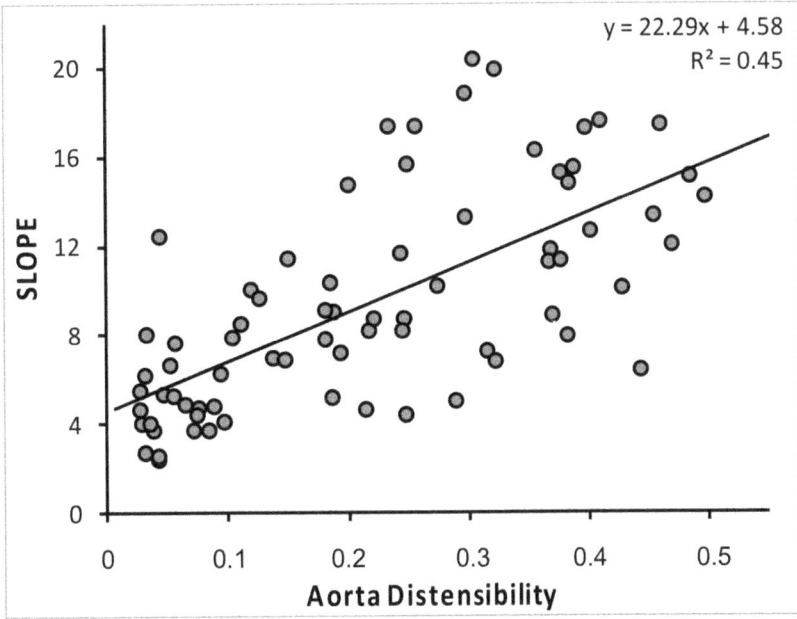

Figure 5. Univariate linear relationship between the slope of the cross-section carotid diameter-pressure curves and aorta distensibility [$1/(carotid–femoral\ PWV)^2$].

Table 4 shows the results of the multivariate stepwise regression analysis with cf-PWV, cr-PWV, AIx, PP amplification, amplification of systolic BP, and carotid arterial distensibility as dependent variables, and age, sex, heart rate, mean BP, height, and weight as independent variables. None of the latter parameters was a determinant of cr-PWV. Age was the main factor determining cf-PWV, Aix, and carotid distensibility. Heart rate was the main variable determining PP amplification and was a significant independent variable also for AIx and carotid distensibility. Sex was a significant determinant only for AIx. Mean BP was the main variable positively associated with systolic BP amplification. Mean BP was also inversely associated with carotid distensibility and directly associated with AIx.

Table 4. Results of stepwise regression analysis with the main parameters for estimating arterial stiffness as dependent variables and anthropometric and clinical parameters as independent variables.

Dependent Variable	r^2	Independent Variable	Regression Coefficient	SE	B	p	r^2 Change(%)
SBP Amplification mmHg	0.29	MAP	0.134	0.045	0.37	0.004	15.3
		HR	0.120	0.046	0.29	0.01	7.4
PP Amplification	0.31	HR	0.365	0.118	0.33	0.003	10.2
		Age	−0.154	0.067	−0.30	0.02	14.9
AIx	0.72	Age	0.534	0.077	0.59	<0.001	52.8
		HR	−0.530	0.136	−0.27	<0.001	6.6
		Sex	14.435	4.235	0.35	0.001	10.1
		MAP	0.381	0.133	0.22	0.006	1.6
cf-PWV	0.66	Age	0.169	0.020	0.79	<0.001	61.4
CCS Distensibility	0.79	Age	−0.030	0.003	−0.76	<0.001	70.8
		Weight	−0.017	0.006	−0.24	0.003	3.9
		MAP	−0.012	0.005	−0.16	0.02	3.0
		HR	−0.011	0.005	−0.13	0.04	1.4

Regression coefficient quantifies the slope of the regression line, and β provides a measure of the relative strength of the association independent of the measurement units. AIx, augmentation index; CCS, carotid cross-sectional; cf-PWV, carotid–femoral pulse wave velocity; HR, heart rate; MAP, mean arterial pressure; PP, pulse pressure; SBP, systolic blood pressure; Sex is 1 = males and 2 = females.

4. Discussion

A number of techniques are currently used to estimate arterial stiffness in a clinical setting, with limited attention to the differences among the methods being used. In such a context, our study offers clear pathophysiological data, based on the simultaneous use of different approaches to the estimate of arterial distensibility, that might help clinicians in correctly interpreting the results of commercially available devices. The close inverse correlation found in our study between cf-PWV, estimated through a "propagative method", and carotid distensibility, estimated through a cross-sectional method, confirms the close link between these two methods. The estimates of aortic and carotid distensibility were also correlated with the major factors which are known to determine alterations in the viscoelastic properties of the large arteries, particularly age and high BP levels.

In spite of these correlations, however, these two approaches offer different perspective on the assessment of mechanical vascular wall properties across the arterial tree.

Overall, cf-PWV accurately reflects the speed of BP wave propagation across the arterial tree from the heart to the periphery [34]. Depending on the PWV itself and on the distance covered, the reflected wave generated at the periphery will overlap with the forward BP wave at different times during the cardiac cycle. In the presence of a low stiffness-low PWV state, the reflected waves are overlapped with the forward waves during the early systolic phase of the cardiac cycle in the peripheral arteries, while in the central arteries, this overlapping occurs during the late systolic phase. Therefore, reflected waves will not contribute to increasing central systolic and PP, while they will amplify peripheral systolic BP and PP. This mechanism explains the PP amplification phenomenon, i.e., why peripheral (brachial) PP is higher than central (aortic or carotid) PP in the presence of elastic arteries.

Indeed, cf-PWV is currently considered as the "gold-standard" measurement of large arteries stiffness [18,45], because, according to the mathematical model proposed by Bramwell and Hill [39], arterial wall distensibility is related to the reverse of the pulse wave propagation velocity squared.

We compared the aortic distensibility estimated by cf-PWV with the assessment of carotid distensibility provided by a carotid cross-sectional approach (wall track system). Although carotid cross-sectional distensibility was obtained only from a specific and well-defined segment of the artery, our study points out that, in the absence of evident atheromatous disease, the hemodynamic conditions and the viscoelastic properties of the common carotid artery are similar to those of the aorta, as shown by the inverse correlation we found between cf-PWV one side and carotid distensibility and AIx on the other side. The mechanical properties of a blood vessel are not linear, i.e., they depend on the pressure distending them, which varies continuously The simultaneous measurement of diameter and pressure variation curves for the definition of carotid cross-sectional distensibility obtained in our study is, thus, an important test, complementary to the tests that are commonly used to study the mechanical properties of the large arteries and the degree of vascular ageing, such as PWV and aortic pulse wave analysis.

In spite of the complementary nature of aortic pulse wave analysis and propagative and non-propagative models, the factors affecting these parameters are different. Overall, cf-PWV is determined by age; AIx by age, gender, heart rate, and BP; PP amplification by heart rate and age; and carotid cross-sectional distensibility is influenced by age, BP, weight, and heart rate.

A further element that has emerged from our study is the inadequacy of the study of the axillo–brachial–radial axis as a window for the general evaluation of the viscoelastic properties of the large arteries. In fact, we found only a weak relationship between cr-PWV on one side, and age, BP, carotid distensibility and compliance and cf-PWV on the other side. The results of our study, therefore, offer additional and complementary evidence supporting and expanding previous observations regarding the fact that the arterial tree is not homogeneous and the various arterial districts can be differently affected either by the aging process, by hypertension or by a combination of both factors [46,47]. Formerly, also, van der Heijden-Spek et al. [48] showed that, after the adjustment for the confounding factor, no relation exists between the age and distensibility of the brachial artery. Moreover, it has been shown that, for the same mean transmural pressure, normotensive and hypertensive patients had the same PWV in the forearm and, therefore, the same distensibility [49]. Evidence is also available that radial artery compliance paradoxically increases in hypertensive patients, compared to normotensive individuals, when assessed at the same BP level [50,51]. This can be related to the specific anatomical characteristics of the arteries of the upper limb, which are prevalently muscular (whereas the aorta has a mixed, prevalently elastic structure, especially in its proximal portion) and not subjected to vascular ageing.

Our study has a few limitations affecting the generalizability of our results. Some caution should be used in the interpretation of the data, due to limited sample of the subgroups, which makes a complete adjustment for confounders in the subgroup analysis impossible. A further limitation consists of the selection of individuals considered in the present study, which is lacking patients with overt cardiovascular disease, to whom the evaluation of arterial stiffness is usually addressed. Larger studies in cardiovascular patients are needed to confirm our data.

5. Conclusions

In this study, we expand the available evidence on the close association between aortic propagative models detecting arterial stiffness (cf-PWV) and local carotid cross-sectional models (based on simultaneous measurement of diameter and pressure variation curves, in order to measure distensibility and compliance). Instead, cr-PWV clearly appeared in our study to be inadequate for the general evaluation of the mechanical properties of large arteries. These data strongly support the complementary nature of some, but not all, of the currently available methods to estimate mechanical arterial wall properties in a clinical setting.

Author Contributions: Conceptualization, P.S. and A.B.; methodology, P.S., A.G. and F.V.; data analysis, P.S., F.V. and C.L.; formal analysis, C.L. and A.K.-S.; investigation, P.S., F.V. and A.K.-S. writing—original draft preparation, P.S. and F.V.; writing—review and editing, G.P. and A.B.; supervision, A.G., G.P. and A.B. All authors have read and agreed to the published version of the manuscript.

Funding: This research received no external funding.

Institutional Review Board Statement: The study was conducted in accordance with the Declaration of Helsinki and approved by the Local Institutional Ethics Committee (CPP Est III 15 December 2006)

Informed Consent Statement: Informed consent was obtained from all subjects involved in the study

Data Availability Statement: The data presented in this study are available upon request from the corresponding author. The data are not publicly available, due to privacy concerns.

Conflicts of Interest: P.S. has been involved as a consultant and expert witness in DiaTecne s.r.l. The other authors declare no conflict of interest.

References

1. Laurent, S.; Boutouyrie, P.; Asmar, R.; Gautier, I.; Laloux, B.; Guize, L.; Ducimetiere, P.; Benetos, A. Aortic stiffness is an independent predictor of all-cause and cardiovascular mortality in hypertensive patients. *Hypertension* **2001**, *37*, 1236–1241 [CrossRef] [PubMed]
2. Boutouyrie, P.; Tropeano, A.I.; Asmar, R.; Gautier, I.; Benetos, A.; Lacolley, P.; Laurent, S. Aortic stiffness is an independent predictor of primary coronary events in hypertensive patients: A longitudinal study. *Hypertension* **2002**, *39*, 10–15. [CrossRef] [PubMed]
3. van Popele, N.M.; Mattace-Raso, F.U.; Vliegenthart, R.; Grobbee, D.E.; Asmar, R.; van der Kuip, D.A.; Hofman, A.; de Feijter, P.J.; Oudkerk, M.; Witteman, J.C. Aortic stiffness is associated with atherosclerosis of the coronary arteries in older adults: The Rotterdam Study. *J. Hypertens.* **2006**, *24*, 2371–2376. [CrossRef] [PubMed]
4. Sequi-Dominguez, I.; Cavero-Redondo, I.; Alvarez-Bueno, C.; Pozuelo-Carrascosa, D.P.; Nunez de Arenas-Arroyo, S.; Martinez-Vizcaino, V. Accuracy of Pulse Wave Velocity Predicting Cardiovascular and All-Cause Mortality. A Systematic Review and Meta-Analysis. *J. Clin. Med.* **2020**, *9*, 2080. [CrossRef] [PubMed]
5. Benetos, A.; Thomas, F.; Joly, L.; Blacher, J.; Pannier, B.; Labat, C.; Salvi, P.; Smulyan, H.; Safar, M.E. Pulse pressure amplification a mechanical biomarker of cardiovascular risk. *J. Am. Coll. Cardiol.* **2010**, *55*, 1032–1037. [CrossRef]
6. Safar, M.E.; Blacher, J.; Pannier, B.; Guerin, A.P.; Marchais, S.J.; Guyonvarch, P.M.; London, G.M. Central pulse pressure and mortality in end-stage renal disease. *Hypertension* **2002**, *39*, 735–738. [CrossRef]
7. London, G.M.; Blacher, J.; Pannier, B.; Guerin, A.P.; Marchais, S.J.; Safar, M.E. Arterial wave reflections and survival in end-stage renal failure. *Hypertension* **2001**, *38*, 434–438. [CrossRef]
8. Blacher, J.; Guerin, A.P.; Pannier, B.; Marchais, S.J.; Safar, M.E.; London, G.M. Impact of aortic stiffness on survival in end-stage renal disease. *Circulation* **1999**, *99*, 2434–2439. [CrossRef]
9. Pannier, B.; Guerin, A.P.; Marchais, S.J.; Safar, M.E.; London, G.M. Stiffness of capacitive and conduit arteries: Prognostic significance for end-stage renal disease patients. *Hypertension* **2005**, *45*, 592–596. [CrossRef]
10. Blacher, J.; Asmar, R.; Djane, S.; London, G.M.; Safar, M.E. Aortic pulse wave velocity as a marker of cardiovascular risk in hypertensive patients. *Hypertension* **1999**, *33*, 1111–1117. [CrossRef]
11. Laurent, S.; Katsahian, S.; Fassot, C.; Tropeano, A.I.; Gautier, I.; Laloux, B.; Boutouyrie, P. Aortic stiffness is an independent predictor of fatal stroke in essential hypertension. *Stroke* **2003**, *34*, 1203–1206. [CrossRef] [PubMed]
12. Cruickshank, K.; Riste, L.; Anderson, S.G.; Wright, J.S.; Dunn, G.; Gosling, R.G. Aortic pulse-wave velocity and its relationship to mortality in diabetes and glucose intolerance: An integrated index of vascular function? *Circulation* **2002**, *106*, 2085–2090. [CrossRef] [PubMed]
13. Meaume, S.; Benetos, A.; Henry, O.F.; Rudnichi, A.; Safar, M.E. Aortic pulse wave velocity predicts cardiovascular mortality in subjects >70 years of age. *Arter. Thromb. Vasc. Biol.* **2001**, *21*, 2046–2050. [CrossRef]
14. Benetos, A.; Gautier, S.; Labat, C.; Salvi, P.; Valbusa, F.; Marino, F.; Toulza, O.; Agnoletti, D.; Zamboni, M.; Dubail, D.; et al. Mortality and cardiovascular events are best predicted by low central/peripheral pulse pressure amplification but not by high blood pressure levels in elderly nursing home subjects: The PARTAGE (Predictive Values of Blood Pressure and Arterial Stiffness in Institutionalized Very Aged Population) study. *J. Am. Coll. Cardiol.* **2012**, *60*, 1503–1511.

5. Weber, T.; Auer, J.; O'Rourke, M.F.; Kvas, E.; Lassnig, E.; Lamm, G.; Stark, N.; Rammer, M.; Eber, B. Increased arterial wave reflections predict severe cardiovascular events in patients undergoing percutaneous coronary interventions. *Eur. Heart J.* **2005**, *26*, 2657–2663. [CrossRef] [PubMed]
6. Chirinos, J.A.; Zambrano, J.P.; Chakko, S.; Veerani, A.; Schob, A.; Willens, H.J.; Perez, G.; Mendez, A.J. Aortic pressure augmentation predicts adverse cardiovascular events in patients with established coronary artery disease. *Hypertension* **2005**, *45*, 980–985. [CrossRef] [PubMed]
7. Mattace-Raso, F.U.; van der Cammen, T.J.; Hofman, A.; van Popele, N.M.; Bos, M.L.; Schalekamp, M.A.; Asmar, R.; Reneman, R.S.; Hoeks, A.P.; Breteler, M.M.; et al. Arterial stiffness and risk of coronary heart disease and stroke: The Rotterdam Study. *Circulation* **2006**, *113*, 657–663. [CrossRef]
8. Townsend, R.R.; Wilkinson, I.B.; Schiffrin, E.L.; Avolio, A.P.; Chirinos, J.A.; Cockcroft, J.R.; Heffernan, K.S.; Lakatta, E.G.; McEniery, C.M.; Mitchell, G.F.; et al. Recommendations for Improving and Standardizing Vascular Research on Arterial Stiffness: A Scientific Statement From the American Heart Association. *Hypertension* **2015**, *66*, 698–722. [CrossRef]
9. Salvi, P. *Pulse Waves. How Vascular Hemodynamics Affects Blood Pressure*, 2nd ed.; Springer Nature: Berlin/Heidelberg, Germany, 2017.
10. Laurent, S.; Caviezel, B.; Beck, L.; Girerd, X.; Billaud, E.; Boutouyrie, P.; Hoeks, A.; Safar, M. Carotid artery distensibility and distending pressure in hypertensive humans. *Hypertension* **1994**, *23*, 878–883. [CrossRef]
11. O'Rourke, M.F.; Gallagher, D.E. Pulse wave analysis. *J. Hypertens. Suppl.* **1996**, *14*, S147–S157. [CrossRef]
12. Avolio, A.P.; Van Bortel, L.M.; Boutouyrie, P.; Cockcroft, J.R.; McEniery, C.M.; Protogerou, A.D.; Roman, M.J.; Safar, M.E.; Segers, P.; Smulyan, H. Role of pulse pressure amplification in arterial hypertension: Experts' opinion and review of the data. *Hypertension* **2009**, *54*, 375–383. [CrossRef] [PubMed]
13. Nichols, W.; O'Rourke, M.; Vlachopoulos, C. *McDonald's Blood Flow in Arteries. Theoretical, Experimental and Clinical Principles*, 6th ed.; Oxford University Press: New York, NY, USA, 2011.
14. Namasivayam, M.; McDonnell, B.J.; McEniery, C.M.; O'Rourke, M.F. Does wave reflection dominate age-related change in aortic blood pressure across the human life span? *Hypertension* **2009**, *53*, 979–985. [CrossRef] [PubMed]
15. McEniery, C.M.; Yasmin, N.; Hall, I.R.; Qasem, A.; Wilkinson, I.B.; Cockcroft, J.R. Normal vascular aging: Differential effects on wave reflection and aortic pulse wave velocity: The Anglo-Cardiff Collaborative Trial (ACCT). *J. Am. Coll. Cardiol.* **2005**, *46*, 1753–1760. [CrossRef] [PubMed]
16. O'Rourke, M.F.; Seward, J.B. Central arterial pressure and arterial pressure pulse: New views entering the second century after Korotkov. *Mayo Clin. Proc.* **2006**, *81*, 1057–1068. [CrossRef]
17. Segers, P.; Rietzschel, E.R.; De Buyzere, M.L.; Vermeersch, S.J.; De Bacquer, D.; Van Bortel, L.M.; De Backer, G.; Gillebert, T.C.; Verdonck, P.R. Noninvasive (input) impedance, pulse wave velocity, and wave reflection in healthy middle-aged men and women. *Hypertension* **2007**, *49*, 1248–1255. [CrossRef]
18. El Assaad, M.A.; Topouchian, J.A.; Asmar, R.G. Evaluation of two devices for self-measurement of blood pressure according to the international protocol: The Omron M5-I and the Omron 705IT. *Blood Press. Monit.* **2003**, *8*, 127–133. [CrossRef]
19. Giannattasio, C.; Salvi, P.; Valbusa, F.; Kearney-Schwartz, A.; Capra, A.; Amigoni, M.; Failla, M.; Boffi, L.; Madotto, F.; Benetos, A.; et al. Simultaneous measurement of beat-to-beat carotid diameter and pressure changes to assess arterial mechanical properties. *Hypertension* **2008**, *52*, 896–902. [CrossRef]
20. van Sloten, T.T.; Schram, M.T.; van den Hurk, K.; Dekker, J.M.; Nijpels, G.; Henry, R.M.; Stehouwer, C.D. Local stiffness of the carotid and femoral artery is associated with incident cardiovascular events and all-cause mortality: The Hoorn study. *J. Am. Coll. Cardiol.* **2014**, *63*, 1739–1747. [CrossRef]
21. Hoeks, A.P.; Brands, P.J.; Smeets, F.A.; Reneman, R.S. Assessment of the distensibility of superficial arteries. *Ultrasound Med. Biol.* **1990**, *16*, 121–128. [CrossRef]
22. Kool, M.J.; van Merode, T.; Reneman, R.S.; Hoeks, A.P.; Struyker Boudier, H.A.; Van Bortel, L.M. Evaluation of reproducibility of a vessel wall movement detector system for assessment of large artery properties. *Cardiovasc. Res.* **1994**, *28*, 610–614. [CrossRef]
23. Salvi, P.; Lio, G.; Labat, C.; Ricci, E.; Pannier, B.; Benetos, A. Validation of a new non-invasive portable tonometer for determining arterial pressure wave and pulse wave velocity: The PulsePen device. *J. Hypertens.* **2004**, *22*, 2285–2293. [CrossRef] [PubMed]
24. Salvi, P.; Scalise, F.; Rovina, M.; Moretti, F.; Salvi, L.; Grillo, A.; Gao, L.; Baldi, C.; Faini, A.; Furlanis, G.; et al. Noninvasive Estimation of Aortic Stiffness Through Different Approaches. *Hypertension* **2019**, *74*, 117–129. [CrossRef] [PubMed]
25. Joly, L.; Perret-Guillaume, C.; Kearney-Schwartz, A.; Salvi, P.; Mandry, D.; Marie, P.Y.; Karcher, G.; Rossignol, P.; Zannad, F.; Benetos, A. Pulse wave velocity assessment by external noninvasive devices and phase-contrast magnetic resonance imaging in the obese. *Hypertension* **2009**, *54*, 421–426. [CrossRef] [PubMed]
26. O'Rourke, M.F.; Staessen, J.A.; Vlachopoulos, C.; Duprez, D.; Plante, G.E. Clinical applications of arterial stiffness; definitions and reference values. *Am. J. Hypertens.* **2002**, *15*, 426–444. [CrossRef]
27. Mackenzie, I.S.; Wilkinson, I.B.; Cockcroft, J.R. Assessment of arterial stiffness in clinical practice. *QJM* **2002**, *95*, 67–74. [CrossRef]
28. Van Bortel, L.M.; Duprez, D.; Starmans-Kool, M.J.; Safar, M.E.; Giannattasio, C.; Cockcroft, J.; Kaiser, D.R.; Thuillez, C. Clinical applications of arterial stiffness, Task Force III: Recommendations for user procedures. *Am. J. Hypertens.* **2002**, *15*, 445–452. [CrossRef]
29. Bramwell, J.C.; Hill, A.V. Velocity of transmission of the pulse-wave and elasticity of the arteries. *Lancet* **1922**, *1*, 891–892. [CrossRef]

40. Mackay, R.S.; Marg, E.; Oechsli, R. Automatic tonometer with exact theory: Various biological applications. *Science* **1960**, *131*, 1668–1669. [CrossRef]
41. Pressman, G.L.; Newgard, P.M. A Transducer for the Continuous External Measurement of Arterial Blood Pressure. *IEEE Trans. Biomed. Eng.* **1963**, *10*, 73–81. [CrossRef]
42. Matthys, K.; Verdonck, P. Development and modelling of arterial applanation tonometry: A review. *Technol. Health Care* **2002**, *10*, 65–76. [CrossRef]
43. Bland, J.M.; Altman, D.G. Statistical methods for assessing agreement between two methods of clinical measurement. *Lancet* **1986**, *1*, 307–310. [CrossRef]
44. Grillo, A.; Simon, G.; Salvi, P.; Rovina, M.; Baldi, C.; Prearo, I.; Bernardi, S.; Fabris, B.; Faini, A.; Parati, G.; et al. Influence of carotid atherosclerotic plaques on pulse wave assessment with arterial tonometry. *J. Hypertens.* **2017**, *35*, 1609–1617. [CrossRef] [PubMed]
45. Laurent, S.; Cockcroft, J.; Van Bortel, L.; Boutouyrie, P.; Giannattasio, C.; Hayoz, D.; Pannier, B.; Vlachopoulos, C.; Wilkinson, I.; Struijker-Boudier, H. Expert consensus document on arterial stiffness: Methodological issues and clinical applications. *Eur. Heart J.* **2006**, *27*, 2588–2605. [CrossRef] [PubMed]
46. Benetos, A.; Laurent, S.; Hoeks, A.P.; Boutouyrie, P.H.; Safar, M.E. Arterial alterations with aging and high blood pressure. A noninvasive study of carotid and femoral arteries. *Arter. Thromb.* **1993**, *13*, 90–97. [CrossRef]
47. Benetos, A.; Asmar, R.; Gautier, S.; Salvi, P.; Safar, M. Heterogeneity of the arterial tree in essential hypertension: A noninvasive study of the terminal aorta and the common carotid artery. *J. Hum. Hypertens.* **1994**, *8*, 501–507.
48. van der Heijden-Spek, J.J.; Staessen, J.A.; Fagard, R.H.; Hoeks, A.P.; Boudier, H.A.; van Bortel, L.M. Effect of age on brachial artery wall properties differs from the aorta and is gender dependent: A population study. *Hypertension* **2000**, *35*, 637–642. [CrossRef]
49. Smulyan, H.; Vardan, S.; Griffiths, A.; Gribbin, B. Forearm arterial distensibility in systolic hypertension. *J. Am. Coll. Cardiol.* **1984**, *3*, 387–393. [CrossRef]
50. Laurent, S.; Girerd, X.; Mourad, J.J.; Lacolley, P.; Beck, L.; Boutouyrie, P.; Mignot, J.P.; Safar, M. Elastic modulus of the radial artery wall material is not increased in patients with essential hypertension. *Arter. Thromb.* **1994**, *14*, 1223–1231. [CrossRef]
51. Laurent, S.; Hayoz, D.; Trazzi, S.; Boutouyrie, P.; Waeber, B.; Omboni, S.; Brunner, H.R.; Mancia, G.; Safar, M. Isobaric compliance of the radial artery is increased in patients with essential hypertension. *J. Hypertens.* **1993**, *11*, 89–98. [CrossRef]

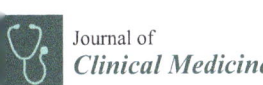

Increased Platelet Reactivity and Proinflammatory Profile Are Associated with Intima–Media Thickness and Arterial Stiffness in Prediabetes

Maurizio Di Marco, Francesca Urbano, Agnese Filippello, Stefania Di Mauro, Alessandra Scamporrino, Nicoletta Miano, Giuseppe Coppolino, Giuseppe L'Episcopo, Stefano Leggio, Roberto Scicali, Salvatore Piro, Francesco Purrello * and Antonino Di Pino

Department of Clinical and Experimental Medicine, University of Catania, 95131 Catania, Italy; maurizio.dimarco@studium.unict.it (M.D.M.); francescaurbano@hotmail.it (F.U.); agnese.filippello@gmail.com (A.F.); 8stefaniadimauro6@gmail.com (S.D.M.); alessandraska@hotmail.com (A.S.); nicoletta.miano@gmail.com (N.M.); giuseppecoppolino93@gmail.com (G.C.); peppe94@gmail.com (G.L.); stefano_leggio@yahoo.it (S.L.); robertoscicali@gmail.com (R.S.); salvatore.piro@unict.it (S.P.); nino_dipino@hotmail.com (A.D.P.)
* Correspondence: francesco.purrello@unict.it; Tel.: +39-095-759-8401

Abstract: Alterations of glucose homeostasis are associated with subclinical vascular damage; however, the role of platelet reactivity in this process has not been fully investigated. In this cross-sectional study, we evaluated the correlation between markers of platelet reactivity and inflammation and markers of vascular disease in subjects with prediabetes. Markers of platelet reactivity such as 11-dehydro-thromboxane B2 urinary levels (11-dh-TXB2) and mean platelet volume (MPV) and inflammatory indexes such as platelet-to-lymphocyte ratio (PLR) were evaluated in subjects with prediabetes ($n = 48$), new-onset type 2 diabetes (NODM, $n = 60$) and controls ($n = 62$). Furthermore, we assessed the cardiovascular risk profile of the study population with arterial stiffness and quality intima–media thickness (qIMT). Subjects with prediabetes and NODM exhibited higher 11-dh-TXB2 urinary levels and MPV and a proinflammatory profile with an increased PLR, high-sensitivity C-reactive protein, ferritin and fibrinogen. Furthermore, after multiple regression analyses, we found that urinary 11-dh-TXB2 was one of the major determinants of IMT and arterial stiffness parameters. In conclusion, subjects with prediabetes exhibit increased platelet reactivity as well as a proinflammatory profile. Furthermore, this condition is associated with early markers of cardiovascular disease.

Keywords: prediabetes; 11-dh-thromboxane; cardiovascular risk; IMT; arterial stiffness

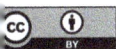

1. Introduction

Prediabetes identifies a clinical condition with a higher risk of developing diabetes and cardiovascular disease [1]. According to the American Diabetes Association (ADA), this category includes subjects with impaired fasting glucose (IFG) and/or impaired glucose tolerance (IGT) and/or HbA1c 5.7–6.4% [2].

It is well known that mechanisms at the base of macrovascular complications of diabetes already act in the prediabetes phase, prior to diagnosis of diabetes, via atherosclerosis [3–5]. Based on these considerations, prediabetes is associated with more advanced vascular damage compared with normoglycemia [6]. In the last few years, several different pathways have been analyzed to explain the link between early alterations of glucose homeostasis and vascular damage, such as the role of advanced glycation end-products and their soluble receptors [7], the increase in small, dense low-density lipoproteins (sdLDLs) [8], low vitamin D plasma levels [9] and micro-RNA (mi-RNA) deregulation [10].

Even though platelets play a pivotal role in the pathogenesis of atherothrombosis, the role of platelet reactivity in this process has not been fully investigated, especially in the setting of prediabetes [11]. This phenomenon has been studied in other conditions related to metabolic syndrome, such as overweight, obesity and insulin resistance [12–14].

Platelet activation is quite a complex mechanism, and platelet reactivity can be evaluated both with morphological and functional parameters, i.e., mean platelet volume (MPV) and 11-dehydro-thromboxane B2 (11-dh-TXB2) urinary excretion. In physiological conditions, in response to external stimuli, platelets increase their thromboxane A2 (TXA2) production, while prostacyclin production is reduced. This phenomenon is regulated by the activity of cyclooxygenases (COXs) [15]. The importance of platelet morphological features can be explained considering that larger platelets are more active because of the presence of a higher quantity of alpha-granules and the production of more thromboxane A2 (TXA2) [16]. TXA2 is chemically instable, and thus it is rapidly converted into thromboxane B2 (TXB2) that, in turn, is metabolized into 11-dh-TXB2. 11-dh-TXB2 is the principal metabolite of TXA2, and different studies have shown the possibility of using its urinary excretion as a biomarker of platelet reactivity [17,18].

Platelets are essential for primary hemostasis and repair of the endothelium; however they also play a key role in the development of vascular inflammation and participate in the process of forming and extending atherosclerotic plaques. The relationship between chronic and acute vascular inflammation is unclear, but platelets are a source of inflammatory mediators; i.e., the F2 isoprostane 8-iso-PGF2α can be produced as a minor product of the cyclooxygenase activity of platelets in response to platelet stimulation with collagen thrombin or arachidonate, and it is also a marker of oxidative stress [18,19]. In addition, it is interesting to consider the platelet-to-lymphocyte ratio (PLR), which is a cheap and easy way to obtain a parameter that takes into account two different aspects of atherosclerosis platelet count and inflammation. This index has been used in the field of oncology, but in the last few years, it has become a promising biomarker in other conditions, particularly in cardiovascular disease [20–22]. In the atherosclerotic process, the inflammatory response and oxidative stress also play important roles, and the activation of platelets by inflammatory triggers may be a critical component of vascular damage [23,24].

In this study, we evaluated platelet reactivity and inflammatory parameters in subjects with prediabetes and new-onset type 2 diabetes (NODM) and examined their association with early markers of cardiovascular disease.

2. Materials and Methods

Study subjects. One hundred seventy subjects with no previous diagnosis of diabetes who attended our university hospital for diabetes and cardiovascular risk evaluation were consecutively recruited in this study. The inclusion criteria were ages ranging from 18–65 years and Caucasian race. All patients underwent a physical examination and review of clinical history, smoking status (active or nonsmokers) and alcohol consumption. The exclusion criteria were as follows: a previous history of diabetes; a previous history of overt cardiovascular events (stroke, ischemic heart disease, chronic obstructive peripheral arteriopathy or heart failure), anemia or hemoglobinopathies; use of medications known to affect glucose metabolism and platelet aggregation (statins, antiplatelet drugs); clinical evidence of advanced liver or renal disease, chronic inflammatory disease or other chronic diseases; and/or recent history of acute illness, malignant disease and drug or alcohol abuse.

BMI was calculated as weight (kg)/(height (m))^2. Blood pressure (BP) was measured with a calibrated sphygmomanometer after 10 min rest. Venous blood samples were drawn from the antecubital vein in the morning after an overnight fast. Baseline venous blood samples were obtained for the measurement of clinical biochemistry parameters. LDL cholesterol concentrations were estimated using the Friedewald formula. All subjects underwent a 75 g oral glucose tolerance test (OGTT) with 0, 30, 60, 90, and 120 min sampling for plasma and insulin, as previously described [25]. Glucose tolerance status was defined on the basis of OGTT according to ADA recommendations [2].

Biochemical analyses. Plasma glucose, serum total cholesterol, triglycerides, high-density lipoprotein (HDL) cholesterol and high-sensitivity C-reactive protein (hs-CRP) were measured using available enzymatic methods, as previously described [26].

The concentrations of urinary 11-dh-TXB2 and 8-iso-PGF2α were measured with an enzyme-linked immunosorbent assay commercial kit (Cayman Chemical, Ann Arbor, MI, USA). Data are expressed as ng/mg creatinine. Analyses were performed in a blinded manner. Thus, the biologist who analyzed the samples was not aware of the clinical characteristics of the subjects. The commercially available ELISA kits were used according to the manufacturer's instructions.

HbA1c was measured via high-performance liquid chromatography using a National Glycohemoglobin Standardization Program and was standardized to the Diabetes Control and Complications Trial (DCCT) assay reference [27]. Chromatography was performed using a certified automated analyzer (HPLC; HLC-723G7 hemoglobin HPLC analyzer; Tosoh Corp.) (normal range 4.25–5.9%).

Carotid ultrasound examination. Ultrasound scans were performed using a high-resolution B-mode ultrasound system equipped with a linear array transducer. All ultrasound examinations were performed by a single physician who was blinded to the clinical and laboratory characteristics of the subjects. Longitudinal B-mode (60 Hz, 128 radiofrequency lines) images of the right common carotid artery 2 cm below the carotid bulb were obtained using a high-precision echo tracking device (MyLab Alpha, Esaote, Maastricht, The Netherlands) paired with a high-resolution linear array transducer (13 MHz) to acquire quality intima–media thickness (qIMT) using the built-in echo tracking software.

Pulse wave velocity. The SphygmoCor CvMS (AtCor Medical, Sydney, Australia) system was used for the determination of the pulse wave velocity (PWV), as previously described [28]. This system uses a tonometer, and two different pressure waves obtained at the common carotid artery (proximal recording site) and at the femoral artery (distal recording site). An electrocardiogram was used to determine the start of the pulse wave. The PWV was determined as the difference in travel time of the pulse wave between the two different recording sites and the heart, divided by the travel distance of the pulse waveform. The PWV was calculated on the mean basis of 10 consecutive pressure waveforms to cover a complete respiratory cycle.

Pulse wave analysis. All measurements were made from the right radial artery by applanation tonometry using a Millar tonometer (SPC-301; Millar Instruments, Houston, TX, USA) [29]. The measurements were performed by a single investigator with the subject in the supine position. The data were collected directly with a desktop computer and processed with SphygmoCorCvMS (AtCor Medical, Sydney, Australia). The aortic waveform has two systolic pressure peaks; the latter one is caused by wave reflection from the periphery. With arterial stiffening, both the PWV and the amplitude of the reflected wave are increased such that the reflected wave arrives earlier and adds to (or augments) the central systolic pressure. The aortic waveform in pulse wave analysis was subjected to further analysis for the calculation of the aortic augmentation pressure (AugP), augmentation index (AugI—calculated by dividing augmentation by pulse pressure), central BP, ejection duration (duration of the systolic period in milliseconds) and Buckberg subendocardial viability ratio (SEVR; area of diastole divided by area of systole during one cardiac cycle in the aorta). Pulse pressure is the difference between the systolic and diastolic BPs.

Statistical analyses. The sample size was calculated based on 11-dh-TXB2 using a level of significance (α) set to 5% and a power ($1 - \beta$) set to 80%. The estimated sample size was 48 subjects per group.

Statistical comparisons of clinical and biomedical parameters were performed using Stat View 6.0 for Windows. The data are presented as the mean ± standard deviation (SD) or median and interquartile range (IQR). Each variable's distributional characteristics, including normality, were assessed by the Kolmogorov–Smirnov test. ANOVA for clinical and biological data was performed to test the differences among groups, and the Bonferroni post hoc test for multiple comparisons was further performed. The χ2 test was used for categorical variables. A p value less than 0.05 was considered significant. When necessary, numerical variables were logarithmically transformed to reduce skewness.

Simple regression analysis was performed to relate 11-dh-TXB2, MPV and PLR to the following variables: age, sex, BMI, systolic and diastolic BP, HDL cholesterol, triglycerides, LDL cholesterol, homeostasis model assessment insulin resistance index (HOMA-IR), HbA1c and fasting glucose.

In order to identify variables independently associated with variations in qIMT, PWV and AugP, we performed two multivariate regression models: the first model included cardiovascular risk factors (age, sex, BMI, systolic and diastolic BP, LDL cholesterol, HDL cholesterol, HbA1c, fasting glucose, HOMA-IR); variables reaching significance in the first model were included in a second model including variables related to platelet activation and inflammation (11-dh-TXB2, platelet count, MPV, 8-iso-PGF2α, PLR, hs-CRP, fibrinogen).

The variance inflation factor (VIF) was used to check for the problem of multicollinearity among the predictor variables in multiple regression analysis. Any variable with a VIF that exceeded 4 was excluded from the model, as recommended in the literature (no variable was detected with a VIF greater than 4) [30].

The study was approved by the local ethics committee. Informed consent was obtained from each participant.

3. Results

The study population (170 subjects) was divided into three groups based on fasting glucose, OGTT and HbA1c levels: 62 control subjects (36%) (control group) (NFG and NT and HbA1c < 5.7%), 48 subjects with prediabetes (28%) (prediabetes group) (IFG and/or impaired glucose tolerance (IGT) and/or HbA1c 5.7–6.4%) and 60 subjects with NODM (35%) (NODM group) (fasting glucose $\geq$ 126 mg/dL and/or 2 h glucose post-OGTT $\geq$ 200 mg/dL and/or HbA1c $\geq$ 6.5%). The clinical and biochemical characteristics of the study subjects are presented in Table 1. The prediabetic patients were not older than the controls and had a similar BMI. Subjects with prediabetes were younger than subjects with NODM; however, there were no differences concerning BMI and diastolic BP. In addition, subjects with NODM showed a higher HOMA index than those of the prediabetic and control groups.

3.1. Platelet Reactivity and Inflammation Indexes in Subjects with Prediabetes

MPV was in prediabetic subjects significantly higher than that in controls (9.1 ± 0.8 vs. 8.7 ± 1.1 fL, $p < 0.05$) and showed no significant differences from that in subjects with NODM. No differences were found in 8-iso-PGF2α urinary levels between the three groups.

The platelet count in the subjects with prediabetes was higher than that in controls without reaching statistical significance (230 ± 64.2 vs. 251.5 ± 69 10^3/μL, $p = 0.15$) but was similar to that in subjects with NODM.

In the simple regression analysis, 11-dh-TXB2 urinary levels were associated with age ($r = 0.197$, $p = 0.01$) and systolic blood pressure ($r = 0.14$, $p < 0.05$). Moreover, MPV was associated with fasting glucose ($r = 0.25$, $p = 0.001$), HbA1c ($r = 0.16$, $p < 0.05$) and HOMA-IR ($r = 0.25$, $p = 0.0018$).

Hs-CRP was significantly higher in prediabetic subjects in comparison with controls (0.21 (0, 12–0.54) vs. 0.09 (0.07–0.29) mg/dL, $p < 0.05$) and in diabetic subjects than in controls (0.28 (0.19–0.59) vs. 0.09 (0.07–0.29) mg/dL, $p < 0.05$). Ferritin was significantly higher in the prediabetes group in comparison with the control group (119 (73–120) vs. 68 (73–200) ng/mL, $p < 0.05$) and in the NODM group than in the control group (108 (40.5–192.5) vs. 68 (73–200) ng/mL, $p < 0.05$). Fibrinogen in the prediabetes group was significantly higher than that in the control group (350 ± 71.3 vs. 324 ± 73.1 mg/dL, $p < 0.05$) and showed no significant differences from that in the NODM group. PLR was higher in the prediabetes group than in the control group without reaching statistical significance (138 ± 54 vs. 121.2 ± 38, $p = 0.16$), and it was significantly higher in the NODM group than in the control group (144 ± 87 vs. 121.2 ± 38, $p < 0.05$) (Table 2).

Table 1. Clinical and metabolic characteristics of the study population according to glucose tolerance.

	Controls ($n = 62$)	Prediabetes ($n = 48$)	New-Onset Type 2 Diabetes (NODM) ($n = 60$)
Age (years)	51.35 ± 7.84	51.75 ± 7.75	54.7 ± 6.84 *,#
BMI (kg/m²)	27.54 ± 3.95	30.39 ± 6.18	30.25 ± 5.22
SBP (mmHg)	118.83 ± 11.91	123.37 ± 14.54	131.17 ± 15.05 *,#
DBP (mmHg)	74.83 ± 9.61	78.54 ± 9.73 *	81.33 ± 8.53 *
Total cholesterol (mg/dL)	225 ± 36.23	233.46 ± 36.32	216.62 ± 23.94
HDL (mg/dL)	59.55 ± 17.74	54.83 ± 13.8	58.63 ± 37.95
TG (mg/dL)	93 (61–118)	114 (84.5–163.5)	108 (78–132)
LDL (mg/dL)	137.00 ± 44.61	153.22 ± 34.44	139.9 ± 24.13
eGFR (mL/min/1.73 m²)	99.25 ± 15.05	98.52 ± 15.55	103.40 ± 21.48
Fasting glucose (mg/dL)	85.58 ± 6.61	98.46 ± 16.99 *	127.30 ± 39.33 *,#
Plasma insulin (mIU/L)	7.10 (5.70–9.30)	9.20 (5.80–11.50) *	10.40 (6.50–19.70) *
HOMA-IR	1.46 (1.15–1.95)	2.11 (1.54–3.1) *	3.2 (1.77–5.45) *,#
HbA1c (%)	5.36 ± 0.23	5.87 ± 0.38 *	6.90 ± 1.19 *,#
ACR (mg/g creatinine)	7 (6–8)	8 (5–10)	10 (8–18) *,#
Hypertension (%)	23%	28%	45% *,#
Use of ACEis or ARBs (%)	13%	25% *	33% *
Use of CCBs (%)	3%	6%	13% *
Use of other antihypertensive drugs (%)	0%	4% *	3% *
Active smokers (%)	20%	36%	31%
Sex (M/F)	26/36	30/18 *	42/18 *

The data are presented as the mean ± SD or median (IQR). BMI: body mass index; SBP: systolic blood pressure; DBP: diastolic blood pressure; TG: triglycerides; eGFR: estimated glomerular filtration rate; HOMA-IR: homeostasis model assessment insulin resistance; ACR: albuminuria-to-creatininuria ratio; ACEis: angiotensin-converting enzyme inhibitors; ARBs: angiotensin receptor blockers; CCBs: calcium channel blockers. * $p < 0.05$ vs. controls; # $p < 0.05$ vs. prediabetes.

Table 2. Inflammation and platelet activation indexes in the study population according to glucose tolerance.

	Controls ($n = 62$)	Prediabetes ($n = 48$)	New-Onset Type 2 Diabetes (NODM) ($n = 60$)
hs-CRP (mg/dL)	0.09 (0.07–0.29)	0.21 (0.12–0.54) *	0.28 (0.19–0.59) *
WBC (10⁶/μL)	6.1 ± 1.8	7.2 ± 1.8 *	7.5 ± 1.8 *
Ferritin (ng/mL)	68 (25–125)	119 (73–200) *	108 (40.5–192.5) *
Fibrinogen (mg/dL)	324 ± 23.1	350 ± 71.3 *	348.9 ± 42.8
Platelet count (10³/μL)	230 ± 64.2	251.5 ± 69	255.2 ± 85.4 *,#
MPV (fL)	8.7 ± 1.1	9.1 ± 0.8 *	9.1 ± 0.8 *
PLR	121.2 ± 38	138 ± 54	144 ± 87 *
11-dh-TXB2 (ng/mg creatine)	10.6 (6.3–27.6)	16.5 (9.9–27.8) *	18.2 (8.5;36.6) *,#
8-iso-PGF$_{2\alpha}$ (ng/mg creatine)	9.7 (6.4–18.3)	9.9 (5.6–13.7)	10.7 (6.8–18.2)

The data are presented as the mean ± SD or median (IQR). Hs-CRP: high-sensitivity C-reactive protein; WBC: white blood cells; MPV: mean platelet volume; PLR: platelet-to-lymphocyte ratio; 11-dh-TXB2: 11-dehydrothromboxane B2 urinary levels; 8-Iso-PGF$_{2\alpha}$: isoprostane PGF$_{2\alpha}$ urinary levels. * $p < 0.05$ vs. controls; # $p < 0.05$ vs. prediabetes.

PLR was associated with diastolic BP ($r = 0.28$, $p = 0.0002$), HbA1c ($r = 0.16$, $p = 0.04$) and HOMA-IR ($r = 0.15$, $p < 0.05$) in the simple regression analysis.

3.2. Intima–Media Thickness and Arterial Stiffness in Subjects with Prediabetes

We found several differences in intima–media thickness and arterial stiffness parameters between the study groups (Table 3).

Table 3. Arterial stiffness and thickness parameters according to glucose tolerance.

	Controls (n = 62)	Prediabetes (n = 48)	New-Onset Type 2 Diabetes (NODM) (n = 60)
qIMT (mm)	0.69 ± 0.11	0.75 ± 0.12 *	0.76 ± 0.12 *
PWV (m/sec)	7.4 ± 1	7.9 ± 1.5 *	8.1 ± 1.9 *,#
AugP (mmHg)	10 ± 4.8	12 ± 8 *	12.7 ± 5.5 *
AugI (%)	26 ± 8.2	28.8 ± 13.1	30.5 ± 9.7 *
SEVR (%)	159.8 ± 27.7	160 ± 25.5	150.4 ± 25.5 *,#
Atherosclerotic plaque presence (%)	19%	27%	28%

The data are presented as the mean ± SD. qIMT: quality intima–media thickness; PWV: pulsed wave velocity; AugP: augmentation pressure; AugI: augmentation index; SEVR: subendocardial viability ratio. * $p < 0.05$ vs controls; # $p < 0.05$ vs. prediabetes.

qIMT in the prediabetes group was significantly higher than that in the control group (0.75 ± 0.12 vs. 0.69 ± 0.11 mm, $p < 0.05$) and had no differences from that in the NODM group.

In the multiple regression analysis using two models (see Section 2), qIMT exhibited a significant correlation with age ($p < 0.0001$) and fasting glucose ($p = 0.01$) in the first model. In the second model, the variables that remained significantly associated with qIMT were age ($p < 0.0001$), 11-dh-TXB2 urinary levels ($p < 0.05$), 8-iso-PGF2α urinary levels ($p = 0.04$) and fibrinogen ($p < 0.05$) (Table 4).

Table 4. Multiple regression analysis evaluating qIMT, AugP and PWV as dependent variables.

	Coefficient β	p Value
qIMT		
Multiple regression—Model 1 *		
Age (years)	8.9	<0.0001
FG (mg/dl)	1.48	0.01
Multiple regression—Model 2 **		
Age (years)	0.007	<0.0001
11-dh-TXB2 (ng/mg creatinine)	0.002	<0.05
Fibrinogen (mg/dL)	0.0003	<0.05
8-iso-PGF$_{2\alpha}$ (ng/mg creatinine)	−0.003	0.04
AugP		
Multiple regression—Model 1 *		
Male sex	−5.97	<0.0001
HbA$_{1c}$ (%)	1.65	0.02
HDL (mg/dL)	−0.04	0.03
Multiple regression—Model 2 **		
Male sex	−7.74	<0.0001
HbA$_{1c}$ (%)	2.46	0.02
HDL (mg/dL)	−0.05	0.01
11-dh-TXB2 (ng/mg creatinine)	0.107	<0.05
PWV		
Multiple regression—Model 1 *		
Male sex	0.56	0.03
SBP (mmHg)	0.04	<0.0001
HDL (mg/dL)	−0.12	0.01
Multiple regression—Model 2 **		
Male sex	0.88	0.03
SBP (mmHg)	0.03	0.005
11-dh-TXB2 (ng/mg creatinine)	0.031	0.0002

* Model 1 was adjusted for age, sex, BMI, systolic BP, HDL cholesterol, LDL cholesterol, HbA$_{1c}$, fasting glycemia and HOMA-IR. ** Model 2 was adjusted for 11-dh-TXB2 urinary levels, fibrinogen, MPV, platelet count, hs-CRP, 8-iso-PGF$_{2\alpha}$ urinary levels and PLR. FG: fasting glycemia; 11-dh-TXB2: 11-dehydro-thromboxane B2 urinary levels; 8-iso-PGF$_{2\alpha}$: isoprostane PGF$_{2\alpha}$ urinary levels; BMI: body mass index; PLR: platelet-to-lymphocyte ratio; hs-CRP: high-sensitivity C-reactive protein; SBP: systolic blood pressure.

PWV was significantly higher in the prediabetes group vs. the control group (7.9 ± 1.5 vs. 7.4 ± 1 m/s, $p < 0.05$) and in NODM vs. the prediabetes group and the control group (8.1 ± 1.9 vs. 7.9 ± 1.5 and 7.4 ± 1 m/s, $p < 0.05$). AugP was significantly higher in the prediabetes group than in the control group (12 ± 8 vs. 10 ± 4.8 mmHg, $p < 0.05$) and in NODM in comparison with the control group (12.7 ± 5.5 vs. 10 ± 4.8 mmHg, $p < 0.05$). AugI was higher in the prediabetes group than in the control group without reaching statistical significance (28.8 ± 13.1 vs. 26 ± 8.2%, $p = 0.08$), while it was significantly higher in the NODM group (30.5 ± 9.7 vs. 26 ± 8.2%, $p < 0.05$).

As regards the multiple regression analysis, in the first model, PWV showed a statistically significant association with male sex ($p = 0.03$), systolic BP ($p < 0.0001$) and HDL cholesterol ($p = 0.01$), while in the second model the variables that remained significantly related to PWV were male sex ($p = 0.03$), systolic BP ($p = 0.005$) and 11-dh-TXB2 urinary levels ($p = 0.0002$). Furthermore, AugP in the first model showed a correlation with male sex ($p < 0.0001$), HbA1c ($p = 0.02$) and HDL cholesterol ($p = 0.03$). In the second model, the variables significantly associated with AugP were male sex ($p < 0.0001$), HbA1c ($p = 0.02$), HDL cholesterol ($p = 0.01$) and 11-dh-TXB2 urinary levels ($p < 0.05$).

4. Discussion

In this study, we measured biomarkers of platelet reactivity and inflammation in subjects with prediabetes. Furthermore, we evaluated the association of these factors with qIMT and arterial stiffness, which are well known as early markers of cardiovascular disease and predictive of cardiovascular events.

We found that 11-dh-TXB2 urinary levels were significantly higher in the prediabetes group compared with the control group, as well as MPV; moreover, we found no differences between these parameters in the prediabetes group compared with the NODM group; these data provide evidence of an in vivo increased platelet activation in subjects with early alterations of glucose homeostasis.

Few studies are available concerning the 11-dh-TXB2 marker in subjects with prediabetes. Previous studies highlighted the association between prediabetes and platelet over-reactivity and resistance to antiplatelet therapy [31]. Santilli et al. found an enhanced thromboxane biosynthesis in subjects with impaired glucose tolerance (IGT), a subset of prediabetic subjects. Moreover, they observed that, among IGT subjects, those experiencing conversion to overt diabetes were characterized by a progressive rise in urinary thromboxane metabolite excretion rate [32]

The increase in 11-dh-TXB2, which is a direct marker of platelet activation, was already described in patients with type 1 and type 2 diabetes mellitus. Zaccardi et al. found that asymptomatic young subjects with type 1 diabetes showed persistently enhanced TXA2-dependent platelet activation and oxidant stress in vivo, and this phenomenon was related to female sex and microvascular and oxidative damages [18]. Al-Sofiani et al. demonstrated that type 2 diabetic patients have higher in vivo platelet activation compared with subjects without diabetes both before and after antiplatelet therapy, and they hypothesized that endothelial dysfunction may play a role in this platelet hyperactivity [33]. In addition, Lopez et al. highlighted that type 2 diabetes is associated not only with an increase in platelet reactivity biomarkers, but also with a poor response to antiaggregant therapy [34].

Platelet hyperactivity was observed in other conditions often associated with diabetes and prediabetes, such as obesity, dyslipidemia and hypertension. Davì et al. reported that urinary 11-dh-TXB2 is significantly increased in otherwise healthy obese women, as compared to non-obese controls [35]. Furthermore, the same study group found that successful short-term weight loss was associated with a statistically significant reduction in thromboxane urinary metabolites, identifying insulin resistance as one of the major determinants of platelet reactivity in subjects with obesity [36]. A large body of evidence strongly supports a reciprocal relationship between insulin resistance and endothelial function, sustaining the hypothesis that endothelial dysfunction may be the link between insulin resistance and platelet activation [37]

In addition, previous studies demonstrated that increased total and LDL cholesterol levels are correlated with a higher 11-dh-TXB2 excretion rate, suggesting that platelet activation can be a main determinant of hypercholesterolemia-induced cardiovascular risk [38]. As regards hypertension, Dolegowska et al. highlighted the mutual connections between platelet activation and mean arterial pressure, hypothesizing a potential platelet involvement in atherosclerosis development [39].

Thus, higher urinary thromboxane metabolite excretion is associated with atherosclerosis risk factors and is partially reversible after improved disease control, suggesting that the primary abnormalities, such as hyperglycemia, insulin resistance and hypercholesterolemia, may be responsible for enhanced and persistent thromboxane biosynthesis. In this regard, it is of relevance that disease-modifying strategies, such as lifestyle intervention, different antidiabetic agents and statins, may blunt, at least in part, urinary thromboxane metabolites [38]. Moreover, urinary thromboxane metabolite excretion could be a predictive biomarker of adverse cardiovascular outcomes, as demonstrated in patients with established atherosclerotic cardiovascular disease [40].

The higher MPV in subjects with prediabetes is consistent with other studies such as the one by Inoue et al. that analyzed a Japanese cohort [41]. Furthermore, we found that MPV was directly associated with HbA1c and HOMA-IR, as previously described [42,43]. Insulin resistance is a common denominator of several metabolic conditions related to platelet hyperactivity. This is consistent with the fact that platelets exhibit insulin receptors. Therefore, insulin resistance may cause the lack of the physiological action exerted by insulin on platelet function, such as reduction of the pro-aggregatory properties of agonists, and the activation of endothelial nitric oxide (NO) synthase, with increased NO formation and intraplatelet concentrations of cyclic adenosine monophosphate (cAMP) [36].

As previously reported [44], we highlighted a significant alteration of arterial stiffness and thickness parameters in our prediabetic subjects. Furthermore, we found that 11-dh-TXB2 urinary levels were associated with carotid atherosclerosis and arterial stiffness. Thus, these data suggest a link between platelet over-activation and atherosclerosis in prediabetes, confirming the high cardiovascular risk of this condition. This is clinically relevant, considering the incidence of macrovascular complications is already increased in prediabetes and in new-onset type 2 diabetes [45].

In addition, we found an increase in different inflammatory parameters, such as white blood cell count, hs-CRP, ferritin and fibrinogen. Moreover, even though it did not reach statistical significance, probably because of the sample size, we found an increase in PLR in prediabetic subjects, and we found a significant increase in PLR in diabetic patients compared with controls; furthermore, this parameter was associated with HbA1c and HOMA-IR in the simple regression analysis. This observation is consistent with previous studies in different populations and suggests that prediabetes is a proinflammatory condition [46,47]. Our group previously explored this hypothesis, demonstrating an impaired inflammatory profile in subjects with early glucose intolerance status and metabolic syndrome [6,48]. PLR can be a key factor for emphasizing the interplay between two major components of atherothrombosis: thrombosis and inflammation. Previous studies demonstrated that higher platelet and lower lymphocyte counts are associated with adverse cardiovascular outcomes. Thus, an elevated PLR may have an additive role in predicting major adverse cardiovascular outcomes [22].

This study presents some strengths and limitations. The major strength of the study is the exclusion of patients undergoing therapies known to affect platelet activation such as statins and antiplatelet drugs. Therefore, our results cannot be affected by drugs. As regards limitations, this was a cross-sectional study, and a longitudinal causal relationship cannot be established between changes in plasma platelet activation biomarkers and arterial stiffness and thickness. In addition, there are some differences in the sex distribution between the study groups.

As regards the evaluation of arterial stiffness, we used PWV. However, another indicator has emerged in recent years. The cardio-ankle vascular index (CAVI), which reflects the stiffness of the arterial tree from the beginning of the aorta to the ankle, is easy to measure and operator-independent. Thus, it could be a promising alternative to PWV. In addition, CAVI has been used in the prediabetic and diabetic populations [49,50].

5. Conclusions

In conclusion, subjects with prediabetes exhibit increased platelet reactivity as well as a proinflammatory profile. Furthermore, this condition is associated with early markers of cardiovascular disease independently of classical risk factors.

Author Contributions: Conceptualization, M.D.M. and A.D.P.; methodology, A.D.P.; software, M.D.M.; validation, S.P., F.P. and R.S.; formal analysis, A.S. and F.U.; investigation, N.M.; resources, G.C. and G.L.; data curation, S.L.; writing—original draft preparation, M.D.M.; writing—review and editing, A.D.P.; visualization, F.P.; supervision, F.P.; project administration, S.D.M.; funding acquisition, A.F. All authors have read and agreed to the published version of the manuscript.

Funding: This research received no external funding.

Institutional Review Board Statement: The study was conducted in accordance with the Declaration of Helsinki, and the protocol was approved by the Ethics Committee of ethics committee Catania 2 (702/CE, SMP-01, 23 September 2016, n. 28/2016/CECT2).

Informed Consent Statement: Informed consent was obtained from all subjects involved in the study.

Data Availability Statement: Data for this study are available under request.

Acknowledgments: A.D.P. is the guarantor of this work and, as such, had full access to all the data in the study and takes responsibility for the integrity of the data and the accuracy of the data analysis. All authors approved the final version. This study was in keeping with the objectives of the project "DEGENER-action", Department of Clinical and Experimental Medicine, University of Catania.

Conflicts of Interest: The authors declare no conflict of interest.

References

1. Tabák, A.G.; Herder, C.; Rathmann, W.; Brunner, E.J.; Kivimäki, M. Prediabetes: A High-Risk State for Diabetes Development. *Lancet* **2012**, *379*, 2279–2290. [CrossRef]
2. American Diabetes Association Professional Practice Committee. Classification and Diagnosis of Diabetes: Standards of Medical Care in Diabetes—2022. *Diabetes Care* **2022**, *45*, S17–S38. [CrossRef] [PubMed]
3. Brunner, E.J.; Shipley, M.J.; Witte, D.R.; Fuller, J.H.; Marmot, M.G. Relation Between Blood Glucose and Coronary Mortality Over 33 Years in the Whitehall Study. *Diabetes Care* **2006**, *29*, 26–31. [CrossRef] [PubMed]
4. Barr, E.L.M.; Zimmet, P.Z.; Welborn, T.A.; Jolley, D.; Magliano, D.J.; Dunstan, D.W.; Cameron, A.J.; Dwyer, T.; Taylor, H.R.; Tonkin, A.M.; et al. Risk of Cardiovascular and All-Cause Mortality in Individuals with Diabetes Mellitus, Impaired Fasting Glucose, and Impaired Glucose Tolerance: The Australian Diabetes, Obesity, and Lifestyle Study (AusDiab). *Circulation* **2007**, *116*, 151–157. [CrossRef]
5. Açar, B.; Ozeke, O.; Karakurt, M.; Ozen, Y.; Özbay, M.B.; Unal, S.; Karanfil, M.; Yayla, C.; Cay, S.; Maden, O.; et al. Association of Prediabetes with Higher Coronary Atherosclerotic Burden Among Patients with First Diagnosed Acute Coronary Syndrome. *Angiology* **2019**, *70*, 174–180. [CrossRef]
6. Di Pino, A.; Urbano, F.; Scicali, R.; Di Mauro, S.; Filippello, A.; Scamporrino, A.; Rabuazzo, A.M. 1-h Postload Glycemia Is Associated with Low Endogenous Secretory Receptor for Advanced Glycation End Product Levels and Early Markers of Cardiovascular Disease. *Cells* **2019**, *8*, 910. [CrossRef]
7. Di Pino, A.; Urbano, F.; Zagami, R.M.; Filippello, A.; Di Mauro, S.; Piro, S.; Purrello, F.; Rabuazzo, A.M. Low Endogenous Secretory Receptor for Advanced Glycation End-Products Levels Are Associated with Inflammation and Carotid Atherosclerosis in Prediabetes. *J. Clin. Endocrinol. Metab.* **2016**, *101*, 1701–1709. [CrossRef]
8. Gerber, P.A.; Thalhammer, C.; Schmied, C.; Spring, S.; Amann-Vesti, B.; Spinas, G.A.; Berneis, K. Small, Dense LDL Particles Predict Changes in Intima Media Thickness and Insulin Resistance in Men with Type 2 Diabetes and Prediabetes—A Prospective Cohort Study. *PLoS ONE* **2013**, *8*, e72363. [CrossRef]
9. Zagami, R.M.; Di Pino, A.; Urbano, F.; Piro, S.; Purrello, F.; Rabuazzo, A.M. Low Circulating Vitamin D Levels Are Associated with Increased Arterial Stiffness in Prediabetic Subjects Identified According to HbA1c. *Atherosclerosis* **2015**, *243*, 395–401. [CrossRef]
10. Mononen, N.; Lyytikäinen, L.P.; Seppälä, I.; Mishra, P.P.; Juonala, M.; Waldenberger, M.; Klopp, N.; Illig, T.; Leiviskä, J.; Loo, B.M.; et al. Whole Blood MicroRNA Levels Associate with Glycemic Status and Correlate with Target MRNAs in Pathways Important to Type 2 Diabetes. *Sci. Rep.* **2019**, *9*, 1–12. [CrossRef]
11. Davì, G.; Patrono, C. Platelet Activation and Atherothrombosis. *N. Engl. J. Med.* **2007**, *357*, 2482–2494. [CrossRef] [PubMed]
12. Samad, F.; Ruf, W. Inflammation, Obesity, and Thrombosis. *Blood* **2013**, *122*, 3415–3422. [CrossRef] [PubMed]
13. Puccini, M.; Rauch, C.; Jakobs, K.; Friebel, J.; Hassanein, A.; Landmesser, U.; Rauch, U. Being Overweight or Obese Is Associated with an Increased Platelet Reactivity Despite Dual Antiplatelet Therapy with Aspirin and Clopidogrel. *Cardiovasc. Drugs Ther.* **2022**, 1–5. [CrossRef] [PubMed]

14. Varol, E.; Akcay, S.; Ozaydin, M.; Erdogan, D.; Dogan, A.; Altinbas, A. Mean Platelet Volume Is Associated with Insulin Resistance in Non-Obese, Non-Diabetic Patients with Coronary Artery Disease. *J. Cardiol.* **2010**, *56*, 154–158. [CrossRef]
15. Gremmel, T.; Frelinger, A.L.; Michelson, A.D. Platelet Physiology. *Semin. Thromb. Hemost.* **2016**, *42*, 191–204. [CrossRef]
16. Martin, J.F.; Kristensen, S.D.; Mathur, A.; Grove, E.L.; Choudry, F.A. The Causal Role of Megakaryocyte-Platelet Hyperactivity in Acute Coronary Syndromes. *Nat. Rev. Cardiol.* **2012**, *9*, 658–670. [CrossRef]
17. Ciabattoni, G.; Pugliese, F.; Davì, G.; Pierucci, A.; Simonetti, B.M.; Patrono, C. Fractional Conversion of Thromboxane B2 to Urinary 11-Dehydrothromboxane B2 in Man. *Biochim. Biophys. Acta* **1989**, *992*, 66–70. [CrossRef]
18. Zaccardi, F.; Rizzi, A.; Petrucci, G.; Ciaffardini, F.; Tanese, L.; Pagliaccia, F.; Cavalca, V.; Ciminello, A.; Habib, A.; Squellerio, I.; et al. In Vivo Platelet Activation and Aspirin Responsiveness in Type 1 Diabetes. *Diabetes* **2016**, *65*, 503–509. [CrossRef]
19. Patrono, C.; Fitzgerald, G.A. Isoprostanes: Potential Markers of Oxidant Stress in Atherothrombotic Disease. *Arterioscler. Thromb. Vasc. Biol.* **1997**, *17*, 2309–2315. [CrossRef]
20. Krenn-Pilko, S.; Langsenlehner, U.; Thurner, E.M.; Stojakovic, T.; Pichler, M.; Gerger, A.; Kapp, K.S.; Langsenlehner, T. The Elevated Preoperative Platelet-to-Lymphocyte Ratio Predicts Poor Prognosis in Breast Cancer Patients. *Br. J. Cancer* **2014**, *110*, 2524–2530. [CrossRef]
21. Miyazaki, T.; Yamasaki, N.; Tsuchiya, T.; Matsumoto, K.; Kunizaki, M.; Taniguchi, D.; Nagayasu, T. Inflammation-Based Scoring Is a Useful Prognostic Predictor of Pulmonary Resection for Elderly Patients with Clinical Stage I Non-Small-Cell Lung Cancer. *Eur. J. Cardio-Thorac. Surg.* **2015**, *47*, e140–e145. [CrossRef] [PubMed]
22. Kurtul, A.; Ornek, E. Platelet to Lymphocyte Ratio in Cardiovascular Diseases: A Systematic Review. *Angiology* **2019**, *70*, 802–818. [CrossRef] [PubMed]
23. Huilcaman, R.; Venturini, W.; Fuenzalida, L.; Cayo, A.; Segovia, R.; Valenzuela, C.; Brown, N.; Moore-Carrasco, R. Platelets, a Key Cell in Inflammation and Atherosclerosis Progression. *Cells* **2022**, *11*, 1014. [CrossRef] [PubMed]
24. Marchio, P.; Guerra-Ojeda, S.; Vila, J.M.; Aldasoro, M.; Victor, V.M.; Mauricio, M.D. Targeting Early Atherosclerosis: A Focus on Oxidative Stress and Inflammation. *Oxidative Med. Cell. Longev.* **2019**, *2019*, 8563845. [CrossRef] [PubMed]
25. Calanna, S.; Urbano, F.; Piro, S.; Zagami, R.M.; Di Pino, A.; Spadaro, L.; Purrello, F.; Rabuazzo, A.M. Elevated Plasma Glucose-Dependent Insulinotropic Polypeptide Associates with Hyperinsulinemia in Metabolic Syndrome. *Eur. J. Endocrinol.* **2012**, *166*, 917–922. [CrossRef]
26. Di Pino, A.; Currenti, W.; Urbano, F.; Mantegna, C.; Purrazzo, G.; Piro, S.; Purrello, F.; Rabuazzo, A.M. Low Advanced Glycation End Product Diet Improves the Lipid and Inflammatory Profiles of Prediabetic Subjects. *J. Clin. Lipidol.* **2016**, *10*, 1098–1108. [CrossRef]
27. Mosca, A.; Goodall, I.; Hoshino, T.; Jeppsson, J.O.; John, W.G.; Little, R.R.; Miedema, K.; Myers, G.L.; Reinauer, H.; Sacks, D.B.; et al. Global Standardization of Glycated Hemoglobin Measurement: The Position of the IFCC Working Group. *Clin. Chem. Lab. Med.* **2007**, *45*, 1077–1080. [CrossRef]
28. Di Pino, A.; Scicali, R.; Marchisello, S.; Zanoli, L.; Ferrara, V.; Urbano, F.; Filippello, A.; di Mauro, S.; Scamporrino, A.; Piro, S.; et al. High Glomerular Filtration Rate Is Associated with Impaired Arterial Stiffness and Subendocardial Viability Ratio in Prediabetic Subjects. *Nutr. Metab. Cardiovasc. Dis.* **2021**, *31*, 3393–3400. [CrossRef]
29. Di Pino, A.; Alagona, C.; Piro, S.; Calanna, S.; Spadaro, L.; Palermo, F.; Urbano, F.; Purrello, F.; Rabuazzo, A.M. Separate Impact of Metabolic Syndrome and Altered Glucose Tolerance on Early Markers of Vascular Injuries. *Atherosclerosis* **2012**, *223*, 458–462. [CrossRef]
30. Pan, Y.; Jackson, R.T. Ethnic Difference in the Relationship between Acute Inflammation and Serum Ferritin in US Adult Males. *Epidemiol. Infect.* **2008**, *136*, 421–431. [CrossRef]
31. Jia, W.; Jia, Q.; Zhang, Y.; Zhao, X.; Wang, Y. Effect of Prediabetes on Asprin or Clopidogrel Resistance in Patients with Recent Ischemic Stroke/TIA. *Neurol. Sci.* **2021**, *42*, 2829–2835. [CrossRef] [PubMed]
32. Santilli, F.; Zaccardi, F.; Liani, R.; Petrucci, G.; Simeone, P.; Pitocco, D.; Tripaldi, R.; Rizzi, A.; Formoso, G.; Pontecorvi, A.; et al. In Vivo Thromboxane-Dependent Platelet Activation Is Persistently Enhanced in Subjects with Impaired Glucose Tolerance. *Diabetes Metab. Res. Rev.* **2020**, *36*, e3232. [CrossRef] [PubMed]
33. Al-Sofiani, M.E.; Yanek, L.R.; Faraday, N.; Kral, B.G.; Mathias, R.; Becker, L.C.; Becker, D.M.; Vaidya, D.; Kalyani, R.R. Diabetes and Platelet Response to Low-Dose Aspirin. *J. Clin. Endocrinol. Metab.* **2018**, *103*, 4599–4608. [CrossRef]
34. Lopez, L.R.; Guyer, K.E.; La Torre, I.G.D.; Pitts, K.R.; Matsuura, E.; Ames, P.R. Platelet Thromboxane (11-Dehydro-Thromboxane B2) and Aspirin Response in Patients with Diabetes and Coronary Artery Disease. *World J. Diabetes* **2014**, *5*, 115–127. [CrossRef] [PubMed]
35. Davì, G.; Guagnano, M.T.; Ciabattoni, G.; Basili, S.; Falco, A.; Marinopiccoli, M.; Nutini, M.; Sensi, S.; Patrono, C. Platelet Activation in Obese Women Role of Inflammation and Oxidant Stress. *JAMA* **2002**, *288*, 2008–2014. [CrossRef] [PubMed]
36. Santilli, F.; Vazzana, N.; Liani, R.; Guagnano, M.T.; Davì, G. Platelet Activation in Obesity and Metabolic Syndrome. *Obes. Rev.* **2012**, *13*, 27–42. [CrossRef]
37. Basili, S.; Pacini, G.; Guagnano, M.T.; Manigrasso, M.R.; Santilli, F.; Pettinella, C.; Ciabattoni, G.; Patrono, C.; Davì, G. Insulin Resistance as a Determinant of Platelet Activation in Obese Women. *J. Am. Coll. Cardiol.* **2006**, *48*, 2531–2538. [CrossRef]
38. Simeone, P.; Boccatonda, A.; Liani, R.; Santilli, F. Significance of Urinary 11-Dehydro-Thromboxane B2 in Age-Related Diseases: Focus on Atherothrombosis. *Ageing Res. Rev.* **2018**, *48*, 51–78. [CrossRef]

29. Dolegowska, B.; Blogowski, W.; Kedzierska, K.; Safranow, K.; Jakubowska, K.; Olszewska, M.; Rac, M.; Chlubek, D.; Ciechanowski, K. Platelets Arachidonic Acid Metabolism in Patients with Essential Hypertension. *Platelets* **2009**, *20*, 242–249. [CrossRef]
30. Wang, N.; Vendrov, K.C.; Simmons, B.P.; Schuck, R.N.; Stouffer, G.A.; Lee, C.R. Urinary 11-Dehydro-Thromboxane B2 Levels Are Associated with Vascular Inflammation and Prognosis in Atherosclerotic Cardiovascular Disease. *Prostaglandins Lipid Mediat.* **2018**, *134*, 24–31. [CrossRef]
31. Inoue, H.; Saito, M.; Kouchi, K.; Asahara, S.; Nakamura, F.; Kido, Y. Association between Mean Platelet Volume in the Pathogenesis of Type 2 Diabetes Mellitus and Diabetic Macrovascular Complications in Japanese Patients. *J. Diabetes Investig.* **2020**, *11*, 938–945. [CrossRef] [PubMed]
32. Lippi, G.; Salvagno, G.L.; Nouvenne, A.; Meschi, T.; Borghi, L.; Targher, G. The Mean Platelet Volume Is Significantly Associated with Higher Glycated Hemoglobin in a Large Population of Unselected Outpatients. *Prim. Care Diabetes* **2015**, *9*, 226–230. [CrossRef] [PubMed]
33. Oshima, S.; Higuchi, T.; Okada, S.; Takahashi, O. The Relationship between Mean Platelet Volume and Fasting Plasma Glucose and HbA1c Levels in a Large Cohort of Unselected Health Check-Up Participants. *J. Clin. Med. Res.* **2018**, *10*, 345–350. [CrossRef] [PubMed]
34. Di Pino, A.; Scicali, R.; Calanna, S.; Urbano, F.; Mantegna, C.; Rabuazzo, A.M.; Purrello, F.; Piro, S. Cardiovascular Risk Profile in Subjects with Prediabetes and New-Onset Type 2 Diabetes Identified by HbA1c According to American Diabetes Association Criteria. *Diabetes Care* **2014**, *37*, 1447–1453. [CrossRef] [PubMed]
35. Yadav, R.; Jain, N.; Raizada, N.; Jhamb, R.; Rohatgi, J.; Madhu, S.V. Prevalence of Diabetes Related Vascular Complications in Subjects with Normal Glucose Tolerance, Prediabetes, Newly Detected Diabetes and Known Diabetes. *Diabetes Metab. Syndr. Clin. Res. Rev.* **2021**, *15*, 102226. [CrossRef] [PubMed]
36. Al Akl, N.S.; Khalifa, O.; Errafii, K.; Arredouani, A. Association of Dyslipidemia, Diabetes and Metabolic Syndrome with Serum Ferritin Levels: A Middle Eastern Population-Based Cross-Sectional Study. *Sci. Rep.* **2021**, *11*, 1–9. [CrossRef]
37. Ghule, A.; Kamble, T.K.; Talwar, D.; Kumar, S.; Acharya, S.; Wanjari, A.; Gaidhane, S.A.; Agrawal, S. Association of Serum High Sensitivity C-Reactive Protein with Pre-Diabetes in Rural Population: A Two-Year Cross-Sectional Study. *Cureus* **2021**, *13*, e19088. [CrossRef]
38. Zanoli, L.; di Pino, A.; Terranova, V.; Di Marca, S.; Pisano, M.; di Quattro, R.; Ferrara, V.; Scicali, R.; Rabuazzo, A.M.; Fatuzzo, P.; et al. Inflammation and Ventricular-Vascular Coupling in Hypertensive Patients with Metabolic Syndrome. *Nutr. Metab. Cardiovasc. Dis.* **2018**, *28*, 1222–1229. [CrossRef]
39. Sumin, A.N.; Bezdenezhnykh, N.A.; Bezdenezhnykh, A.V.; Artamonova, G.V. Cardio-Ankle Vascular Index in the Persons with Pre-Diabetes and Diabetes Mellitus in the Population Sample of the Russian Federation. *Diagnostics* **2021**, *11*, 474. [CrossRef]
40. Gomez-Sanchez, L.; Garcia-Ortiz, L.; PatinoAlonso, M.C.; Recio-Rodriguez, J.I.; Feuerbach, N.; Marti, R.; Agudo-Conde, C.; Rodriguez-Sanchez, E.; Maderuelo-Fernandez, J.A.; Ramos, R.; et al. Glycemic markers and relation with arterial stiffness in Caucasian subjects of the MARK study. *PLoS ONE* **2017**, *12*, e0175982. [CrossRef]

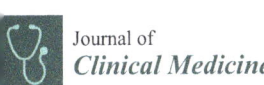

Review

The Importance of Arterial Stiffness Assessment in Patients with Familial Hypercholesterolemia

Beáta Kovács [1], Orsolya Cseprekál [2], Ágnes Diószegi [1], Szabolcs Lengyel [1], László Maroda [3], György Paragh [1], Mariann Harangi [1,*] and Dénes Páll [1,3]

[1] Division of Metabolism, Institute of Internal Medicine, Faculty of Medicine, University of Debrecen, 4032 Debrecen, Hungary; kovibea01@gmail.com (B.K.); dioszegi.agnes@med.unideb.hu (Á.D.); szabolcs.lengyel@med.unideb.hu (S.L.); paragh@belklinika.com (G.P.); pall.denes@med.unideb.hu (D.P.)
[2] Department of Surgery, Transplantation and Gastroenterology, Semmelweis University, 1085 Budapest, Hungary; cseprekal.orsolya@med.semmelweis-univ.hu
[3] Department of Medical Clinical Pharmacology, Faculty of Medicine, University of Debrecen, 4032 Debrecen, Hungary; maroda.laszlo@unideb.hu
* Correspondence: harangi@belklinika.com; Tel.: +36-52-255-525

Abstract: Cardiovascular diseases are still the leading cause of mortality due to increased atherosclerosis worldwide. In the background of accelerated atherosclerosis, the most important risk factors include hypertension, age, male gender, hereditary predisposition, diabetes, obesity, smoking and lipid metabolism disorder. Arterial stiffness is a firmly established, independent predictor of cardiovascular risk. Patients with familial hypercholesterolemia are at very high cardiovascular risk. Non-invasive measurement of arterial stiffness is suitable for screening vascular dysfunction at subclinical stage in this severe inherited disorder. Some former studies found stiffer arteries in patients with familial hypercholesterolemia compared to healthy controls, while statin treatment has a beneficial effect on it. If conventional drug therapy fails in patients with severe familial hypercholesterolemia, PCSK9 inhibitor therapy should be administered; if these agents are not available, performing selective LDL apheresis could be considered. The impact of recent therapeutic approaches on vascular stiffness is not widely studied yet, even though the degree of accelerated athero and arteriosclerosis correlates with cardiovascular risk. The authors provide an overview of the diagnosis of familial hypercholesterolemia and the findings of studies on arterial dysfunction in patients with familial hypercholesterolemia, in addition to presenting the latest therapeutic options and their effects on arterial elasticity parameters.

Keywords: familial hypercholesterolemia; selective LDL apheresis; PCSK9 inhibitor monoclonal antibody; arterial stiffness

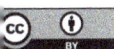

1. Introduction

Cardiovascular diseases are still the leading cause of mortality worldwide, which is primarily due to increased atherosclerosis. In the background, the most important risk factors include hypertension, age, male gender, hereditary predisposition, diabetes, obesity, smoking and lipid metabolism disorders [1]. The proportion of people with high cholesterol levels is the highest in Europe in a worldwide comparison: it affects one in every two people [2,3]. Lipid metabolism is a complex process, with several known diseases that can significantly influence the lipid parameters of the serum, including cholesterol levels (secondary hypercholesterolemia). In two thirds of the cases, genetic factors are responsible for a pathological functioning of lipid metabolism (primary hypercholesterolemia). Polygenic forms are the most common, stemming from a cumulative effect of minor genetic deviances and gene variants, but more rarely, severe lipid metabolism disorders can be attributed to the mutations of individual genes [4].

2. Genotype and Phenotype of Familial Hypercholesterolemia

Diagnosing primary hypercholesterolemia is based on hereditary features as well as the lack of secondary factors. The group of patients suffering from familial hypercholesterolemia (FH) is prominent due to the prevalence of the disease and the severity of related cardiovascular complications. The disease, which was formerly described as a result of an inactivating mutation of the low-density lipoprotein (LDL) receptor (LDLR), is today accounted for as familial hypercholesterolemia syndrome, including both the classic form of the disease as well as a form caused by the loss-of-function mutation of apolipoprotein B100 (ApoB100), formerly termed familial defective apoB syndrome, in addition to other severe types of hypercholesterolemia similarly exhibiting autosomal dominant inheritance, some of which have been found to be related to gain-of-function mutations of the proprotein convertase subtilisin/kexin type 9 (PCSK9) gene [5]. In 2014, STAP1 (signal transducing adaptor family member 1) was reported as a novel FH candidate gene [6]. However, functional validation studies have not been reported, and possible mechanisms by which STAP1 could influence plasma lipid levels have not been explored. Indeed, no marked changes have been demonstrated in plasma lipid profiles of carriers of STAP1 variants compare to controls as well as in a mouse model [7]. Moreover, global loss of Stap1 in mice did not result in an abnormal lipid phenotype [8]. Accordingly, following these negative findings the combined studies exclude STAP1 as an FH gene [9]. The rather rare autosomal recessive form is caused by the mutation of LDL receptor adaptor protein 1 (LDLRAP1) [10] (Table 1).

Table 1. Genetic deviations in the background of FH syndrome [4].

Inheritance	Chromosome	Gene	Name	Prevalence
	19p13	LDLR	Familial hypercholesterolemia (FH)	60–80%
Autosomal dominant	2p24–p23	ApoB100	Familial defective ApoB syndrome (FDB)/(FH2)	1–5%
	1p32	PCSK9	PCSK9 gain-of-function (FH3)	0–3%
		several genes	Polygenic forms	20–40%
Autosomal recessive	1p35	LDLRAP1	Autosomal recessive hypercholesterolemia	rare

ApoB100: apolipoprotein B100; FH: familial hypercholesterolemia; FDB: familiar defective ApoB; LDLR: low-density lipoprotein receptor; LDLRAP1: LDLR adaptor protein 1; PCSK9: proprotein convertase subtilisin/kexin type 9.

It must be noted that in clinically diagnosed FH patients without mutations in the classical genes, elevated LDL-C levels might have a polygenic cause. Such patients often carry a cluster of common polymorphisms affecting several loci associated with markedly raised LDL-C levels, comparable to those observed in patients carrying FH-causative mutations. Even in patients with monogenic FH, a polygenic contribution may subsist, contributing to the variable phenotypic expression [11]. Both monogenic FH and polygenic hypercholesterolemia are found to be associated with greater risk of cardiovascular disease (CVD) than hypercholesterolemia without a known genetic cause, with monogenic FH associated with the greatest risk [12].

2.1. Heterozygous FH

Genetically, the less severe heterozygous form of FH is more common than it has been previously believed. Its prevalence in the European population is currently estimated at approximately 1:300, but it may reach 1:200 [13]. According to the findings of a Hungarian research project conducted a few years ago on a large patient population, the prevalence of FH in Hungary, similarly to several European countries, is around 1:340 [14]. The study found that in addition to a substantial rise in total cholesterol and LDL-cholesterol (LDL-C) levels, the level of triglyceride did not increase in general, and the level of high-density lipoprotein-cholesterol (HDL-C) approximated the upper normal domain. Lipid abnormalities are acquired already in childhood, so screening the entire population for cholesterol levels no later than at age 8–11 has been proposed [13–15].

The LDL-C level is also significantly high in heterozygous cases between 4.9 and 11.6 mmol/L. As a result of the early and extremely high total cholesterol, atherosclerosis is already pronounced in childhood, and without treatment it may well lead to coronary artery disease before the patient is 35, but other vascular diseases—cerebrovascular disease or lower extremity arterial disease—have a greater risk. There is also a risk of developing tendonous xanthomata above extensor tendons, xanthelasmata on the eyelids, and corneal arcus on the iris. These are conspicuous deviations, which may help in diagnosing the disease.

Diagnosing FH is assisted by the Dutch Lipid Clinic Network criteria, which rests on three pillars: clinical symptoms, deviations in laboratory findings, and—in the case of ambiguous laboratory and clinical symptoms—a genetic test [16] (Table 2). Treatment relies on the efficient administering of statins in high doses, which in most cases is complemented by ezetimibe. As the patients are at high or extremely high cardiovascular risk, in order to reach lipid targets, it may become necessary to introduce PCSK9-inhibitor monoclonal antibodies, too [17]. Inclisiran, a small interfering RNA (siRNA) therapy, is another non-statin medication available for cholesterol management [18]. Cardiovascular screening for patients and their family members is obligatory in the case of FH [19].

Table 2. Dutch Lipid Clinic Network diagnostic criteria [16].

Family History	Earl-Onset CAD or PAD First-Degree Relative	1 point
	Presence of Xanthomata or Corneal Arcus in First-Degree Relative	2 points
Clinical history	CAD in women under 60, in men under 55	2 points
	stroke or PAD in women under 60, in men under 55	1 point
Physical examination	presence of tendonous xanthomata at any age	6 points
	presence of corneal arcus under 45	4 points
Laboratory tests	LDL > 8.5 mmol/L	8 points
	LDL 6.5–8.4 mmol/L	5 points
	LDL 5.0–6.4 mmol/L	3 points
	LDL 4.0–4.9 mmol/L	1 point
	note: HDL and TG levels norm.	
DNA analysis	detectable mutation in the LDL receptor gene	8 points
The diagnosis is verified if score is higher than 8 points		
The diagnosis is probable: 6–8 points		
The diagnosis is possible: 3–5 points		

CAD: coronary artery disease; HDL: high-density lipoprotein; LDL: low-density lipoprotein; PAD: peripheral artery disease; TG: triglyceride.

2.2. Homozygous FH

The homozygous form of FH is a rare but rather severe disease, characterized by extreme increased LDL-C (above 12.9 mmol/L) from birth. Progressive atherosclerosis causes myocardial infarction and vascular complications in other parts of the body even in childhood, but cases of aortic valve stenosis as well as subvalvular aortic stenosis have also been recorded. Prevalence is 1:1,000,000, but due to premature mortality it is supposedly higher [20].

To examine the interconnections between the genotype and the phenotype, we need to pose the question whether the severe clinical phenotype is unequivocally tied to the homozygous mutation of a single gene. True homozygous cases, in which the same pathogenic mutation occurs in identical candidate genes in both DNA strands, result in a severe clinical disease, but similarly severe clinical diseases can be caused by compound and double heterozygous forms, too, in which a pathogenic mutation develops in different sections of the given gene, or in two different candidate genes. Therefore, when a homozygous form is suspected, it is reasonable to perform a genetic test.

3. Treatments of Familial Hypercholesterolemia

3.1. Pharmacological Treatment

The basis of the treatment is administering high-dose, intensive statin, then, if that should prove insufficient, it is combined with ezetimibe. If the LDL-C target is not accomplished, PCSK9-inhibitor treatment should be provided as a third stage [19]. In the case of homozygous as well as severe homozygous FH, the impact of statin, ezetimibe and PCSK9-inhibitors is for the most part inefficient. In the case of homozygous FH, the administering of lomitapid, a microsomal transfer protein inhibitor [21], or mipomersen, an ApoB100 synthesis inhibitor antisense oligonucleotide [22] is recommended.

In addition to these, in the case of severe heterozygous and homozygous cases, it may become necessary to provide selective LDL apheresis treatment.

3.2. Selective LDL Apheresis Treatment

LDL apheresis treatment involves the removal of atherogenic lipid fractions by a selective extracorporeal procedure. During apheresis, the particles containing ApoB100 are removed selectively, which can acutely reduce total and LDL-C levels by a further 50–75% beyond pharmacological treatment. In addition to that, it reduces the level of lipoprotein (a) (Lp(a)) [23], known as an individual cardiovascular risk factor also in FH patients [24,25], as well as very low-density lipoprotein levels (VLDL), also containing ApoB, by 70% [26]. During apheresis, the level of protein-like components causing cardiovascular diseases is decreased in the serum; thus, the treatment has an evidently beneficial anti-atherosclerotic impact [27]. The serum levels of inflammatory cytokines and oxidative stress are reduced [28]. Vasodilation increases, and beneficial hemorheological changes are affected [29,30].

In accordance with international recommendations (by the Food and Drug Administration), in Europe it is recommended to perform LDL apheresis in the following patient groups: *functional FH homozygote, LDL-C > 13 mmol/L, functional FH heterozygote, LDL-C > 7.8 mmol/L, functional FH heterozygote with documented ischemic heart disease and LDL-C > 5.2 mmol/L*. Alongside the recommended diet and lipid lowering pharmacological treatment at the maximum tolerated dose, LDL-C levels must exceed the specified target throughout the course of 6 months. Alternative indication is provided by findings that show *below 40% LDL-C decrease in heterozygous FH patients* alongside lipid lowering pharmacological treatment at the maximum tolerated dose. Further indication is provided by an over 60 mg/dL Lp(a) level at documented ischemic heart disease, with over 4 mmol/L LDL-C level despite the administered pharmacological treatment. The above treatments have yielded favorable results, but due to limited funding the number of patients systematically treated in Europe is unfortunately still low [31].

4. Significance of Cardiovascular Risk Assessment

Cardiovascular morbidity and mortality are significantly enhanced in patients with different types of FH; therefore; they all would require individual cardiovascular risk assessment at the earliest possible stage of the disease course [32]. Not all FH patients are at the same cardiovascular risk [33]. The main predictors of morbidity and mortality in this patient population are known to be the age HDL-s, gender, hypertension, and smoking, which all together make up the Montreal FH risk prediction score [34]. Those individual biomarkers do not provide direct information about the hard outcomes and moreover, their cumulative effect could only be declared only if hard endpoints have already occurred. Biomarkers and comorbidities result in an intermediate state of decreased arterial elasticity as a surrogate endpoint of cardiovascular hard outcome in this patient population [35]. Signs of accelerated athero- and arteriosclerosis may occur in early childhood in special types of FH, which refer to the hazard of later functional and structural arterial damage. AHA for instance classified homozygous FH as a Tier I risk group from early childhood [36].

Early risk assessment and patient education are crucial factors to prevent later fatal outcomes. Arterial stiffness measurement contributes to understanding cardiovascular morbidity and mortality risk beyond traditional risk factors or blood pressure measurement [37]. There are several methods to assess arterial stiffness. Due to the fact that there are plenty of measurement tools to assess central and peripheral vascular elasticity, none of them has been approved as a standard method to routinely measure stiffness as a surrogate marker [38]. Nonetheless, ESH suggests the non-invasive measurement of central PWV as the gold standard method to assess preclinical organ damage in patients at high cardiovascular risk [39]. Some studies proved that beyond traditional risk assessment tools, and it may offer additional value and refinement of strategies applied thus far.

Measuring arterial stiffness as a surrogate marker is of paramount importance and will further help lengthen the survival of FH patients.

5. Arterial Stiffness

Suitable non-invasive methods in early stages of atherosclerosis and related artery wall disorders include measuring arterial stiffness. Increased arterial wall stiffness is a result of complex structural changes in the tunica media of the great arteries and of their increased and progressive calcification. Severe arterial stiffness precedes the development of atherosclerosis, which then causes the symptoms. Functional parameters that are independent predictors of cardiovascular diseases include applied pulse wave velocity (PWV) and augmentation index (Aix), which are suitable for both screening and monitoring the efficiency of the treatment [40]. In the past years, the 24-h monitoring of stiffness has become increasingly widespread. Internationally these measurements are most often performed by devices using the oscillometric method, such as Vasotens® (BPLab GmBH Schwalbach am Taunus, Hessen, Germany) and Mobil-O-Graph® (IEM, Stolberg, Germany). Arterial stiffness parameters—pulse wave velocity, augmentation index, central blood pressure—are recorded throughout 24 h with the help of an upper arm blood pressure monitor. The development of early-onset artery wall dysfunction with increased cardiovascular risk was first diagnosed in diseases with chronic inflammation and lipid metabolism disorder. Artery wall dysfunction and related chronic inflammation involve a change in the marker levels of several inflammatory proteins and other serum markers [41].

6. Relationship between Cholesterol and Arterial Stiffness

The link between serum cholesterol level and arterial stiffness may be explained by several potential mechanisms [42]. The more obvious and probably the most important is the development of atherosclerosis, which has been consistently associated with increased arterial stiffness in subjects with and without severe hypercholesterolemia. However, cholesterol and especially oxidatively modified LDL (oxLDL) have further, non-atheromatous effects on the arterial wall, leading to arterial stiffening. OxLDL promotes peroxynitrite formation and increased oxidative stress, which may lead to the direct damage of elastin, the main elastic element of the arterial wall [43]. Furthermore, oxLDL has pro-inflammatory effects characterized by increased serum levels of C-reactive protein (CRP), which was associated with arterial stiffness in apparently healthy individuals [44].

Inflammatory cytokines enhance the expression of some inducible enzymes, such as matrix metalloproteinase-9 (MMP-9), that may damage the structural components of the arterial wall. MMP-9 is a gelatinase secreted by immigrating inflammatory cells of the vascular wall, capable of digesting elastin leading to the remodeling of the arterial wall [45]. Local inflammation and inflammatory lipids may also promote calcium deposition in the medial elastic fibers, resulting in arterial calcification [46]. In addition to structural changes, hypercholesterolemia induces functional dysregulation of the vascular endothelium found to be associated with arterial stiffness. High serum levels of cholesterol are significantly associated with reduced bioavailability of nitric oxide, impaired L-arginine/nitric oxide pathway and increased asymmetric dimethyl arginine production, leading to impaired endothelial vasodilatation [47]. On the other hand, vascular dysfunction may also be caused by the overproduction of vasoconstrictor agents, including endothelin-1 [48].

The relationship between serum lipid levels and arterial stiffness have been examined in several former studies. Most of them demonstrated a significant positive relationship between large artery stiffness and total or LDL-cholesterol [49–52]. It must be noted that many of these studies included a relatively low number of patients with other cardiovascular risk factors. Therefore, careful interpretation of the data is essential. FH represents an extreme form of total and LDL cholesterol elevation; therefore, it may serve as an excellent model to prove the link between LDL cholesterol and arterial stiffness.

7. Assessing Arterial Stiffness in Familial Hypercholesterolemia

Patients with familial hypercholesterolemia have an extremely high risk of atherosclerosis and early-onset vascular ageing, which can be measured by the increase of arterial stiffness. This is due to high cholesterol levels, including the presence of high serum LDL-C values as well as high Lp(a), more prevalent than in the general population, and higher levels of oxidized LDL and chronic artery wall inflammation due to increased oxidative stress [53]. In the case of FH, a low-fat diet and a conventional lipid lowering treatment have limited efficiency and due to the already existing arterial complication, often it is not possible to do physical exercise to the desired effect. All of these may be exacerbated by conventional cardiovascular risk factors, such as age, excess weight, diabetes, hypertension, and smoking. These may be accompanied by other unfavorable genetic factors as well [54] (Figure 1).

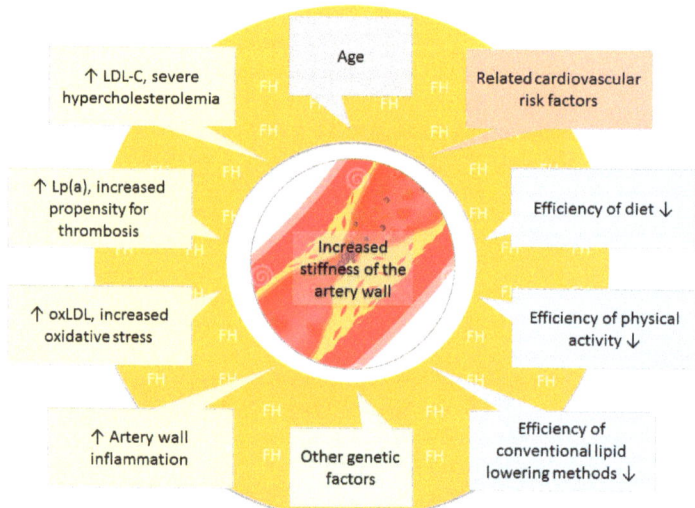

Figure 1. Factors leading to increased vascular stiffness in familial hypercholesterolemia. LDL-C: low density lipoprotein-cholesterol, Lp(a): lipoprotein (a); oxLDL: oxidized low-density lipoprotein.

As a result of accelerated atherosclerosis, sooner or later all patients develop coronary stenosis; however, its extent and the severity of the resulting clinical symptoms have a broader spectrum. Even though the injurious effects of arterial stiffness on the population of non-FH patients have been registered by several studies, the available data on the clinical impact of arterial stiffness on FH patients is insufficient.

In a small cross-sectional comparative study, brachial-ankle pulse wave velocity (baPWV) was measured in 35 heterozygous FH subjects and 17 healthy control subjects. Although baPWV disi not differ significantly between FH patients and controls (12.5 ± 2.9 vs. 11.9 ± 2.3 m/s), among FH patients, the baPWV and carotid IMT were higher in cases with high cholesterol burden than those without. Similarly, the baPWV and carotid IMT were also higher in cases with elevated hs-CRP than those without [55].

In a former case control study of 22 patients with FH and matched healthy controls, PWV values were compared before and after lipoprotein apheresis (LA) treatment. Baseline PWV was similar between the two groups (controls 8.2 ± 0.9 m/s vs. FH 7.7 ± 0.8 m/s, $p = 0.12$). Moreover, baseline PWV did not change following LA (pre 8.8 ± 1.2 m/s vs. post 9.2 ± 1.2 m/s, $p = 0.19$) [56].

Another study involved 60 patients without documented cardiovascular events and clinical symptoms of cardiovascular diseases: 21 patients with elevated plasma LDL-C levels and genetically confirmed FH, 19 patients with elevated LDL-C levels and without FH mutations and 20 healthy controls. In each patient, echo-tracking and photoplethysmography were used to assess the parameters of arterial stiffness. They found that arterial stiffness parameters were similar between the groups [57].

A study conducted on the population of 125 FH patients as per the guidelines displayed significantly higher Aix values in comparison to those of a control group of identical age and gender (9.6 ± 17.2 vs. $2.6 \pm 10.3\%$; $p = 0.011$), based on which the measuring of Aix value is recommended in patient tracking [58].

In a study conducted on 66 untreated FH patients and 57 first-degree non-FH relatives, when measuring carotid β-stiffness index and carotid-femoral PWV it was found that while FH patients' β-index (6.3 (4.8–8.2) vs. 5.2 (4.2–6.4); $p = 0.005$) and local PWV values (5.4 (4.5–6.4) vs. 4.7 (4.2–5.4) m/s; $p = 0.005$) were significantly higher than in the case of their non-FH relatives, there was no substantial deviation in carotid-femoral PWV values (6.76 (7.0–7.92) vs. 6.48 (6.16–7.12) m/s; $p = 0.138$). Based on all the above, the measurement of carotid arterial stiffness, especially in the case of younger patients, may indicate the extent of calcification sooner than does arterial stiffness of the aorta [59].

A Japanese group of researchers recorded changes in brachial-tibial pulse wave velocity (baPWV) as well as the development of coronary artery disease in 245 medicated FH individuals. The patients were selected on the basis of clinical criteria for FH specified by the Japan Atherosclerosis Society. According to these, two out of three clinical criteria need to be met for a diagnosis of FH, namely, LDL-C $\geq$ 180 mg/dL, the presence of tendonous xanthoma or xanthoma tuberosum, as well as an FH-positive family history or early-onset CAD diagnosed in second-degree relatives. Cardiovascular risk factors (age, male gender, hypertension, diabetes, smoking) have been assessed as well as deviances in lipid parameters (total cholesterol, triglycerides, HDL) and the presence of CAD. In the latter case, the diagnosis was established on the basis of coronary CT angiography by taking into account only over 50% stenosis of the main coronary arteries. Measurement of brachial-tibial pulse wave velocity was performed with a Colin VP-1000, Omron® device. The goal of the study was to establish a connection between arterial stiffness and the risk of CAD in the given population. The findings proved that in the case of FH arterial stiffness, including baPWV as a biomarker indicating high cardiovascular risk, showed correlation with CAD [60].

Parameters of arterial stiffness as well as aortic root thickness by cardiac MRI have also been tested on heterozygous FH children. Testing 33 children aged 7–18, it was found that in comparison to a non-FH group of identical age, the PWV values of FH children were significantly higher (4.5 ± 0.8 vs. 3.5 ± 0.3 m/s; $p < 0.001$), and the wall thickness of the ascending aorta was higher (1.37 ± 0.18 vs. 1.3 ± 0.02 mm; $p < 0.05$), which suggests the importance of early statin treatment [61].

However, some further studies in children and young patients with FH with low patient numbers could not demonstrated significant differences compared to control subjects [35,62,63].

Indeed, a recent meta-analysis of 8 studies involving 317 patients with FH and 244 non-FH individuals did not suggest a significantly altered PWV in FH patients versus controls, although the authors admit that different scores for FH diagnosis as well as different methods for PWV estimation were used in different studies included and there was a lack of information about the duration and type of lipid-lowering therapy [64].

Taken together, larger studies evaluating PWV in FH patients compared with controls in order to elucidate the impact of FH on arterial stiffness as measured by PWV are definitely needed. A very recent position paper of the Associations of Preventive Paediatrics of Serbia, Mighty Medic and International Lipid Expert Panel focusing on risk assessment and clinical management of children and adolescents with heterozygous FH stated that depending on the availability of noninvasive equipment for PWV measurement and staff experience, it would be clinically meaningful to perform PWV measurements in all children with FH and evaluate their changes over time. PWV values above 97th could be a possible guide for treatment initiation in ambiguous clinical cases (Level B evidence). The paper prefers oscillometric devices; it suggests the usage of Mobile-O-Graph device due to the simplicity of measurement [65].

Whether the parameters for establishing arterial stiffness can be replaced by measuring inflammatory parameters of atherosclerosis is an important question. According to the findings of a study conducted on 89 FH patients and a control group of 31, PWV values were higher in FH patients ($p < 0.05$), but no significant connections to serum inflammatory parameters have been found (C-reactive proteins and white blood count) [66].

8. Effect of Traditional Oral Lipid-Lowering Treatment on Arterial Stiffness

Several human studies have investigated the effect of HMG-CoA reductase inhibitor statins on arterial stiffness. It is well documented that in addition to cholesterol reduction, a number of other pleiotropic effects have been described with statins that may improve atherogenesis independently of cholesterol reduction, including their anti-inflammatory and antioxidant effects, leading to improved endothelial function [67,68]. With the exception of one short-term, cross-over study, which could not find any impact of pravastatin on carotid, brachial and femoral artery stiffness [69], most of these former studies reported significant reduction in stiffness parameters after higher doses of atorvastatin and cerivastatin treatment [70–73]. Even a long-term, but low-dose pravastatin treatment could improve the aortic pulse wave velocity, especially in patients with the greatest lowering of cholesterol [74]. It must be noted that most statins had significant adjuvant effects on peripheral systolic blood pressure [72,75]. On the contrary, 20-week treatment with statins (rosuvastatin or atorvastatin) combined with regular exercise significantly improved exercise capacity and brachial artery PWV, but had no effect on blood pressure [76]. In patients with coronary artery disease compared with simvastatin/ezetimibe, rosuvastatin was found to more effectively improve arterial wall stiffness [77]. Although the beneficial effect of statin on stiffness parameters in various patient populations are well established, to date, their effects on stiffness parameters in FH patients has not been investigated.

Recently, the impact of PCSK9 plasma levels on mechanical vascular impairment was verified [78]. The exact mechanism is not fully clarified, but PCSK9 might promote atherogenesis by stimulating oxidative stress and the production of proinflammatory cytokine production of the atherosclerotic lesions [79]. It must be highlighted that statins, especially the lipophilic agents significantly increase the circulating level of PCSK9. Furthermore, statin-induced PCSK9 increase may limit the absolute magnitude of statin LDL-C lowering effect, by limiting the statin-driven LDLR upregulation [80].

9. Changes in Arterial Stiffness and PCSK9-Inhibitor Monoclonal Antibody Treatment

In the past few years, new product groups have appeared in the range of FH therapeutic medicines. Breakthrough products included the aforementioned ApoB synthesis inhibitors, microsomal transfer protein inhibitors and especially PCSK9-inhibitors. Currently, the efficiency, side effect profiles and effect of PCSK9-inhibitor monoclonal antibodies on the cardiovascular endpoints are very similar. In the RUTHERFORD study, 168 heterozygous FH patients were treated with 350 mg and 420 mg evolocumab every 4 weeks alongside statin treatment. In the case of 350 mg, LDL-C decreased by 43%, in the case of 420 mg by 55%. After 12 weeks, 44% and 65% of the patients, respectively, reached the desired 1.8 mmol/L target value. Triglyceride levels decreased by 15% and 20%, respectively, while HDL-C increased by 7%, and Lp(a) fell by 23% and 32%, respectively, as a result of evolocumab treatment. In the case of administering 140 mg every 2 weeks, LDL-C decreased by 66% [81]. Therefore, the impact on total cholesterol and LDL-C is conclusive; however, the impact on Lp(a) level lags that of LDL apheresis.

Changes in lipid parameters and pulse wave velocity due to complementary treatment using PCSK9-inhibitors or ezetimibe were studied in a 6-week tracking study. The research project involved ninety-eight certified FH patients who had previously undergone other cardiovascular risk assessment. All patients had genetically certified FH. The patients had received high-dose statin (atorvastatin 40–80 mg, rosuvastatin 20–40 mg) and/or ezetimibe treatment at least 6 months prior to the commencement of the study, but still they had not reached the desired LDL-C targets. In the study, 53 patients were administered statin+ezetimibe+PCSK9-inhibitors (alirocumab 75 mg/150 mg or evolocumab 140 mg). Forty-five patients were administered ezetimibe alongside the statin already administered. PWV measurements had been taken prior to the complementary pharmacological treatment and 6 months after the optimized treatment. Measurements were conducted with the SphygmoCor CVMS® device. In the case of patients in the PCSK9 group, a more significant decrease was recorded not only in LDL-C values, but also in pulse wave velocity (-51% vs. -22.8%, $p < 0.001$ and -15% vs. -8.5%, $p < 0.01$) [82].

The effect of six-month add-on PCSK9 inhibitor monoclonal antibodies on circulating PCSK9 and PWV was detected in a cohort of FH subjects. The PCSK9 plasma level was correlated with PWV at baseline. Furthermore, reduction of PCSK9 plasma level seems to be associated with a significant mechanical vascular improvement after PCSK9 inhibitor monoclonal antibody therapy. Therefore, PCSK9 could be a novel cardiovascular biomarker of the mechanical vascular homeostasis through lipid and non-lipid pathways, and it could identify subjects at high CVD risk with a limited LDL-C lowering benefit after high-intensity statin therapy in FH [78].

10. The Impact of LDL Apheresis Treatment on Vascular Parameters

The impact of LDL apheresis treatment on arterial stiffness is the least documented in spite of the fact that in acute cases this extracorporeal procedure yields the most substantial metabolic and hemodynamic changes. Professional literature on the subject is also rather scarce. A German research team examined the impact of lipoprotein apheresis treatment on the parameters of endothelial function (circulating endothelial cells, circulating endothelial progenitor cells, flow-mediated vasodilation, microalbuminuria) as well as left ventricular ejection fraction and changes in homocystein levels. Heterozygous FH patients were examined: 21 patients were administered statin at the maximum tolerated dose, while 8 patients proved to be statin intolerant. Direct adsorption of lipoproteins (DALI) was provided on a weekly basis. Primarily in the case of the statin intolerant patient's immediate improvement was recorded in vascular contractility even after a single treatment. Regular apheresis throughout a course of 6 months clearly had a favorable effect on the metabolic parameters under survey and improved endothelial function, which is one of the key causes of clinical improvement [83].

11. Conclusions

In familial hypercholesterolemia, complex molecular and hemodynamic changes are involved in the development of cardiovascular complications. Even though an increasing amount of clinical data is available, the exact role of serum cholesterol in the changing elasticity of different arterial sections is still not clear. Several combined pharmacological treatments are available for remedying metabolic deviations, but in clinically severe cases, complex pharmacological and non-medicinal treatments, such as selective LDL apheresis, can be used jointly. Similarly, little is known about changes in arterial stiffness induced by new generations of medicines, such as PCSK9-inhibitor monoclonal antibodies, siRNAs and selective LDL apheresis treatments. Atherosclerosis and related artery wall dysfunction can be screened for by non-invasive arterial stiffness measurements. Today oscillometric ABPM devices are available for performing a 24-h measurement of arterial stiffness; these are used primarily in scientific research but not widespread in clinical practice. Since these devices are suitable for measuring biomarkers indicating high cardiovascular risk, such measurements may contribute to screening especially high-risk patients with familial hypercholesterolemia and to improving the efficiency of their treatment.

Author Contributions: B.K. contributed with the processing of data from professional literature, O.C., S.L., L.M. and Á.D. edited the manuscript, M.H. generated the figures and compiled the manuscript and G.P. and D.P. proofread the final version. All authors have read and agreed to the published version of the manuscript.

Funding: The project is co-financed by the European Union under the European Regional Development Fund. The funding number is the GINOP-2.3.2-15-2016-00062.

Conflicts of Interest: The authors declare no conflict of interest.

Abbreviations

ABPM	ambulatory blood pressure monitoring
Aix	augmentation index
ApoB100	apolipoprotein B100
CAD	coronary artery disease
CRP	C-reactive protein
CVD	cardiovascular disease
DALI	direct adsorption of lipoproteins
FH	familial hypercholesterolemia
HDL-C	high-density lipoprotein cholesterol
LDL	low-density lipoprotein
LDL-C	low-density lipoprotein cholesterol
LDLR	LDL receptor
LDLRAP1	LDL receptor adaptor protein 1
Lp (a)	lipoprotein (a)
MMP-9	matrix metalloprotease-9
oxLDL	oxidized LDL
PAD	peripheral artery disease
PCSK9	proprotein convertase subtilisin/kexin type 9
siRNA	small interfering ribonucleic acid
TG	triglycerides
PWV	pulse wave velocity
STAP1	signal transducing adaptor family member 1
VLDL	very low-density lipoprotein

References

1. Goldstein, J.L.; Hazzard, W.R.; Schrott, H.G.; Bierman, E.L.; Motulsky, A.G. Hyperlipidemia in coronary heart disease. I. Lipid levels in 500 survivors of myocardial infarction. *J. Clin. Investig.* **1973**, *52*, 1533–1543. [CrossRef] [PubMed]
2. Ang, T.W.; ten Have, H.; Solbakk, J.H.; Nys, H. UNESCO Global Ethics Observatory: Database on ethics related legislation and guidelines. *J. Med. Ethics* **2008**, *34*, 738–741. [CrossRef] [PubMed]
3. Catapano, A.L.; Wiklund, O.; Society, E.A. Think Again About Cholesterol Survey. *Atheroscler. Suppl.* **2015**, *20*, 1–5. [CrossRef]
4. Paththinige, C.S.; Sirisena, N.D.; Dissanayake, V. Genetic determinants of inherited susceptibility to hypercholesterolemia-a comprehensive literature review. *Lipids Health Dis.* **2017**, *16*, 103. [CrossRef]
5. Di Taranto, M.D.; Giacobbe, C.; Fortunato, G. Familial hypercholesterolemia: A complex genetic disease with variable phenotypes. *Eur. J. Med. Genet.* **2019**, *63*, 103831. [CrossRef] [PubMed]
6. Fouchier, S.W.; Dallinga-Thie, G.M.; Meijers, J.C.; Zelcer, N.; Kastelein, J.J.; Defesche, J.C.; Hovingh, G.K. Mutations in STAP1 are associated with autosomal dominant hypercholesterolemia. *Circ. Res.* **2014**, *115*, 552–555. [CrossRef]
7. Loaiza, N.; Hartgers, M.L.; Reeskamp, L.F.; Balder, J.W.; Rimbert, A.; Bazioti, V.; Wolters, J.C.; Winkelmeijer, M.; Jansen, H.P.G.; Dallinga-Thie, G.M.; et al. Taking One Step Back in Familial Hypercholesterolemia: STAP1 Does Not Alter Plasma LDL (Low-Density Lipoprotein) Cholesterol in Mice and Humans. *Arterioscler. Thromb. Vasc. Biol.* **2020**, *40*, 973–985. [CrossRef]
8. Kanuri, B.; Fong, V.; Haller, A.; Hui, D.Y.; Patel, S.B. Mice lacking global Stap1 expression do not manifest hypercholesterolemia. *BMC Med. Genet.* **2020**, *21*, 234. [CrossRef]
9. Hegele, R.A.; Knowles, J.W.; Horton, J.D. Delisting. *Arterioscler. Thromb. Vasc. Biol.* **2020**, *40*, 847–849. [CrossRef]
10. Tada, H.; Kawashiri, M.A.; Ohtani, R.; Noguchi, T.; Nakanishi, C.; Konno, T.; Hayashi, K.; Nohara, A.; Inazu, A.; Kobayashi, J.; et al. A novel type of familial hypercholesterolemia: Double heterozygous mutations in LDL receptor and LDL receptor adaptor protein 1 gene. *Atherosclerosis* **2011**, *219*, 663–666. [CrossRef]
11. Olmastroni, E.; Gazzotti, M.; Arca, M.; Averna, M.; Pirillo, A.; Catapano, A.L.; Casula, M.; Bertolini, S.; Calandra, S.; Tarugi, P.; et al. Twelve Variants Polygenic Score for Low-Density Lipoprotein Cholesterol Distribution in a Large Cohort of Patients With Clinically Diagnosed Familial Hypercholesterolemia With or Without Causative Mutations. *J. Am. Heart Assoc.* **2022**, *11*, e023668. [CrossRef] [PubMed]
12. Trinder, M.; Francis, G.A.; Brunham, L.R. Association of Monogenic vs Polygenic Hypercholesterolemia With Risk of Atherosclerotic Cardiovascular Disease. *JAMA Cardiol.* **2020**, *5*, 390–399. [CrossRef] [PubMed]
13. Bowman, F.L.; Molster, C.M.; Lister, K.J.; Bauskis, A.T.; Garton-Smith, J.; Vickery, A.W.; Watts, G.F.; Martin, A.C. Identifying Perceptions and Preferences of the General Public Concerning Universal Screening of Children for Familial Hypercholesterolaemia. *Public Health Genom.* **2019**, *22*, 25–35. [CrossRef] [PubMed]
14. Paragh, G.; Harangi, M.; Karányi, Z.; Daróczy, B.; Németh, Á.; Fülöp, P. Identifying patients with familial hypercholesterolemia using data mining methods in the Northern Great Plain region of Hungary. *Atherosclerosis* **2018**, *277*, 262–266. [CrossRef] [PubMed]
15. Wiegman, A. Lipid Screening, Action, and Follow-up in Children and Adolescents. *Curr. Cardiol. Rep.* **2018**, *20*, 80. [CrossRef] [PubMed]
16. Al-Rasadi, K.; Al-Waili, K.; Al-Sabti, H.A.; Al-Hinai, A.; Al-Hashmi, K.; Al-Zakwani, I.; Banerjee, Y. Criteria for Diagnosis of Familial Hypercholesterolemia: A Comprehensive Analysis of the Different Guidelines, Appraising their Suitability in the Omani Arab Population. *Oman Med. J.* **2014**, *29*, 85–91. [CrossRef]
17. Bajnok, L. Newer evidences and recommendations in lipidology. *Orvosi Hetil.* **2018**, *159*, 1303–1309. [CrossRef]
18. Wright, R.S.; Ray, K.K.; Raal, F.J.; Kallend, D.G.; Jaros, M.; Koenig, W.; Leiter, L.A.; Landmesser, U.; Schwartz, G.G.; Friedman, A.; et al. Pooled Patient-Level Analysis of Inclisiran Trials in Patients With Familial Hypercholesterolemia or Atherosclerosis. *J. Am. Coll. Cardiol.* **2021**, *77*, 1182–1193. [CrossRef]
19. Mach, F.; Baigent, C.; Catapano, A.L.; Koskinas, K.C.; Casula, M.; Badimon, L.; Chapman, M.J.; De Backer, G.G.; Delgado, V.; Ference, B.A.; et al. 2019 ESC/EAS Guidelines for the management of dyslipidaemias: Lipid modification to reduce cardiovascular risk. *Eur. Heart J.* **2019**, *294*, 80–82. [CrossRef]
20. Sjouke, B.; Kusters, D.M.; Kindt, I.; Besseling, J.; Defesche, J.C.; Sijbrands, E.J.; Roeters van Lennep, J.E.; Stalenhoef, A.F.; Wiegman, A.; de Graaf, J.; et al. Homozygous autosomal dominant hypercholesterolaemia in the Netherlands: Prevalence, genotype-phenotype relationship, and clinical outcome. *Eur. Heart J.* **2015**, *36*, 560–565. [CrossRef]
21. Cuchel, M.; Meagher, E.A.; du Toit Theron, H.; Blom, D.J.; Marais, A.D.; Hegele, R.A.; Averna, M.R.; Sirtori, C.R.; Shah, P.K.; Gaudet, D.; et al. Efficacy and safety of a microsomal triglyceride transfer protein inhibitor in patients with homozygous familial hypercholesterolaemia: A single-arm, open-label, phase 3 study. *Lancet* **2013**, *381*, 40–46. [CrossRef]
22. Akdim, F.; Stroes, E.S.; Sijbrands, E.J.; Tribble, D.L.; Trip, M.D.; Jukema, J.W.; Flaim, J.D.; Su, J.; Yu, R.; Baker, B.F.; et al. Efficacy and safety of mipomersen, an antisense inhibitor of apolipoprotein B, in hypercholesterolemic subjects receiving stable statin therapy. *J. Am. Coll. Cardiol.* **2010**, *55*, 1611–1618. [CrossRef] [PubMed]
23. Nordestgaard, B.G.; Chapman, M.J.; Humphries, S.E.; Ginsberg, H.N.; Masana, L.; Descamps, O.S.; Wiklund, O.; Hegele, R.A.; Raal, F.J.; Defesche, J.C.; et al. Familial hypercholesterolaemia is underdiagnosed and undertreated in the general population: Guidance for clinicians to prevent coronary heart disease: Consensus statement of the European Atherosclerosis Society. *Eur. Heart J.* **2013**, *34*, 3478–3490. [CrossRef]

24. Németh, Á.; Daróczy, B.; Juhász, L.; Fülöp, P.; Harangi, M.; Paragh, G. Assessment of Associations Between Serum Lipoprotein (a) Levels and Atherosclerotic Vascular Diseases in Hungarian Patients With Familial Hypercholesterolemia Using Data Mining and Machine Learning. *Front. Genet.* **2022**, *13*, 849197. [CrossRef] [PubMed]
25. Alonso, R.; Andres, E.; Mata, N.; Fuentes-Jiménez, F.; Badimón, L.; López-Miranda, J.; Padró, T.; Muñiz, O.; Díaz-Díaz, J.L.; Mauri, M.; et al. Lipoprotein(a) levels in familial hypercholesterolemia: An important predictor of cardiovascular disease independent of the type of LDL receptor mutation. *J. Am. Coll. Cardiol.* **2014**, *63*, 1982–1989. [CrossRef] [PubMed]
26. Stoffel, W.; Demant, T. Selective removal of apolipoprotein B-containing serum lipoproteins from blood plasma. *Proc. Natl. Acad. Sci. USA* **1981**, *78*, 611–615. [CrossRef]
27. Varga, V.E.; Lőrincz, H.; Zsíros, N.; Fülöp, P.; Seres, I.; Paragh, G.; Balla, J.; Harangi, M. Impact of selective LDL apheresis on serum chemerin levels in patients with hypercholesterolemia. *Lipids Health Dis.* **2016**, *15*, 182. [CrossRef]
28. Varga, V.E.; Lőrincz, H.; Szentpéteri, A.; Juhász, L.; Seres, I.; Paragh, G.; Balla, J.; Harangi, M. Changes in serum afamin and vitamin E levels after selective LDL apheresis. *J. Clin. Apher.* **2018**, *33*, 569–575. [CrossRef]
29. Raal, F.; Scott, R.; Somaratne, R.; Bridges, I.; Li, G.; Wasserman, S.M.; Stein, E.A. Low-density lipoprotein cholesterol-lowering effects of AMG 145, a monoclonal antibody to proprotein convertase subtilisin/kexin type 9 serine protease in patients with heterozygous familial hypercholesterolemia: The Reduction of LDL-C with PCSK9 Inhibition in Heterozygous Familial Hypercholesterolemia Disorder (RUTHERFORD) randomized trial. *Circulation* **2012**, *126*, 2408–2417. [CrossRef]
30. Stefanutti, C.; Morozzi, C.; Petta, A. Lipid and low-density-lipoprotein apheresis. Effects on plasma inflammatory profile and on cytokine pattern in patients with severe dyslipidemia. *Cytokine* **2011**, *56*, 842–849. [CrossRef]
31. Harangi, M.; Juhász, L.; Nádró, B.; Paragh, G. Az LDL-aferezis helye a dyslipidaemia kezelésében a 2017-ben érvényes magyar és európai irányelvek alapján. *Metabolizmus* **2017**, *15*, 79–84.
32. Paquette, M.; Baass, A. Predicting cardiovascular disease in familial hypercholesterolemia. *Curr. Opin. Lipidol.* **2018**, *29*, 299–306. [CrossRef] [PubMed]
33. Mata, P.; Alonso, R.; Pérez de Isla, L. Atherosclerotic cardiovascular disease risk assessment in familial hypercholesterolemia: Does one size fit all? *Curr. Opin. Lipidol.* **2018**, *29*, 445–452. [CrossRef] [PubMed]
34. Paquette, M.; Dufour, R.; Baass, A. The Montreal-FH-SCORE: A new score to predict cardiovascular events in familial hypercholesterolemia. *J. Clin. Lipidol.* **2017**, *11*, 80–86. [CrossRef]
35. Riggio, S.; Mandraffino, G.; Sardo, M.A.; Iudicello, R.; Camarda, N.; Imbalzano, E.; Alibrandi, A.; Saitta, C.; Carerj, S.; Arrigo, T.; et al. Pulse wave velocity and augmentation index, but not intima-media thickness, are early indicators of vascular damage in hypercholesterolemic children. *Eur. J. Clin. Investig.* **2010**, *40*, 250–257. [CrossRef] [PubMed]
36. Kavey, R.E.; Allada, V.; Daniels, S.R.; Hayman, L.L.; McCrindle, B.W.; Newburger, J.W.; Parekh, R.S.; Steinberger, J. Cardiovascular risk reduction in high-risk pediatric patients: A scientific statement from the American Heart Association Expert Panel on Population and Prevention Science; the Councils on Cardiovascular Disease in the Young, Epidemiology and Prevention, Nutrition, Physical Activity and Metabolism, High Blood Pressure Research, Cardiovascular Nursing, and the Kidney in Heart Disease; and the Interdisciplinary Working Group on Quality of Care and Outcomes Research: Endorsed by the American Academy of Pediatrics. *Circulation* **2006**, *114*, 2710–2738. [CrossRef] [PubMed]
37. Townsend, R.R. Arterial Stiffness: Recommendations and Standardization. *Pulse* **2017**, *4*, 3–7. [CrossRef]
38. Nemcsik, J.; Cseprekál, O.; Tislér, A. Measurement of Arterial Stiffness: A Novel Tool of Risk Stratification in Hypertension. *Adv. Exp. Med. Biol.* **2017**, *956*, 475–488. [CrossRef]
39. Williams, B.; Mancia, G.; Spiering, W.; Agabiti Rosei, E.; Azizi, M.; Burnier, M.; Clement, D.L.; Coca, A.; de Simone, G.; Dominiczak, A.; et al. 2018 ESC/ESH Guidelines for the management of arterial hypertension. *Eur. Heart J.* **2018**, *39*, 3021–3104. [CrossRef]
40. Omboni, S.; Posokhov, I.N.; Kotovskaya, Y.V.; Protogerou, A.D.; Blacher, J. Twenty-Four-Hour Ambulatory Pulse Wave Analysis in Hypertension Management: Current Evidence and Perspectives. *Curr. Hypertens. Rep.* **2016**, *18*, 72. [CrossRef]
41. Rajendran, P.; Jayakumar, T.; Nishigaki, I.; Ekambaram, G.; Nishigaki, Y.; Vetriselvi, J.; Sakthisekaran, D. Immunomodulatory Effect of Mangiferin in Experimental Animals with Benzo(a)Pyrene-induced Lung Carcinogenesis. *Int. J. Biomed. Sci.* **2013**, *9*, 68–74. [PubMed]
42. Wilkinson, I.; Cockcroft, J.R. Cholesterol, lipids and arterial stiffness. In *Atherosclerosis, Large Arteries and Cardiovascular Risk*; Safar, M., Frohlich, E., Eds.; Karger: Basel, Switzerland, 2007; Volume 44, pp. 261–277.
43. Paik, D.C.; Ramey, W.G.; Dillon, J.; Tilson, M.D. The nitrite/elastin reaction: Implications for in vivo degenerative effects. *Connect. Tissue Res.* **1997**, *36*, 241–251. [CrossRef] [PubMed]
44. Yasmin; McEniery, C.M.; Wallace, S.; Mackenzie, I.S.; Cockcroft, J.R.; Wilkinson, I.B. C-reactive protein is associated with arterial stiffness in apparently healthy individuals. *Arterioscler. Thromb. Vasc. Biol.* **2004**, *24*, 969–974. [CrossRef] [PubMed]
45. Yasmin; McEniery, C.M.; Wallace, S.; Dakham, Z.; Pulsalkar, P.; Pusalkar, P.; Maki-Petaja, K.; Ashby, M.J.; Cockcroft, J.R.; Wilkinson, I.B. Matrix metalloproteinase-9 (MMP-9), MMP-2, and serum elastase activity are associated with systolic hypertension and arterial stiffness. *Arterioscler. Thromb. Vasc. Biol.* **2005**, *25*, 372. [CrossRef]
46. Niederhoffer, N.; Lartaud-Idjouadiene, I.; Giummelly, P.; Duvivier, C.; Peslin, R.; Atkinson, J. Calcification of medial elastic fibers and aortic elasticity. *Hypertension* **1997**, *29*, 999–1006. [CrossRef]
47. Chowienczyk, P.J.; Watts, G.F.; Cockcroft, J.R.; Ritter, J.M. Impaired endothelium-dependent vasodilation of forearm resistance vessels in hypercholesterolaemia. *Lancet* **1992**, *340*, 1430–1432. [CrossRef]

28. Sakurai, K.; Cominacini, L.; Garbin, U.; Fratta Pasini, A.; Sasaki, N.; Takuwa, Y.; Masaki, T.; Sawamura, T. Induction of endothelin-1 production in endothelial cells via co-operative action between CD40 and lectin-like oxidized LDL receptor (LOX-1). *J. Cardiovasc. Pharmacol.* **2004**, *44* (Suppl. S1), S173–S180. [CrossRef]
29. Dart, A.M.; Lacombe, F.; Yeoh, J.K.; Cameron, J.D.; Jennings, G.L.; Laufer, E.; Esmore, D.S. Aortic distensibility in patients with isolated hypercholesterolaemia, coronary artery disease, or cardiac transplant. *Lancet* **1991**, *338*, 270–273. [CrossRef]
30. Hopkins, K.D.; Lehmann, E.D.; Gosling, R.G.; Parker, J.R.; Sönksen, P.H. Biochemical correlates of aortic distensibility in vivo in normal subjects. *Clin. Sci.* **1993**, *84*, 593–597. [CrossRef]
31. Cameron, J.D.; Jennings, G.L.; Dart, A.M. The relationship between arterial compliance, age, blood pressure and serum lipid levels. *J. Hypertens.* **1995**, *13*, 1718–1723. [CrossRef]
32. Giannattasio, C.; Mangoni, A.A.; Failla, M.; Stella, M.L.; Carugo, S.; Bombelli, M.; Sega, R.; Mancia, G. Combined effects of hypertension and hypercholesterolemia on radial artery function. *Hypertension* **1997**, *29*, 583–586. [CrossRef] [PubMed]
33. Márk, L.; Harangi, M.; Paragh, G. The labyrinth of residual risk: Reduction of the remaining lipid and inflammation risk in the prevention of atherosclerosis. *Rvosi Hetil.* **2018**, *159*, 124–130. [CrossRef] [PubMed]
34. Mundal, L.; Igland, J.; Ose, L.; Holven, K.B.; Veierød, M.B.; Leren, T.P.; Retterstøl, K. Cardiovascular disease mortality in patients with genetically verified familial hypercholesterolemia in Norway during 1992–2013. *Eur. J. Prev. Cardiol.* **2017**, *24*, 137–144. [CrossRef]
35. Cheng, H.M.; Ye, Z.X.; Chiou, K.R.; Lin, S.J.; Charng, M.J. Vascular stiffness in familial hypercholesterolaemia is associated with C-reactive protein and cholesterol burden. *Eur. J. Clin. Investig.* **2007**, *37*, 197–206. [CrossRef] [PubMed]
36. Ellins, E.A.; New, K.J.; Datta, D.B.; Watkins, S.; Haralambos, K.; Rees, A.; Aled Rees, D.; Halcox, J.P. Validation of a new method for non-invasive assessment of vasomotor function. *Eur. J. Prev. Cardiol.* **2016**, *23*, 577–583. [CrossRef] [PubMed]
37. Lewandowski, P.; Romanowska-Kocejko, M.; Węgrzyn, A.; Chmara, M.; Żuk, M.; Limon, J.; Wasąg, B.; Rynkiewicz, A.; Gruchała, M. Noninvasive assessment of endothelial function and vascular parameters in patients with familial and nonfamilial hypercholesterolemia. *Pol. Arch. Med. Wewn.* **2014**, *124*, 516–524. [CrossRef] [PubMed]
38. Plana, N.; Ferré, R.; Merino, J.; Aragonès, G.; Girona, J.; Heras, M.; Masana, L. Heterozygous familial hypercholesterolaemic patients have increased arterial stiffness, as determined using the augmentation index. *J. Atheroscler. Thromb.* **2011**, *18*, 1110–1116. [CrossRef]
39. Ershova, A.I.; Meshkov, A.N.; Rozhkova, T.A.; Kalinina, M.V.; Deev, A.D.; Rogoza, A.N.; Balakhonova, T.V.; Boytsov, S.A. Carotid and Aortic Stiffness in Patients with Heterozygous Familial Hypercholesterolemia. *PLoS ONE* **2016**, *11*, e0158964. [CrossRef]
40. Tada, H.; Kawashiri, M.A.; Nohara, A.; Inazu, A.; Mabuchi, H.; Yamagishi, M. Assessment of arterial stiffness in patients with familial hypercholesterolemia. *J. Clin. Lipidol.* **2018**, *12*, 397–402.e392. [CrossRef]
41. Tran, A.; Burkhardt, B.; Tandon, A.; Blumenschein, S.; van Engelen, A.; Cecelja, M.; Zhang, S.; Uribe, S.; Mura, J.; Greil, G.; et al. Pediatric heterozygous familial hypercholesterolemia patients have locally increased aortic pulse wave velocity and wall thickness at the aortic root. *Int. J. Cardiovasc. Imaging* **2019**, *35*, 1903–1911. [CrossRef]
42. Vlahos, A.P.; Naka, K.K.; Bechlioulis, A.; Theoharis, P.; Vakalis, K.; Moutzouri, E.; Miltiadous, G.; Michalis, L.K.; Siamopoulou-Mavridou, A.; Elisaf, M.; et al. Endothelial dysfunction, but not structural atherosclerosis, is evident early in children with heterozygous familial hypercholesterolemia. *Pediatr. Cardiol.* **2014**, *35*, 63–70. [CrossRef] [PubMed]
43. Waluś-Miarka, M.; Wojciechowska, W.; Miarka, P.; Kloch-Badełek, M.; Woźniakiewicz, E.; Czarnecka, D.; Sanak, M.; Małecki, M.; Idzior-Waluś, B. Intima-media thickness correlates with features of metabolic syndrome in young people with a clinical diagnosis of familial hypercholesterolaemia. *Kardiol. Pol.* **2013**, *71*, 566–572. [CrossRef] [PubMed]
44. Reiner, Ž.; Simental-Mendía, L.E.; Ruscica, M.; Katsiki, N.; Banach, M.; Al Rasadi, K.; Jamialahmadi, T.; Sahebkar, A. Pulse wave velocity as a measure of arterial stiffness in patients with familial hypercholesterolemia: A systematic review and meta-analysis. *Arch. Med. Sci.* **2019**, *15*, 1365–1374. [CrossRef] [PubMed]
45. Bjelakovic, B.; Stefanutti, C.; Reiner, Ž.; Watts, G.F.; Moriarty, P.; Marais, D.; Widhalm, K.; Cohen, H.; Harada-Shiba, M.; Banach, M. Risk Assessment and Clinical Management of Children and Adolescents with Heterozygous Familial Hypercholesterolaemia. A Position Paper of the Associations of Preventive Pediatrics of Serbia, Mighty Medic and International Lipid Expert Panel. *J. Clin. Med.* **2021**, *10*, 4930. [CrossRef] [PubMed]
46. Martinez, L.R.; Miname, M.H.; Bortolotto, L.A.; Chacra, A.P.; Rochitte, C.E.; Sposito, A.C.; Santos, R.D. No correlation and low agreement of imaging and inflammatory atherosclerosis' markers in familial hypercholesterolemia. *Atherosclerosis* **2008**, *200*, 83–88. [CrossRef] [PubMed]
47. Bedi, O.; Dhawan, V.; Sharma, P.L.; Kumar, P. Pleiotropic effects of statins: New therapeutic targets in drug design. *Naunyn Schmiedebergs Arch. Pharmacol.* **2016**, *389*, 695–712. [CrossRef] [PubMed]
48. Oesterle, A.; Laufs, U.; Liao, J.K. Pleiotropic Effects of Statins on the Cardiovascular System. *Circ. Res.* **2017**, *120*, 229–243. [CrossRef]
49. Kool, M.; Lustermans, F.; Kragten, H.; Struijker Boudier, H.; Hoeks, A.; Reneman, R.; Rila, H.; Hoogendam, I.; Van Bortel, L. Does lowering of cholesterol levels influence functional properties of large arteries? *Eur. J. Clin. Pharmacol.* **1995**, *48*, 217–223. [CrossRef]
50. Raison, J.; Rudnichi, A.; Safar, M.E. Effects of atorvastatin on aortic pulse wave velocity in patients with hypertension and hypercholesterolaemia: A preliminary study. *J. Hum. Hypertens.* **2002**, *16*, 705–710. [CrossRef]

71. Kontopoulos, A.G.; Athyros, V.G.; Pehlivanidis, A.N.; Demitriadis, D.S.; Papageorgiou, A.A.; Boudoulas, H. Long-term treatment effect of atorvastatin on aortic stiffness in hypercholesterolaemic patients. *Curr. Med. Res. Opin.* **2003**, *19*, 22–27. [CrossRef]
72. Ferrier, K.E.; Muhlmann, M.H.; Baguet, J.P.; Cameron, J.D.; Jennings, G.L.; Dart, A.M.; Kingwell, B.A. Intensive cholesterol reduction lowers blood pressure and large artery stiffness in isolated systolic hypertension. *J. Am. Coll. Cardiol.* **2002**, *39*, 1020–1025. [CrossRef]
73. Matsuo, T.; Iwade, K.; Hirata, N.; Yamashita, M.; Ikegami, H.; Tanaka, N.; Aosaki, M.; Kasanuki, H. Improvement of arterial stiffness by the antioxidant and anti-inflammatory effects of short-term statin therapy in patients with hypercholesterolemia *Heart Vessel.* **2005**, *20*, 8–12. [CrossRef] [PubMed]
74. Muramatsu, J.; Kobayashi, A.; Hasegawa, N.; Yokouchi, S. Hemodynamic changes associated with reduction in total cholesterol by treatment with the HMG-CoA reductase inhibitor pravastatin. *Atherosclerosis* **1997**, *130*, 179–182. [CrossRef]
75. Poulter, N.R.; Wedel, H.; Dahlöf, B.; Sever, P.S.; Beevers, D.G.; Caulfield, M.; Kjeldsen, S.E.; Kristinsson, A.; McInnes, G.T.; Mehlsen, J.; et al. Role of blood pressure and other variables in the differential cardiovascular event rates noted in the Anglo-Scandinavian Cardiac Outcomes Trial-Blood Pressure Lowering Arm (ASCOT-BPLA). *Lancet* **2005**, *366*, 907–913. [CrossRef]
76. Toyama, K.; Sugiyama, S.; Oka, H.; Iwasaki, Y.; Sumida, H.; Tanaka, T.; Tayama, S.; Jinnouchi, H.; Ogawa, H. Combination treatment of rosuvastatin or atorvastatin, with regular exercise improves arterial wall stiffness in patients with coronary artery disease. *PLoS ONE* **2012**, *7*, e41369. [CrossRef] [PubMed]
77. Liu, B.; Che, W.; Yan, H.; Zhu, W.; Wang, H. Effects of rosuvastatin vs. simvastatin/ezetimibe on arterial wall stiffness in patients with coronary artery disease. *Intern. Med.* **2013**, *52*, 2715–2719. [CrossRef]
78. Toscano, A.; Cinquegrani, M.; Scuruchi, M.; Di Pino, A.; Piro, S.; Ferrara, V.; Morace, C.; Lo Gullo, A.; Imbalzano, E.; Purrello, F.; et al. PCSK9 Plasma Levels Are Associated with Mechanical Vascular Impairment in Familial Hypercholesterolemia Subjects without a History of Atherosclerotic Cardiovascular Disease: Results of Six-Month Add-On PCSK9 Inhibitor Therapy *Biomolecules* **2022**, *12*, 562. [CrossRef]
79. Ruscica, M.; Tokgözoğlu, L.; Corsini, A.; Sirtori, C.R. PCSK9 inhibition and inflammation: A narrative review. *Atherosclerosis* **2019**, *288*, 146–155. [CrossRef]
80. Sahebkar, A.; Simental-Mendía, L.E.; Guerrero-Romero, F.; Golledge, J.; Watts, G.F. Effect of statin therapy on plasma proprotein convertase subtilisin kexin 9 (PCSK9) concentrations: A systematic review and meta-analysis of clinical trials. *Diabetes Obes. Metab.* **2015**, *17*, 1042–1055. [CrossRef]
81. Bambauer, R.; Bambauer, C.; Lehmann, B.; Latza, R.; Schiel, R. LDL-apheresis: Technical and clinical aspects. *Sci. World J.* **2012**, *2012*, 314283. [CrossRef]
82. Mandraffino, G.; Scicali, R.; Rodríguez-Carrio, J.; Savarino, F.; Mamone, F.; Scuruchi, M.; Cinquegrani, M.; Imbalzano, E.; Di Pino, A.; Piro, S.; et al. Arterial stiffness improvement after adding on PCSK9 inhibitors or ezetimibe to high-intensity statins in patients with familial hypercholesterolemia: A Two-Lipid Center Real-World Experience. *J. Clin. Lipidol.* **2020**, *14*, 231–240. [CrossRef] [PubMed]
83. Sinzinger, H.; Steiner, S.; Derfler, K. Pleiotropic effects of regular lipoprotein-apheresis. *Atheroscler. Suppl.* **2017**, *30*, 122–127. [CrossRef] [PubMed]

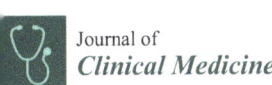

Review

Arterial Stiffness in Thyroid and Parathyroid Disease: A Review of Clinical Studies

Andrea Grillo [1,2,*], Vincenzo Barbato [1], Roberta Maria Antonello [1], Marco Fabio Cola [1], Gianfranco Parati [3,4], Paolo Salvi [3], Bruno Fabris [1,2] and Stella Bernardi [1,2]

1. Department of Medicine, Surgery and Health Sciences, University of Trieste, 34149 Trieste, Italy; barbato.vinc@gmail.com (V.B.); rma.roby@gmail.com (R.M.A.); marcofabio.cola@asugi.sanita.fvg.it (M.F.C.); b.fabris@fmc.units.it (B.F.); stella.bernardi@asugi.sanita.fvg.it (S.B.)
2. SC Medicina Clinica, ASUGI (Azienda Sanitaria Universitaria Giuliano Isontina), Cattinara Hospital, 34149 Trieste, Italy
3. Department of Cardiology, Istituto Auxologico Italiano, IRCCS, 20122 Milan, Italy; gianfranco.parati@unimib.it (G.P.); psalvi.md@gmail.com (P.S.)
4. Department of Medicine and Surgery, University of Milano-Bicocca, 20126 Milan, Italy
* Correspondence: andr.grillo@gmail.com

Abstract: Growing evidence shows that arterial stiffness measurement provides important prognostic information and improves clinical stratification of cardiovascular risk. Thyroid and parathyroid diseases are endocrine diseases with a relevant cardiovascular burden. The objective of this review was to consider the relationship between arterial stiffness and thyroid and parathyroid diseases in human clinical studies. We performed a systematic literature review of articles published in PubMed/MEDLINE from inception to December 2021, restricted to English languages and to human adults. We selected relevant articles about the relationship between arterial stiffness and thyroid and parathyroid diseases. For each selected article, data on arterial stiffness were extracted and factors that may have an impact on arterial stiffness were identified. We considered 24 papers concerning hypothyroidism, 9 hyperthyroidism and 16 primary hyperparathyroidism and hypoparathyroidism. Most studies evidenced an increase in arterial stiffness biomarkers in hypothyroidism, hyperthyroidism and primary hyperparathyroidism, even in subclinical and mild forms, although heterogeneity of measurement methods and of study designs prevented a definitive conclusion, suggesting that the assessment of arterial stiffness may be considered in the clinical evaluation of cardiovascular risk in these diseases.

Keywords: arterial stiffness; thyroid; parathyroid; cardiovascular disease

1. Introduction

Growing evidence shows that arterial stiffness measurement provides important prognostic information and improves clinical stratification of cardiovascular disease [1,2]. The stiffening of arteries is notably linked to aging, but a number of risk factors and diseases may affect this process, which is usually referred as arteriosclerosis [3]. The biological mechanisms underlying arterial stiffening involve the degradation of elastin layers in the tunica media of the large arteries and the proportional increase in collagen fiber content, along with smooth muscle cell hyperplasia, fibrosis and calcification of the media [4]. The process of stiffening interacts with atheromatous plaque formation and inflammation in the development and progression of cardiovascular disease [5]. The use of arterial stiffness markers is considered of clinical interest to assess cardiovascular risk in particular among patients not presenting the classical risk factors (e.g., smoking, obesity, diabetes), in which evaluation of arterial damage may improve risk stratification [6].

Thyroid and parathyroid diseases should be considered as endocrine diseases with relevant implications in the cardiovascular system. Patients with overt hyperthyroidism or hypothyroidism show several alterations, caused either by effects of thyroid hormones in the heart and in the vasculature or by cardiovascular risk factors (including blood pressure, dyslipidemia and inflammation), which may increase cardiovascular risk and lead to cardiovascular morbidity and mortality [7,8]. Similarly, patients with primary hyperparathyroidism often present cardiovascular abnormalities and an increased cardiovascular risk [9]. Less evidence supports the cardiovascular significance of subclinical hyper- or hypothyroidism or mild hyperparathyroidism, although detrimental cardiovascular consequences may affect these conditions as well [10–12].

In recent years, numerous clinical studies have investigated the relationship between thyroid and parathyroid diseases and arterial stiffness markers. New evidence explains the molecular and physiological pathways leading to vascular disease in conditions of hormonal excess or deficiency. The use of arterial stiffness measures has been proposed to improve clinical management of these conditions in several clinical studies.

In this review, we aimed to perform a literature search for the effects of thyroid and parathyroid hormone excess or deficiency on the structural and functional alterations of the arterial wall which leads to arterial stiffening, focusing on clinical studies conducted in humans.

2. Material and methods

A PubMed/MEDLINE search was performed to select peer-reviewed articles published from inception to 31 December 2021. The complete search string included inclusive keywords regarding arterial stiffness (e.g., "arterial stiffness", "arterial compliance", "pulse wave velocity", "PWV", "augmentation index", "AIx") and inclusive keywords regarding the evaluated hormones and their imbalance ("hypothyroidism" or "thyroid hormones" or "thyrotoxicosis" or "levothyroxine" or "Hashimoto" or "Graves" or "Basedow" or "dysthyroidism" "hyperparathyroidism" or "PTH"). Papers written in languages other than English, not pertinent with the present review, or whose full text was not available were excluded. The pertinent references were evaluated and eventually included in the final manuscript. We considered all papers in open-access and non-open access journals. The included papers were summarized and their results discussed in the text, offering an overview of current literature. Clinical studies in adult humans were organized in Tables (Table 1: hypothyroidism, Table 2: hyperthyroidism, Table 3: primary hyperparathyroidism). The manuscript was organized in the following major chapters: (1) Thyroid: hypo- and hyper-thyroidism; (2) Parathyroid.

3. Results

3.1. Thyroid

Our literature search identified 33 papers regarding dysthyroidism and its impact on arterial stiffness. Twenty-five studies evaluated arterial stiffness in patients with overt and/or subclinical hypothyroidism, while nine studies evaluated patients with overt and/or subclinical hyperthyroidism (one study evaluated patients with Hashimoto thyroiditis including both hyperthyroid and hypothyroid patients). From an overall evaluation, variable results about the impact of thyroid hormones on arterial stiffness are reported. In addition, arterial stiffness was assessed using different measurement methods, varying from ultrasounds to tonometry. Considered measures of arterial stiffness included pulse wave velocity (PWV), augmentation index and other surrogate measures. PWV is the velocity at which the pressure pulsation propagates through the circulatory system, and is defined as the distance travelled by the pulse wave divided by the time [2], and the carotid-femoral PWV is the gold standard for measuring stiffness of the aorta [3]. Variability in methodologies, together with the differences in study populations and in inclusion/exclusion criteria among studies, may explain the heterogeneity of results.

3.1.1. Overt and Subclinical Hypothyroidism

The prevalence of subclinical hypothyroidism, defined as a serum thyroid stimulating hormone (TSH) level above the upper normal limit despite normal levels of serum free thyroxine (fT4), in the general population is 5–15% [13]. Of these, 2–5% progress to overt hypothyroidism [14]. Clinical and subclinical hypothyroidism are related to cardiovascular diseases, in particular atherosclerosis and ischemic heart disease [15]. Over the past years, the hypothesis that even in euthyroid subjects thyroid function may affect cardiovascular health has been supported by different authors [16–18]. A large Chinese population-based, cross-sectional study, including 812 euthyroid subjects without major cardiovascular risk factors, showed a significant and independent association of fT4 with baPWV in euthyroid subjects [19].

Regarding subclinical hypothyroidism, evidence observing an increase in arterial stiffness is conflicting and heterogeneous, both in methods used to evaluate arterial stiffness and in results. A number of small studies were conducted to evaluate arterial stiffness in subclinical hypothyroidism, in small cohorts of patients and with different methodologies. Earlier studies mainly considered the evaluation of brachial-ankle PWV, which was found to be increased [20] but not correlated to TSH [21]. Further studies confirmed the increase in aortic stiffness, measured either with brachial-ankle or heart-femoral PWV [21,22] and observed a decrease in stiffness after l-thyroxine replacement [23,24]. The increase in stiffness was confirmed by other methodologies, as the evaluation of β-stiffness index in the carotid artery [25–27], or the augmentation index [28,29], while the evaluation of global aortic distensibility gave contrasting results [30,31]. Considering the response to treatment, the augmentation index tended to reduce with levothyroxine replacement therapy [32].

More recent studies explored the relationship between the PWV in aorta and subclinical hypothyroidism. Three studies found an increase in aortic PWV in this condition [33–35], although one study conducted in a large sample and with gold-standard measurement (carotid-femoral PWV) [36] did not find an association between subclinical hypothyroidism and aortic stiffness. The CAVI, a blood pressure-independent stiffness index of the aorta, which is related to central and peripheral arterial stiffness and to 24 h blood pressure [37], was found to be increased in subclinical hypothyroidism [38], with a possible benefit after acute aerobic exercise [39].

Similarly to subclinical, most studies conducted in overt hypothyroidism found an increase in arterial stiffness, which has been evaluated across studies with a variety of biomarkers. Earlier studies evaluated markers related to reflected waves, as augmentation index [40,41]. Timing and magnitude of reflected waves was determined by hypothyroidism and improved after replacement therapy, indicating a positive effect on arterial stiffness [40]. Other studies focused on biomarkers of structural arterial stiffening, as β index [25,42,43], pulsatility index in carotid arteries [44] or brachial-ankle PWV [21]. One large study conducted in a large population, with brachial-ankle PWV, did not find a significant difference between hypothyroid and euthyroid subjects, which adds heterogeneity in the results [45]. More recently, studies that evaluated the gold-standard measure of aortic stiffness, the carotid-femoral PWV [33,44] or the heart-femoral PWV [35], found an increase in arterial stiffness markers in patients with overt hypothyroidism.

One study conducted in thyroidectomized patients on long-term replacement therapy, did not find an increase in arterial stiffness, suggesting that targeting TSH in the reference range does not seem to cause adverse cardiovascular effects [46].

Table 1. Experimental studies evaluating arterial stiffness and hypothyroidism.

AUTHOR	YEAR, COUNTRY	STUDY DESIGN	DISEASE	OUTCOME MEASURE	STUDY POPULATION	RESULTS
Demellis et al. [42]	2002, Greece	Paired and unpaired case–control study	Hypothyroidism	β index	15 hypothyroid patients, 15 hypertensive patients, 15 hypothyroid and hypertensive patients, 30 controls	Increased aortic stiffness in patients with hypothyroidism and hypertension, reversible by hormone replacement in 50%.
Obuobie et al. [29]	2002, United Kingdom	Paired and unpaired case–control study	Hypothyroidism	AIx, CBP, reflected waves time	12 hypothyroid patients before and after levothyroxine replacement treatment	Hypothyroid patients had significantly higher AIx and CBP and lower reflected waves time than controls; 6 months of levothyroxine replacement therapy reversed the abnormalities.
Dagre et al. [41]	2005, Greece	Cross-sectional study	Hypothyroidism	Augmentation pressure	15 overt hypothyroidism, 50 controls with varying mean TSH serum levels	Serum TSH values were positively correlated with augmentation pressure.
Hamano et al. [21]	2005, Japan	Cross-sectional study	Subclinical hypothyroidism, overt hypothyroidism	baPWV	7 overt hypothyroidism (before and after treatment with L-thyroxin), 28 subclinical hypothyroidism	baPWV was not correlated to TSH. After replacement therapy, fT4 increased and baPWV decreased.
Nagasaki et al. [43]	2005, Japan	Paired and unpaired case–control study	Hypothyroidism before and after levothyroxine replacement therapy	β index, cIMT	30 hypothyroid patients before and after 1 year of treatment	β index higher in hypothyroid patients than controls. After 1 year of treatment significant decreases of β index.
Nagasaki et al. [20]	2006, Japan	Case–control study	Subclinical hypothyroidism	baPWV	50 subclinical hypothyroidism, 50 controls	BaPWV was increased but not correlated with T3, T4 or TSH.
Owen et al. [28]	2006, United Kingdom	Paired and unpaired case–control study	Subclinical hypothyroidism	AIx, CBP, reflected waves time	19 subclinical hypothyroidism (before and after treatment with L-thyroxin), 10 controls	Increased AIx in subclinical hypothyroidism which improved with L-thyroxin

Table 1. Cont.

AUTHOR	YEAR, COUNTRY	STUDY DESIGN	DISEASE	OUTCOME MEASURE	STUDY POPULATION	RESULTS
Nagasaki et al. [22]	2007, Japan	Prospective observational study	Subclinical hypothyroidism	hfPWV, faPWV, baPWV	40 subclinical hypothyroidism, 50 controls	hfPWV, faPWV and baPWV were significantly higher in patients with subclinical hypothyroidism compared to controls.
Nagasaki et al. [24]	2007, Japan	Paired case–control study	Subclinical hypothyroidism	baPWV	42 subclinical hypothyroidism, evaluated before and after levothyroxine (L-T(4))	Replacement therapy decreased baPWV.
Nagasaki et al. [25]	2007, Japan	Paired and unpaired case–control study	Hypothyroidism	β index	46 hypothyroid patients (of which 35 evaluated before and after levothyroxine replacement therapy), 46 controls	β index was significantly higher in hypothyroid patients than in controls. After one year of replacement therapy, β index reduced.
Peleg et al. [32]	2008, Israel	Paired case–control study	Subclinical hypothyroidism	AIx	30 patients with subclinical hypothyroidism treated with levothyroxine and assessed at baseline and after 1, 4 and 7 months	The AIx significantly reduced with treatment.
Nagasaki et al. [23]	2009, Japan	Double-blind,	Subclinical hypothyroidism in Hashimoto thyroiditis, before and after levothyroxine replacement treatment	baPWV	95 subclinical hypothyroidism before and after levothyroxine replacement treatment, 42 controls	The baseline baPWV values in patients with subclinical hypothyroidism were significantly higher than in normal subjects. BaPWV showed a significant decrease with treatment. Changes in baPWV and TSH were not correlated.

Table 1. *Cont.*

AUTHOR	YEAR, COUNTRY	STUDY DESIGN	DISEASE	OUTCOME MEASURE	STUDY POPULATION	RESULTS
Tian et al. [26]	2010, China	Case-control study	Subclinical hypothyroidism	β index	93 subclinical hypothyroidism, 90 controls	β index was significantly higher in patients with subclinical hypothyroidism than in normal controls
	2013, Turkey	Case-control study	Subclinical hypothyroidism	ASI, aortic distensibility	43 subclinical hypothyroidism, 48 controls	Aortic distensibility was significantly lower, and ASI was significantly higher in subclinical hypothyroidism than in controls. TSH level was positively correlated with ASI.
Kilic et al. [30]	2013, Turkey	Case-control study	Subclinical hypothyroidism	cIMT, Aortic distensibility	32 subclinical hypothyroidism, 29 controls	No difference in aortic distensibility between subclinical hypothyroidism and controls.
Masaki et al. [38]	2014, Japan	Cross-sectional study	Subclinical Hypothyroidism	CAVI	83 subclinical hypothyroidism, 83 controls	CAVI was increased and associated with high NT-proBNP in subclinical hypothyroidism.
Owecki et al. [44]	2015, Poland	Case-control study	Treated hypothyroidism and euthyroid autoimmune thyroiditis	Pulsatility index in carotid arteries	31 treated hypothyroidism, 26 euthyoroid thytoiditis	Overt hypothyroidism have increased pulsatility index in common and internal carotid arteries than euthyroid patients with autoimmune thoiditis
Tudoran [33]	2015, Romania	Paired and unpaired case–control study	Subclinical hypothyroidism, overt hypothyroidism	PWV, AIx	41 overt hypothyroidism, 15 subclinical hypothyroidism, 15 controls. Before and after treatment with L-thyroxin.	All patients had higher PWV and AIx compared with controls. After treatment, PWV and of AIx reduced in the majority of patients.

Table 1. Cont.

AUTHOR	YEAR, COUNTRY	STUDY DESIGN	DISEASE	OUTCOME MEASURE	STUDY POPULATION	RESULTS
Feng et al. [27]	2016, China	Cross-sectional study	Hypothyroidism	β index, PWV, distensibility coefficient of carotid arteries	Autoimmune throiditis: 59 hyperthyroidism, 61 hypothyroidism, 60 euthyroidism and controls.	PWV and distensibility coefficients may discriminate hypo- and hyper-throidism patients.
Laugesen et al. [46]	2016, Demark	Cross-sectional study	Thyroidectomized patients	cfPWV, AIx	30 thyroidectomized patients on long-term replacement therapy	PWV and AIx were not significantly higher in patients compared to controls
Peixoto de Miranda et al. [36]	2017, Brazil	Cross-sectional study	Subclinical hypothyroidism	cfPWV	463 subclinical hypothyroidism, 7878 controls	Subclinical hypothyroidism was not associated with increased cf-PWV.
Masaki et al. [39]	2019, Japan	Prospective observational study	Subclinical hypothyroidism	CAVI	53 subclinical hypothyroidism, 55 controls	The CAVI and serum TSH levels significantly decreased after acute aerobic exercise in the subclinical hypothyroidism group and euthyroid group.
Tanriverdi et al. [34]	2019, Turkey	Cross-sectional study	Subclinical hypothyroidism	PWV	32 subclinical hypothyroidism, 28 controls	PWV was significantly higher in the subclinical hypothyroidism group.

TSH: thyroid stimulating factor; CAVI: cardio-ankle vascular stiffness; PWV: pulse wave velocity; cfPWV: carotid-femoral pulse wave velocity; hfPWV: heart-femoral pulse wave velocity; faPWV: femoral-ankle pulse wave velocity; baPWV: brachial-ankle pulse wave velocity; AIx: augmentation index; ASI: arterial stiffness index; cIMT: carotid intima-media thickness; CBP: central blood pressure.

3.1.2. Overt and Subclinical Hyperthyroidism

Studies conducted in patients with overt hyperthyroidism suggest an increase in structural arterial stiffness biomarkers. An increase in β index in carotid arteries was found, which was reduced by antithyroid drug or radioiodine treatment [47,48]. Additionally, a marker of total arterial compliance (Pulse pressure/stroke volume) was found to be reduced in hyperthyroidism and normalized after beta-blockers therapy [49]. Considering a surrogate biomarker of central arterial stiffness derived from 24 h blood pressure monitoring, the ambulatory arterial stiffness index (AASI), one study did not find a significant difference between patients with overt or subclinical hyperthyroidism [50]. Data on subclinical hyperthyroidism (defined as a low or undetectable TSH, with normal fT3 and fT4) are scarce, considering that only one other work [51] has evaluated patients with this condition after thyroidectomy and l-thyroxine suppressive therapy, finding an increase in the β aortic stiffness by echocardiography.

Two studies evaluated the algorithm-derived PWV calculated from Mobil-O-Graph device in patients with hyperthyroidism, finding an increase in PWV in the office setting [52], which is not surprising considering that the PWV estimated by this method is strictly dependent on actual blood pressure values [53]. Interestingly, in another study the Mobil-O-Graph-derived PWV was not different in hyperthyroidism patients compared to blood-pressure matched controls [54], although the circadian profile of PWV was altered.

The evaluation of markers of reflected waves magnitude and the analysis of central pressure waves gave variable results among studies. In thyrotoxicosis, Obuobie et al. found a decrease in AIx despite an increase in central pulse pressure [40], thus suggesting a lowered central arterial stiffness. Conversely, Bodlaj et al. [55] found an increase in aortic AIx in hyperthyroidism patients with Graves' disease. A negative correlation between AIx and TSH, and a positive correlation between AIx and free thyroid hormones (fT3, fT4) was also described by Yildiz et al. [52]. Interpretation of these contrasting results probably resides in the close dependence of reflected waves timing with heart rate, which is acutely affected by thyroid hormones [56]. Alterations in functional markers of arterial stiffness can acutely affect the cardiovascular system, producing possible adverse organ damage, but the long-term effects of these transient changes remain to be elucidated.

Table 2. Experimental studies evaluating arterial stiffness and hyperthyroidism.

AUTHOR	YEAR, COUNTRY	STUDY DESIGN	DISEASE	OUTCOME MEASURE	STUDY POPULATION	RESULTS
Inaba et al. [47]	2002, Japan	Paired case–control study	Hyperthyroidism (Graves' disease)	β index (common carotid artery)	27 patients with GD before and after antithyroid drug therapy	Increased β index in hyperthyroidism, reduced by antithyroid drug therapy.
Obuobie et al. [40]	2002, United Kingdom	Paired and unpaired case–control study	Thyrotoxicosis	AIx	20 thyrotoxic patients (before and after treatment with (131)I and 20 controls	Lower AIx and higher central PP at baseline. AIx reduced at 6 months following treatment with radioiodine therapy
Palmieri et al. [49]	2004, Italy	Paired and unpaired case–control study	Thyrotoxicosis (Graves' disease)	PP/stroke volume (total arterial stiffness)	20 thyrotoxic patients (before and after treatment with bisoprolol) and 20 controls	Thyrotoxicosis is associated with increased total arterial stiffness. Beta blockade normalized total arterial stiffness.
Bodlaj et al. [55]	2007, Austria	Paired case–control study	Hyperthyroidism (Graves' disease)	AIx, SEVR	59 patients with Graves' disease before (hyperthyroidism) and after antithyroid drug treatment (euthyroidism)	AIx was higher and SEVR lower in hyperthyroidism, restored after antithyroid drug (ATD) treatment.
Gazdag et al. [51]	2014, Hungary	Cross-sectional study	Thyroidectomized patients for differentiated thyroid cancer	ASI	24 differentiated thyroid cancer after total thyroidectomy and radioiodine ablation, evaluated on TSH suppressive L-T4 therapy, and 4 weeks after L-T4 withdrawal, 24 controls	Aortic stiffness was increased both in hypothyroidism and subclinical hyperthyroidism compared to controls.
Kang et al. [48]	2015, China	Paired and unpaired case–control study	Hyperthyroidism	β index, PWV, IMT	70 hyperthyroidism before and after (131)I treatment, 74 controls	β index and PWV were higher in patients than in the control group. After treatment, PWV and β were lower than baseline.

Table 2. *Cont.*

AUTHOR	YEAR, COUNTRY	STUDY DESIGN	DISEASE	OUTCOME MEASURE	STUDY POPULATION	RESULTS
İyidir et al. [50]	2017, Turkey	Cross-sectional study	Overt and subclinical hyperthyroidism	AASI	23 overt hyperthyroidism, 36 subclinical hyperthyroidism, 25 controls	AASI did not differ between overt and subclinical hyperthyroidism, but there was a positive relationship between AASI and free thyroid hormone levels.
Yildiz et al. [52]	2019, Turkey	Case-control study	Overt and subclinical hyperthyroidism	PWV, AIx	30 overt hyperthyroid, 28 subclinical hyperthyroid, 14 treated hyperthyroidism, 30 controls	PWV and AIx measurements were significantly higher in the hyperthyroid subclinical hyperthyroid group than in the control group.
Grove-Laugesen et al. [54]	2020, Denmark	Cross-sectional study	Overt hyperthyroidism	PWV (office and 24 h measurement)	55 overt hyperthyroidism (Graves' disease), 55 controls	Patients with Graves' disease showed higher PWV in the 24 h but not in the office setting.

TSH: thyroid stimulating factor; AIx: augmentation index; SEVR: subendocardial variability ratio; PP: pulse pressure; AASI: ambulatory arterial stiffness index; ASI: arterial stiffness index; PWV: pulse wave velocity; IMT: intima-media thickness.

3.2. Parathyroid

Primary hyperparathyroidism (pHPT) is another very common endocrine disorder, affecting between 0.4% and 11% of the population [57]. The highest rates are due to patients—mostly post-menopausal women—with mild pHPT, who exhibit inappropriately high levels of parathyroid hormone (PTH) and normal or only mildly elevated calcium levels [58]. Parathyroidectomy remains the treatment of choice for this condition, and it is recommended in patients with mild pHPT and normal calcium levels in case of young age, or signs of kidney and/or bone damage [59]. Although the kidney and the bone are the main targets of PTH actions, PTH exerts direct actions on the cardiovascular system too, including not only cardiac myocytes but also endothelial and vascular smooth muscle cells, leading to arterial remodeling [60–62].

Based on this background, several works have evaluated the effect of mild pHPT and parathyroidectomy on arterial stiffness. PTH has been found associated with arterial stiffness in the general population [63,64], and mild pHPT has been found associated with an increase of arterial stiffness, as assessed by AIx [65,66] as well as PWV [67–71], additionally to detrimental effects in other forms of vascular organ involvement as aortic intima-media thickness [72] and central blood pressure [73]. By contrast, the studies evaluating the effects of parathyroidectomy upon arterial stiffness have reported conflicting data regarding effects on arterial structure and function [74–78]. Nevertheless, in a recent meta-analysis we found that mild pHPT was associated with an increase of arterial stiffness, which was significantly reduced by parathyroidectomy [79]. These data are in line with the results of another meta-analysis analyzing the effects of parathyroidectomy upon left ventricular mass, where surgery was able to reduce it significantly [80]. These data suggest that surgery could improve arterial stiffness, as well as other signs of cardiovascular organ damage such as left ventricular hypertrophy, and reduce the cardiovascular risk profile in patients with mild pHPT.

Interestingly, hypoparathyroidism has also been associated with an increase of arterial stiffness [81,82], consistent with the higher risk of cardiovascular disease of patients affected by this condition.

Table 3. Experimental studies evaluating arterial stiffness and parathyroid disease in humans.

AUTHOR	YEAR, COUNTRY	STUDY DESIGN	DISEASE	OUTCOME MEASURE	STUDY POPULATION	RESULTS
Barletta et al. [74]	2000, Italy	Prospective case–control study	Mild asymptomatic pHPT	PWV IMT	24 patients with mild asymptomatic pHPT, 20 matched healthy. All patients underwent surgery 1 to 3 months after the study.	Arterial diameters and thickness, blood pressure were not significantly different with respect to normal subjects and were unchanged 6 months after surgery.
Barletta [74]	2000, Italy	Single-blind, placebo-controlled, crossover study	Infusion of PTH	PWV IMT	5 healthy nonsmoker volunteers	There were no significant differences in basal echocardiographic measurements during PTH infusion with respect to placebo and in the hemodynamic response to tilt.
Kosch et al. [75]	2001, Germany	Prospective case–control study	pHPT	PWV IMT	20 patients assessed at baseline and 6 months after PTx and 20 healthy volunteers	No difference found at baseline and 6 months after PTx
Rubin et al. [66]	2005, USA	Cross-sectional case–control study	Mild pHPT	AIx	39 patients, 134 healthy subjects	AIx was also directly correlated with evidence of more active parathyroid disease, including higher PTH levels and lower bone mineral density
Tordjman et al. [78]	2010, Israel	Retrospective cohort study	Hypercalcemic (HC) and normocalcemic (NC) pHPT	PWV AIx	32 patients with NC-pHPT, 81 patients with mild HC-pHPT and a group of non-PHPT control subjects selected to match the patients' population	CV or cerebrovascular disease was more common in the HC-PHPT group. Arterial stiffness parameters did not differ and were unrelated to serum calcium or PTH concentration

Table 3. Cont.

AUTHOR	YEAR, COUNTRY	STUDY DESIGN	DISEASE	OUTCOME MEASURE	STUDY POPULATION	RESULTS
Rosa et al. [68]	2011, Czech Republic	Prospective case–control study	Hypertensive and normotensive patients with pHTP	PWV	28 patients with pHPT and concomitant hypertension, 16 with pHTP without hypertension, 28 essential hypertensive patients and 18 healthy controls	PWV was significantly higher in patients with PH and hypertension when compared with patients with essential hypertension. Similarly, PWV was significantly higher in patients without hypertension in comparison with healthy controls. Specific treatment by PTX significantly decreases PWV, which may be determined primarily by improved BP control after surgery.
Schillaci et al. [67]	2011, Italy	Prospective case–control study	pHTP	PWV	24 patients with pHTP and 48 healthy controls; 17 patients underwent surgical PTx and were examined 4 weeks later.	Aortic PWV was significantly higher among pHTP patients. Aortic PWV decreased after surgery. The change in aortic PWV remained significant also after adjustment for changes in blood pressure
Ring et al. [76]	2012, Sweden	Prospective case–control study.	pHTP patients who underwent surgery	AIx aPWV rIMT cIMT	48 patients with mild pHTP without any known cardiovascular risk factors were studied at baseline and at one year after parathyroidectomy in comparison with 48 healthy age- and gender-matched controls.	Only aoPWV was slightly higher in patients than in the control group at baseline. PTx did not cause any change in indices of vascular function or arterial wall thickness

Table 3. Cont.

AUTHOR	YEAR, COUNTRY	STUDY DESIGN	DISEASE	OUTCOME MEASURE	STUDY POPULATION	RESULTS
Stamatelopoulos et al. [73]	2014, Greece	Cross-sectional case–control study	pHPT and menopause	FMD PWV AIx IMT	102 postmenopausal women with pHPT and 102 women matched 1:1 for age and menopausal status, were consecutively recruited.	Women with pHPT had higher aortic and peripheral BP ($p < 0.05$ for all) but no correlation was observed with subclinical atherosclerosis
Cansu et al. [69]	2016, Turkey	Prospective case–control study	pHTP	AIx PWV IMT	16 normocalcaemic and 17 hypercalcaemic newly diagnosed asymptomatic PHPT patients and 15 age and body mass index (BMI) matched, healthy, normocalcaemic female control subjects; 17 hypercalcaemic patients who underwnt PTx	CIMT and PWV values in the HC and NC patients were higher than in the control group. There was a significant reduction in cIMT at the end of the 6th month after PTx,
Wetzel et al. [71]	2017, Germany	Cross-sectional data from the randomized, double-blind, placebo-controlled trial	pHPT	PWV	76 patients with treatment-naïve PTH levels.	PTH was independently associated with 24 h PWV.
Ejlsmark-Svensson et al. [77]	2019, Denmark	RCT	pHPT patients eligible for PTx.	PWV AIx	69 patients with PHPT; 33 underwent PTx, 36 were allocated in the control group	Changes in PWV, augmentation index and ambulatory 24 h BP did not differ between groups, except for an increase in ambulatory diastolic BP following PTX. However, in patients with baseline levels of ionized calcium > 1.45 mmol/L, PWV decreased significantly in response to PTx compared with the control group

Table 3. Cont.

AUTHOR	YEAR, COUNTRY	STUDY DESIGN	DISEASE	OUTCOME MEASURE	STUDY POPULATION	RESULTS
Underbjerg et al. [82]	2019, Denmark	Cohort study	Ns-HypoPT and pseudohypoparathyroidism	PWV AIx	56 patients with Ns-HypoPT with 30 patients diagnosed with pseudohypoparathyroidism	PWV was significantly higher among patients with Ns-HypoPT, even after adjustment for mean arterial pressure, body mass index, age and gender.
Sumbul et al. [72]	2019, Turkey	Perspective study	pHPT	cIMT aIMT	65 patients and 30 healthy controls.	Aortic IMT is more useful than carotid IMT in showing vascular organ involvement in patients with primary hyperparathyroidism
Buyuksimsek et al. [70]	2020, Turkey	Cross-sectional study	Hypertension and pHTP	PWV	83 hypertensive patients with pHTP and 83 age and gender matched hypertensive controls	PWV significantly increases in newly diagnosed hypertensive patients with PHP and significantly related to serum calcium level.
Pamuk et al. [81]	2020, Turkey	Cross-sectional case–control study	Hypoparathyroidism	PWV	42 patients and 60 matched volunteers	PWV was found higher in the hypoparathyroidism group.

PTH: parathyroid hormone; pHPT: primary hyperparathyroidism; Ns-HypoPT: non-surgical hypoparathyroidism; PTx: parathyroidectomy; PWV: pulse wave velocity; IMT: intima-media thickness; AIx: augmentation index; cIMT: carotid intima-media thickness; aIMT: aortic intima-media thickness; rIMT: radial intima-media thickness; FMD: flow-mediated dilation; BP: blood pressure.

4. Discussion
4.1. Thyroid

Over recent years, the role of thyroid hormones in cardiovascular health has been widely studied. Several mechanisms of action of fT3, fT4 and TSH on arterial stiffness have been hypothesized. Thyroid hormones may affect the cardiovascular system by direct effects on arterial vessels (by regulating smooth muscle cells tone and endothelial function), on the heart (by influencing heart rate, rhythm, myocardial contraction and perfusion) or indirectly by influencing cardiovascular risk factors [7].

Focusing on effects on arterial vessels, thyroid hormones have both genomic and non-genomic mechanisms affecting vascular tone, by ion channel activation and regulation of specific signal transduction pathways.

Firstly, they have a cellular action on endothelium, causing production of nitric oxide via the phosphatidylinositol 3-kinase and serine/threonine protein kinase pathways [83]. Vasodilating effect on vascular smooth muscle cells and on resistance arteries results in widened pulse pressure and decreased systemic vascular resistance [84,85] in conditions of excess of thyroid hormones. Thyroid hormones thus lead to an increase in tissue oxygen consumption and in distending pressures. Higher mechanical stretch and altered perfusion patterns may lead to arterial vascular remodeling and to an increase in arterial, and in particular of aortic, stiffness [84,86].

Secondly, due to its positive inotropic and chronotropic effect, fT3 is directly responsible for acute hemodynamic changes [85], which affect the functional determinants of aortic stiffness [87]. The increase in heart rate and the increase in cardiac output driven by an excess of thyroid hormones lead to an altered hemodynamic adaptation. The resulting increase in mean arterial pressure and the shortening of left ventricular ejection may represent the major hemodynamic determinants of a functional increase in aortic stiffening. Additionally, an increase in heart rate worsens the pressure supply–demand balance, which may cause ischemia of the heart and of tissues with high blood flow supply. These conditions have been widely associated with aortic stiffening [88].

Thirdly, by acting on cardiovascular risk factors, thyroid hormones may indirectly lead to an increase in arterial stiffness. Notably the main determinant of aortic stiffness are blood pressure levels, which may be influenced by thyroid hormones. In hyperthyroidism, caused by inotropic effect on the heart and reduction in systemic vascular resistance, an increase in systolic and pulse pressure is often seen. Hypothyroidism is conversely associated with diastolic hypertension, induced by increased peripheral vascular resistance and by changes in circulating volume [89]. Variations in blood pressure components may acutely and chronically damage the arterial wall thus leading to arterial stiffness. Thyroid hormones are involved in lipid metabolism regulation. Hypothyroidism leads to an increased total cholesterol and LDL cholesterol [90], thus influencing atherosclerotic plaque burden. Non-HDL cholesterol is closely correlated with residual cardiovascular risk and arterial stiffness markers [91], although lipid levels are more linked with atherosclerotic vascular phenotypes, rather than to arteriosclerosis which is the hallmark of arterial stiffness. Thyroid hormones may be also linked to arteriosclerosis through different metabolic pathways: chronic inflammation, oxidative stress, insulin resistance [7].

An additional cause that may affect the promotion of cardiovascular disease in the presence of thyroid disease is the autoimmune process of disease per se [92,93]. Regardless of thyroid hormones level, autoimmune processes in the thyroid gland may cause a low-grade inflammation which plays a relevant role in the atherosclerotic process and in the stiffening of arteries [94]. Subclinical inflammation has been associated with arterial stiffness in the general population [95] with a causative role played by an increase in cytokine levels (Interleukin 1 and 6, tumor necrosis factor-β) and reactive oxygen species in the degradation of elastin, migration of smooth muscle cells and increase in collagen in the arterial wall.

Regarding the effect of treatment of thyroid and parathyroid diseases in relation to thyroid disease, most studies observed an improvement in vascular markers after correction of hormone levels. In hypothyroidism, an improvement in AIx (which is mainly a functional parameter) followed correction with hormone replacement therapy. In hyperthyroidism, treatment with antithyroid drugs may restore both AIx and PWV levels, although the evidence is scarce.

We should consider an important limitation in our work, which is not having considered articles not in the English language. Considering the important heterogeneity of studies considering effects of thyroid hormones on stiffness and the complex interactions of factors determining vascular dysfunction, a further contribution is given by a recent meta-analysis, which found that both hypothyroidism and thyrotoxicosis are associated with an increase of aortic stiffness [96]. The scheme represented in Figure 1 represents the impact of thyroid disease on arterial stiffness and the effects and mutual interactions of all the previously discussed factors.

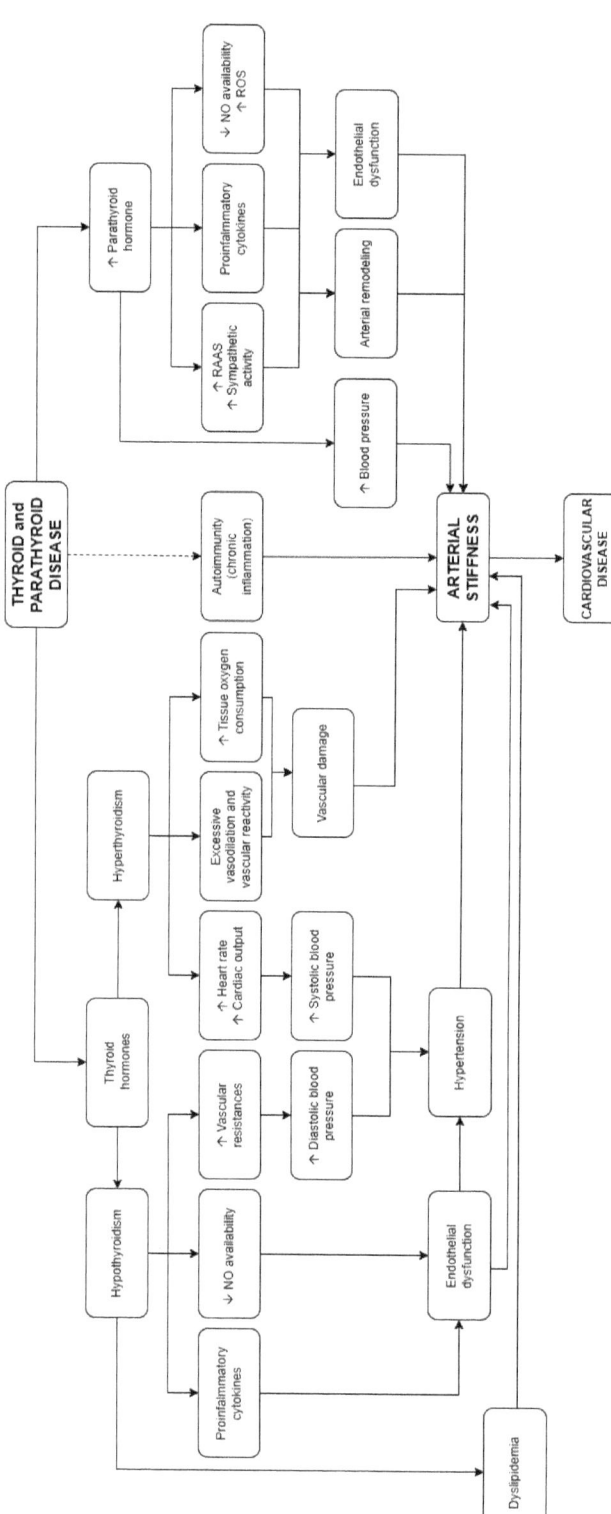

Figure 1. Pathophysiology of arterial stiffness in thyroid and parathyroid disease. RAAS: renin-angiotensin-aldosterone system. NO: nitric oxide. ROS: reactive oxygen species.

4.2. Parathyroid

In pHPT, a prolonged exposure to high levels of PTH may affect the vascular system in different ways, leading to vascular functional and structural changes and to arterial stiffness. Arterial remodeling is induced by PTH with a few mechanisms. A direct effect of PTH on endothelial and vascular smooth muscle cells was hypothesized [97] and confirmed by evidence of a stimulatory effect on nitric oxide synthase, which may contribute to vascular injury and arteriosclerotic progression through reactive oxygen species [60]. PTH may induce expression of other mediators associated with adverse vascular remodeling, as interleukin-6, receptor for advanced glycation end-products and vascular endothelial growth factor [61,98]. An effect mediated by increased intracellular calcium influx was also suggested [99], due to altered calcium metabolism in vascular smooth muscle cells, which may lead to increased arterial resistances [62]. Furthermore, PTH may also have systemic actions, by inducing the activity of renin-angiotensin-aldosterone system as well as the sympathetic nervous system [100,101], which have been notably associated with adverse effects on arterial stiffness [4]. Chronically elevated levels of circulating calcium may also mediate the association between elevated PTH and arterial stiffness. The association of calcium levels with stiffness was also demonstrated at a population level [102] and most likely mediated by the induction of vascular calcifications [103].

An elevation of blood pressure levels, which is a hallmark of pHPT, is associated with functional changes in arterial viscoelastic properties of the large arteries and an increase in the blood pressure-dependent component of arterial stiffness [104]. In experimental conditions, the infusion of physiologic doses of PTH in otherwise healthy adults, is known to produce an increase in blood pressure [105]. The induction of a chronic hypertensive state may also lead to the adverse arterial remodeling typical of hypertension and to arterial stiffness [106].

Regarding possible therapeutic approaches, surgical treatment of pHPT may improve arterial stiffness [79], and thus produce a favorable effect on cardiovascular risk profile in these patients.

The factors and the mechanisms influencing arterial stiffness in pPHT are schematically represented in Figure 1.

5. Conclusions

Our review of clinical studies prompts that thyroid and parathyroid diseases are able to affect arterial stiffness biomarkers, thus leading to possible adverse cardiovascular outcomes. In hypothyroidism, most studies agree that an increase in arterial stiffness is present in both subclinical and overt hypothyroidism, although there is no complete agreement among methodologies evaluating the different aspects of vascular stiffening in the arterial vasculature. Levothyroxine replacement therapy in most studies has shown to lead to an improvement in arterial stiffness markers. Regarding hyperthyroidism, few studies observed an increase in biomarkers of structural arterial stiffening, although a relevant methodological heterogeneity prevents a definite conclusion. The increased heart rate typical of hyperthyroidism significantly alters the blood pressure profile, affecting biomarkers of functional arterial stiffness. In primary hyperparathyroidism, an increase in arterial stiffness is evident also in the mild forms. Arterial stiffening is reversed by parathyroidectomy, suggesting a role of surgery in reducing cardiovascular risk. Regarding methods used to quantify arterial stiffness, most studies focused on PWV, which represents the gold standard method to evaluate this parameter and may thus represent the preferred method in the vascular evaluation of thyroid and parathyroid diseases.

Thyroid and parathyroid diseases are systemic diseases, characterized by an increase of cardiovascular risk, which present an increase in stiffness of the large arteries. Arterial stiffness measurement can be effectively used in the clinical evaluation of these conditions in order to quantify and possibly reduce the risk of cardiovascular events.

Author Contributions: Conceptualization, A.G. and S.B.; methodology, A.G.; data curation, V.B., R.M.A. and M.F.C.; writing—original draft preparation, A.G.; writing—review and editing, B.F., P.S. and G.P.; supervision, S.B. All authors have read and agreed to the published version of the manuscript.

Funding: Research partially supported by the Italian Ministry of Health.

Institutional Review Board Statement: Not applicable.

Informed Consent Statement: Not applicable.

Data Availability Statement: Not applicable.

Conflicts of Interest: The authors declare no conflict of interest.

Abbreviations

AASI	ambulatory arterial stiffness index
fT3	free triiodothyronine
fT4	free thyroxine
pHPT	primary hyperparathyroidism
PTH	parathyroid hormone
PWV	pulse wave velocity
TSH	thyroid stimulating hormone

References

1. Ben-Shlomo, Y.; Spears, M.; Boustred, C.; May, M.; Anderson, S.G.; Benjamin, E.J.; Boutouyrie, P.; Cameron, J.; Chen, C.-H.; Cruickshank, J.K.; et al. Aortic Pulse Wave Velocity Improves Cardiovascular Event Prediction: An Individual Participant Meta-Analysis of Prospective Observational Data from 17,635 Subjects. *J. Am. Coll. Cardiol.* **2014**, *63*, 636–646. [CrossRef] [PubMed]
2. Segers, P.; Rietzschel, E.R.; Chirinos, J.A. How to Measure Arterial Stiffness in Humans. *Arterioscler. Thromb. Vasc. Biol.* **2020**, *40*, 1034–1043. [CrossRef]
3. Laurent, S.; Cockcroft, J.; Van Bortel, L.; Boutouyrie, P.; Giannattasio, C.; Hayoz, D.; Pannier, B.; Vlachopoulos, C.; Wilkinson, I.; Struijker-Boudier, H.; et al. Expert Consensus Document on Arterial Stiffness: Methodological Issues and Clinical Applications. *Eur. Heart J.* **2006**, *27*, 2588–2605. [CrossRef] [PubMed]
4. Chirinos, J.A.; Segers, P.; Hughes, T.; Townsend, R. Large-Artery Stiffness in Health and Disease: JACC State-of-the-Art Review. *J. Am. Coll. Cardiol.* **2019**, *74*, 1237–1263. [CrossRef] [PubMed]
5. Climie, R.E.; Bruno, R.M.; Hametner, B.; Mayer, C.C.; Terentes-Printzios, D. Vascular Age Is Not Only Atherosclerosis, It Is Also Arteriosclerosis. *J. Am. Coll. Cardiol.* **2020**, *76*, 229–230. [CrossRef]
6. Boutouyrie, P.; Bruno, R.-M. The Clinical Significance and Application of Vascular Stiffness Measurements. *Am. J. Hypertens.* **2019**, *32*, 4–11. [CrossRef]
7. Razvi, S.; Jabbar, A.; Pingitore, A.; Danzi, S.; Biondi, B.; Klein, I.; Peeters, R.; Zaman, A.; Iervasi, G. Thyroid Hormones and Cardiovascular Function and Diseases. *J. Am. Coll. Cardiol.* **2018**, *71*, 1781–1796. [CrossRef]
8. Biondi, B.; Cappola, A.R.; Cooper, D.S. Subclinical Hypothyroidism: A Review. *JAMA* **2019**, *322*, 153–160. [CrossRef]
9. Tournis, S.; Makris, K.; Cavalier, E.; Trovas, G. Cardiovascular Risk in Patients with Primary Hyperparathyroidism. *Curr. Pharm. Des.* **2020**, *26*, 5628–5636. [CrossRef]
10. Walker, M.D.; Rundek, T.; Homma, S.; DiTullio, M.; Iwata, S.; Lee, J.A.; Choi, J.; Liu, R.; Zhang, C.; McMahon, D.J.; et al. Effect of Parathyroidectomy on Subclinical Cardiovascular Disease in Mild Primary Hyperparathyroidism. *Eur. J. Endocrinol.* **2012**, *167*, 277–285. [CrossRef]
11. Smedegaard, S.B.; Riis, A.L.; Christiansen, M.K.; Linde, J.K.S. Subclinical Hyperthyroidism and the Risk of Developing Cardiovascular Disease—A Systematic Review. *Dan. Med. J.* **2020**, *67*, A12190701. [PubMed]
12. Manolis, A.A.; Manolis, T.A.; Melita, H.; Manolis, A.S. Subclinical Thyroid Dysfunction and Cardiovascular Consequences: An Alarming Wake-up Call? *Trends Cardiovasc. Med.* **2020**, *30*, 57–69. [CrossRef] [PubMed]
13. Redford, C.; Vaidya, B. Subclinical Hypothyroidism: Should We Treat? *Post Reprod. Health* **2017**, *23*, 55–62. [CrossRef] [PubMed]
14. Surks, M.I.; Ortiz, E.; Daniels, G.H.; Sawin, C.T.; Col, N.F.; Cobin, R.H.; Franklyn, J.A.; Hershman, J.M.; Burman, K.D.; Denke, M.A.; et al. Subclinical Thyroid Disease: Scientific Review and Guidelines for Diagnosis and Management. *JAMA* **2004**, *291*, 228–238. [CrossRef]
15. Tseng, F.-Y.; Lin, W.-Y.; Lin, C.-C.; Lee, L.-T.; Li, T.-C.; Sung, P.-K.; Huang, K.-C. Subclinical Hypothyroidism Is Associated with Increased Risk for All-Cause and Cardiovascular Mortality in Adults. *J. Am. Coll. Cardiol.* **2012**, *60*, 730–737. [CrossRef]

6. Fernández-Real, J.-M.; López-Bermejo, A.; Castro, A.; Casamitjana, R.; Ricart, W. Thyroid Function Is Intrinsically Linked to Insulin Sensitivity and Endothelium-Dependent Vasodilation in Healthy Euthyroid Subjects. *J. Clin. Endocrinol. Metab.* **2006**, *91*, 3337–3343. [CrossRef]
7. Roos, A.; Bakker, S.J.L.; Links, T.P.; Gans, R.O.B.; Wolffenbuttel, B.H.R. Thyroid Function Is Associated with Components of the Metabolic Syndrome in Euthyroid Subjects. *J. Clin. Endocrinol. Metab.* **2007**, *92*, 491–496. [CrossRef]
8. Kim, B.-J.; Kim, T.Y.; Koh, J.-M.; Kim, H.-K.; Park, J.-Y.; Lee, K.-U.; Shong, Y.K.; Kim, W.B. Relationship between Serum Free T4 (FT4) Levels and Metabolic Syndrome (MS) and Its Components in Healthy Euthyroid Subjects. *Clin. Endocrinol.* **2009**, *70*, 152–160. [CrossRef]
9. Wang, J.; Zheng, X.; Sun, M.; Wang, Z.; Fu, Q.; Shi, Y.; Cao, M.; Zhu, Z.; Meng, C.; Mao, J.; et al. Low Serum Free Thyroxine Concentrations Associate with Increased Arterial Stiffness in Euthyroid Subjects: A Population-Based Cross-Sectional Study. *Endocrine* **2015**, *50*, 465–473. [CrossRef]
10. Nagasaki, T.; Inaba, M.; Kumeda, Y.; Hiura, Y.; Shirakawa, K.; Yamada, S.; Henmi, Y.; Ishimura, E.; Nishizawa, Y. Increased Pulse Wave Velocity in Subclinical Hypothyroidism. *J. Clin. Endocrinol. Metab.* **2006**, *91*, 154–158. [CrossRef]
11. Hamano, K.; Inoue, M. Increased Risk for Atherosclerosis Estimated by Pulse Wave Velocity in Hypothyroidism and Its Reversal with Appropriate Thyroxine Treatment. *Endocr. J.* **2005**, *52*, 95–101. [CrossRef] [PubMed]
12. Nagasaki, T.; Inaba, M.; Kumeda, Y.; Hiura, Y.; Yamada, S.; Shirakawa, K.; Ishimura, E.; Nishizawa, Y. Central Pulse Wave Velocity Is Responsible for Increased Brachial-Ankle Pulse Wave Velocity in Subclinical Hypothyroidism. *Clin. Endocrinol.* **2007**, *66*, 304–308. [CrossRef] [PubMed]
13. Nagasaki, T.; Inaba, M.; Yamada, S.; Shirakawa, K.; Nagata, Y.; Kumeda, Y.; Hiura, Y.; Tahara, H.; Ishimura, E.; Nishizawa, Y. Decrease of Brachial-Ankle Pulse Wave Velocity in Female Subclinical Hypothyroid Patients during Normalization of Thyroid Function: A Double-Blind, Placebo-Controlled Study. *Eur. J. Endocrinol.* **2009**, *160*, 409–415. [CrossRef] [PubMed]
14. Nagasaki, T.; Inaba, M.; Yamada, S.; Kumeda, Y.; Hiura, Y.; Nishizawa, Y. Changes in Brachial-Ankle Pulse Wave Velocity in Subclinical Hypothyroidism during Normalization of Thyroid Function. *Biomed. Pharmacother.* **2007**, *61*, 482–487. [CrossRef] [PubMed]
15. Nagasaki, T.; Inaba, M.; Shirakawa, K.; Hiura, Y.; Tahara, H.; Kumeda, Y.; Ishikawa, T.; Ishimura, E.; Nishizawa, Y. Increased Levels of C-Reactive Protein in Hypothyroid Patients and Its Correlation with Arterial Stiffness in the Common Carotid Artery. *Biomed. Pharmacother.* **2007**, *61*, 167–172. [CrossRef] [PubMed]
16. Tian, L.; Gao, C.; Liu, J.; Zhang, X. Increased Carotid Arterial Stiffness in Subclinical Hypothyroidism. *Eur. J. Intern. Med.* **2010**, *21*, 560–563. [CrossRef]
17. Feng, X.; Zhao, L.; Jiang, J.; Ma, W.; Shang, X.; Zhou, Q.; Zhang, H.; Yu, S.; Qi, Y. Discriminatory Value of Carotid Artery Elasticity Changes for the Evaluation of Thyroid Dysfunction in Patients with Hashimoto's Thyroiditis. *J. Clin. Ultrasound* **2016**, *44*, 298–304. [CrossRef]
18. Owen, P.J.D.; Rajiv, C.; Vinereanu, D.; Mathew, T.; Fraser, A.G.; Lazarus, J.H. Subclinical Hypothyroidism, Arterial Stiffness, and Myocardial Reserve. *J. Clin. Endocrinol. Metab.* **2006**, *91*, 2126–2132. [CrossRef]
19. Obuobie, K.; Smith, J.; Evans, L.M.; John, R.; Davies, J.S.; Lazarus, J.H. Increased Central Arterial Stiffness in Hypothyroidism. *J. Clin. Endocrinol. Metab.* **2002**, *87*, 4662–4666. [CrossRef]
20. Kilic, I.D.; Tanriverdi, H.; Fenkci, S.; Akin, F.; Uslu, S.; Kaftan, A. Noninvasive Indicators of Atherosclerosis in Subclinical Hypothyroidism. *Indian J. Endocrinol. Metab.* **2013**, *17*, 271–275. [CrossRef]
21. Yurtdaş, M.; Özcan, T.; Gen, R.; Aydın, M.K. Assessment of the Elasticity Properties of the Ascending Aorta in Patients with Subclinical Hypothyroidism by Tissue Doppler Imaging. *Arq. Bras. Endocrinol. Metabol.* **2013**, *57*, 395–396. [CrossRef] [PubMed]
22. Peleg, R.K.; Efrati, S.; Benbassat, C.; Fygenzo, M.; Golik, A. The Effect of Levothyroxine on Arterial Stiffness and Lipid Profile in Patients with Subclinical Hypothyroidism. *Thyroid* **2008**, *18*, 825–830. [CrossRef]
23. Tudoran, M.; Tudoran, C. Particularities of Endothelial Dysfunction in Hypothyroid Patients. *Kardiol. Pol.* **2015**, *73*, 337–343. [CrossRef]
24. Tanriverdi, A.; Ozcan Kahraman, B.; Ozsoy, I.; Bayraktar, F.; Ozgen Saydam, B.; Acar, S.; Ozpelit, E.; Akdeniz, B.; Savci, S. Physical Activity in Women with Subclinical Hypothyroidism. *J. Endocrinol. Investig.* **2019**, *42*, 779–785. [CrossRef] [PubMed]
25. Mousa, S.; Hemeda, A.; Ghorab, H.; Abdelhamid, A.; Saif, A. Arterial Wall Stiffness And The Risk Of Atherosclerosis in Egyptian Patients with Overt And Subclinical Hypothyroidism. *Endocr. Pract.* **2020**, *26*, 161–166. [CrossRef] [PubMed]
26. Peixoto de Miranda, É.J.F.; Bittencourt, M.S.; Goulart, A.C.; Santos, I.S.; Mill, J.G.; Schmidt, M.I.; Lotufo, P.A.; Benseñor, I.J.M. Lack of Association between Subclinical Hypothyroidism and Carotid–Femoral Pulse Wave Velocity in a Cross-Sectional Analysis of the ELSA–Brasil. *Am. J. Hypertens.* **2016**, *30*, 81–87. [CrossRef]
27. Grillo, A.; Lonati, L.M.; Guida, V.; Parati, G. Cardio-Ankle Vascular Stiffness Index (CAVI) and 24 H Blood Pressure Profiles. *Eur. Heart J. Suppl.* **2017**, *19*, B17–B23. [CrossRef]
28. Masaki, M.; Komamura, K.; Goda, A.; Hirotani, S.; Otsuka, M.; Nakabo, A.; Fukui, M.; Fujiwara, S.; Sugahara, M.; Lee-Kawabata, M.; et al. Elevated Arterial Stiffness and Diastolic Dysfunction in Subclinical Hypothyroidism. *Circ. J.* **2014**, *78*, 1494–1500. [CrossRef]
29. Masaki, M.; Koide, K.; Goda, A.; Miyazaki, A.; Masuyama, T.; Koshiba, M. Effect of Acute Aerobic Exercise on Arterial Stiffness and Thyroid-Stimulating Hormone in Subclinical Hypothyroidism. *Heart Vessel.* **2019**, *34*, 1309–1316. [CrossRef]

40. Obuobie, K.; Smith, J.; John, R.; Davies, J.S.; Lazarus, J.H. The Effects of Thyrotoxicosis and Its Treatment on Central Arterial Stiffness. *Eur. J. Endocrinol.* **2002**, *147*, 35–40. [CrossRef]
41. Dagre, A.G.; Lekakis, J.P.; Papaioannou, T.G.; Papamichael, C.M.; Koutras, D.A.; Stamatelopoulos, S.F.; Alevizaki, M. Arterial Stiffness Is Increased in Subjects with Hypothyroidism. *Int. J. Cardiol.* **2005**, *103*, 1–6. [CrossRef] [PubMed]
42. Dernellis, J.; Panaretou, M. Effects of Thyroid Replacement Therapy on Arterial Blood Pressure in Patients with Hypertension and Hypothyroidism. *Am. Heart J.* **2002**, *143*, 718–724. [CrossRef]
43. Nagasaki, T.; Inaba, M.; Kumeda, Y.; Ueda, M.; Hiura, Y.; Tahara, H.; Ishimura, E.; Onoda, N.; Ishikawa, T.; Nishizawa, Y. Decrease of Arterial Stiffness at Common Carotid Artery in Hypothyroid Patients by Normalization of Thyroid Function. *Biomed. Pharmacother.* **2005**, *59*, 8–14. [CrossRef]
44. Owecki, M.; Sawicka-Gutaj, N.; Owecki, M.K.; Ambrosius, W.; Dorszewska, J.; Oczkowska, A.; Michalak, M.; Fischbach, J.; Kozubski, W.; Ruchała, M. Pulsatility Index in Carotid Arteries Is Increased in Levothyroxine-Treated Hashimoto Disease. *Horm. Metab. Res.* **2015**, *47*, 577–580. [CrossRef] [PubMed]
45. Chen, G.; Wu, J.; Lin, Y.; Huang, B.; Yao, J.; Jiang, Q.; Wen, J.; Lin, L. Associations between Cardiovascular Risk, Insulin Resistance, Beta-Cell Function and Thyroid Dysfunction: A Cross-Sectional Study in She Ethnic Minority Group of Fujian Province in China. *Eur. J. Endocrinol.* **2010**, *163*, 775–782. [CrossRef] [PubMed]
46. Laugesen, E.; Moser, E.; Sikjaer, T.; Poulsen, P.L.; Rejnmark, L. Arterial Stiffness and Central Hemodynamics in Thyroidectomized Patients on Long-Term Substitution Therapy with Levothyroxine. *Thyroid* **2016**, *26*, 779–784. [CrossRef] [PubMed]
47. Inaba, M.; Henmi, Y.; Kumeda, Y.; Ueda, M.; Nagata, M.; Emoto, M.; Ishikawa, T.; Ishimura, E.; Nishizawa, Y. Increased Stiffness in Common Carotid Artery in Hyperthyroid Graves' Disease Patients. *Biomed. Pharmacother.* **2002**, *56*, 241–246. [CrossRef]
48. Kang, C. Using Ultrasound Radio Frequency Technology to Assess Regression of the Structure and Function of the Carotid Artery by Radioiodine Therapy in Hyperthyroidism Patients. *Arch. Med. Sci.* **2015**, *11*, 1236–1243. [CrossRef]
49. Palmieri, E.A.; Fazio, S.; Palmieri, V.; Lombardi, G.; Biondi, B. Myocardial Contractility and Total Arterial Stiffness in Patients with Overt Hyperthyroidism: Acute Effects of beta1-Adrenergic Blockade. *Eur. J. Endocrinol.* **2004**, *150*, 757–762. [CrossRef]
50. İyidir, Ö.T.; Yalcin, M.M.; Altinova, A.E.; Arslan, İ.E.; Ulu, B.U.; Değertekin, C.K.; Törüner, F.S. Evaluation of Ambulatory Arterial Stiffness Index in Hyperthyroidism. *Turk. J. Med. Sci.* **2017**, *47*, 1751–1756. [CrossRef]
51. Gazdag, A.; Nagy, E.V.; Erdei, A.; Bodor, M.; Berta, E.; Szabó, Z.; Jenei, Z. Aortic Stiffness and Left Ventricular Function in Patients with Differentiated Thyroid Cancer. *J. Endocrinol. Investig.* **2015**, *38*, 133–142. [CrossRef] [PubMed]
52. Yildiz, C.; Altay, M.; Yildiz, S.; Çağir, Y.; Akkan, T.; Ünsal, Y.A.; Beyan, E. Arterial Stiffness in Hyperthyroid Patients Is Deteriorated due to Thyroid Hormones. *Arch. Endocrinol. Metab.* **2019**, *63*, 258–264. [CrossRef] [PubMed]
53. Salvi, P.; Furlanis, G.; Grillo, A.; Pini, A.; Salvi, L.; Marelli, S.; Rovina, M.; Moretti, F.; Gaetano, R.; Pintassilgo, I.; et al. Unreliable Estimation of Aortic Pulse Wave Velocity Provided by the Mobil-O-Graph Algorithm-Based System in Marfan Syndrome. *J. Am. Heart Assoc.* **2019**, *8*, e04028. [CrossRef] [PubMed]
54. Grove-Laugesen, D.; Malmstroem, S.; Ebbehoj, E.; Riis, A.L.; Watt, T.; Rejnmark, L.; Würgler Hansen, K. Arterial Stiffness and Blood Pressure in Patients Newly Diagnosed with Graves' Disease Compared with Euthyroid Controls. *Eur. Thyroid J.* **2020**, *9*, 148–156. [CrossRef] [PubMed]
55. Bodlaj, G.; Pichler, R.; Brandstätter, W.; Hatzl-Griesenhofer, M.; Maschek, W.; Biesenbach, G.; Berg, J. Hyperthyroidism Affects Arterial Stiffness, Plasma NT-pro-B-Type Natriuretic Peptide Levels, and Subendocardial Perfusion in Patients with Graves' Disease. *Ann. Med.* **2007**, *39*, 608–616. [CrossRef]
56. Salvi, P.; Grillo, A.; Parati, G. Noninvasive Estimation of Central Blood Pressure and Analysis of Pulse Waves by Applanation Tonometry. *Hypertens. Res.* **2015**, *38*, 646–648. [CrossRef]
57. Yeh, M.W.; Ituarte, P.H.G.; Zhou, H.C.; Nishimoto, S.; Liu, I.-L.A.; Harari, A.; Haigh, P.I.; Adams, A.L. Incidence and Prevalence of Primary Hyperparathyroidism in a Racially Mixed Population. *J. Clin. Endocrinol. Metab.* **2013**, *98*, 1122–1129. [CrossRef]
58. Bilezikian, J.P. Primary Hyperparathyroidism. *J. Clin. Endocrinol. Metab.* **2018**, *103*, 3993–4004. [CrossRef]
59. Bilezikian, J.P.; Brandi, M.L.; Eastell, R.; Silverberg, S.J.; Udelsman, R.; Marcocci, C.; Potts, J.T., Jr. Guidelines for the Management of Asymptomatic Primary Hyperparathyroidism: Summary Statement from the Fourth International Workshop. *J. Clin. Endocrinol. Metab.* **2014**, *99*, 3561–3569. [CrossRef]
60. Rashid, G.; Bernheim, J.; Green, J.; Benchetrit, S. Parathyroid Hormone Stimulates the Endothelial Nitric Oxide Synthase through Protein Kinase A and C Pathways. *Nephrol. Dial. Transplant.* **2007**, *22*, 2831–2837. [CrossRef]
61. Rashid, G.; Bernheim, J.; Green, J.; Benchetrit, S. Parathyroid Hormone Stimulates Endothelial Expression of Atherosclerotic Parameters through Protein Kinase Pathways. *Am. J. Physiol. Renal Physiol.* **2007**, *292*, F1215–F1218. [CrossRef] [PubMed]
62. Schiffl, H.; Lang, S.M. Hypertension Secondary to PHPT: Cause or Coincidence? *Int. J. Endocrinol.* **2011**, *2011*, 974647. [CrossRef] [PubMed]
63. Lee, Y.-H.; Kweon, S.-S.; Choi, J.-S.; Nam, H.-S.; Park, K.-S.; Choi, S.-W.; Ryu, S.-Y.; Oh, S.-H.; Shin, M.-H. Association of Serum Vitamin D and Parathyroid Hormone with Subclinical Atherosclerotic Phenotypes: The Dong-Gu Study. *PLoS ONE* **2017**, *12*, e0186421. [CrossRef] [PubMed]
64. Cheng, Y.-B.; Li, L.-H.; Guo, Q.-H.; Li, F.-K.; Huang, Q.-F.; Sheng, C.-S.; Wang, J.-G.; Staessen, J.A.; Li, Y. Independent Effects of Blood Pressure and Parathyroid Hormone on Aortic Pulse Wave Velocity in Untreated Chinese Patients. *J. Hypertens.* **2017**, *35*, 1841–1848. [CrossRef]

5. Smith, J.C.; Page, M.D.; John, R.; Wheeler, M.H.; Cockcroft, J.R.; Scanlon, M.F.; Davies, J.S. Augmentation of Central Arterial Pressure in Mild Primary Hyperparathyroidism. *J. Clin. Endocrinol. Metab.* **2000**, *85*, 3515–3519. [CrossRef]
6. Rubin, M.R.; Maurer, M.S.; McMahon, D.J.; Bilezikian, J.P.; Silverberg, S.J. Arterial Stiffness in Mild Primary Hyperparathyroidism. *J. Clin. Endocrinol. Metab.* **2005**, *90*, 3326–3330. [CrossRef]
7. Schillaci, G.; Pucci, G.; Pirro, M.; Monacelli, M.; Scarponi, A.M.; Manfredelli, M.R.; Rondelli, F.; Avenia, N.; Mannarino, E. Large-Artery Stiffness: A Reversible Marker of Cardiovascular Risk in Primary Hyperparathyroidism. *Atherosclerosis* **2011**, *218*, 96–101. [CrossRef]
8. Rosa, J.; Raska, I., Jr.; Wichterle, D.; Petrak, O.; Strauch, B.; Somloova, Z.; Zelinka, T.; Holaj, R.; Widimsky, J., Jr. Pulse Wave Velocity in Primary Hyperparathyroidism and Effect of Surgical Therapy. *Hypertens. Res.* **2011**, *34*, 296–300. [CrossRef]
9. Cansu, G.B.; Yılmaz, N.; Özdem, S.; Balcı, M.K.; Süleymanlar, G.; Arıcı, C.; Boz, A.; Sarı, R.; Altunbaş, H.A. Parathyroidectomy in Asymptomatic Primary Hyperparathyroidism Reduces Carotid Intima-Media Thickness and Arterial Stiffness. *Clin. Endocrinol.* **2016**, *84*, 39–47. [CrossRef]
10. Buyuksimsek, M.; Gulumsek, E.; Demirtas, D.; Icen, Y.K.; Sumbul, H.E.; Ogul, A.; Ay, N.; Saler, T.; Koc, M. Carotid-Femoral Pulse Wave Velocity Is Significantly Increased in Newly Diagnosed Hypertensive Patients with Primary Hyperparathyroidism and Significantly Related with Serum Calcium Level. *J. Ultrasound* **2020**, *24*, 439–446. [CrossRef]
11. Wetzel, J.; Pilz, S.; Grübler, M.R.; Fahrleitner-Pammer, A.; Dimai, H.P.; von Lewinski, D.; Kolesnik, E.; Perl, S.; Trummer, C.; Schwetz, V.; et al. Plasma Parathyroid Hormone and Cardiovascular Disease in Treatment-Naive Patients with Primary Hyperparathyroidism: The EPATH Trial. *J. Clin. Hypertens.* **2017**, *19*, 1173–1180. [CrossRef]
12. Sumbul, H.E.; Koc, A.S. The Abdominal Aortic Intima-Media Thickness Increases in Patients with Primary Hyperparathyroidism. *Exp. Clin. Endocrinol. Diabetes* **2019**, *127*, 387–395. [CrossRef] [PubMed]
13. Stamatelopoulos, K.; Athanasouli, F.; Pappa, T.; Lambrinoudaki, I.; Papamichael, C.; Polymeris, A.; Georgiopoulos, G.; Vemmou, A.; Sarika, L.; Terpos, E.; et al. Hemodynamic Markers and Subclinical Atherosclerosis in Postmenopausal Women with Primary Hyperparathyroidism. *J. Clin. Endocrinol. Metab.* **2014**, *99*, 2704–2711. [CrossRef]
14. Barletta, G.; De Feo, M.L.; Del Bene, R.; Lazzeri, C.; Vecchiarino, S.; La Villa, G.; Brandi, M.L.; Franchi, F. Cardiovascular Effects of Parathyroid Hormone: A Study in Healthy Subjects and Normotensive Patients with Mild Primary Hyperparathyroidism. *J. Clin. Endocrinol. Metab.* **2000**, *85*, 1815–1821. [CrossRef] [PubMed]
15. Kosch, M.; Hausberg, M.; Barenbrock, M.; Posadzy-Malaczynska, A.; Kisters, K.; Rahn, K.H. Arterial Distensibility and Pulse Wave Velocity in Patients with Primary Hyperparathyroidism before and after Parathyroidectomy. *Clin. Nephrol.* **2001**, *55*, 303–308. [PubMed]
16. Ring, M.; Farahnak, P.; Gustavsson, T.; Nilsson, I.-L.; Eriksson, M.J.; Caidahl, K. Arterial Structure and Function in Mild Primary Hyperparathyroidism Is Not Directly Related to Parathyroid Hormone, Calcium, or Vitamin D. *PLoS ONE* **2012**, *7*, e39519. [CrossRef] [PubMed]
17. Ejlsmark-Svensson, H.; Rolighed, L.; Rejnmark, L. Effect of Parathyroidectomy on Cardiovascular Risk Factors in Primary Hyperparathyroidism: A Randomized Clinical Trial. *J. Clin. Endocrinol. Metab.* **2019**, *104*, 3223–3232. [CrossRef]
18. Tordjman, K.M.; Yaron, M.; Izkhakov, E.; Osher, E.; Shenkerman, G.; Marcus-Perlman, Y.; Stern, N. Cardiovascular Risk Factors and Arterial Rigidity Are Similar in Asymptomatic Normocalcemic and Hypercalcemic Primary Hyperparathyroidism. *Eur. J. Endocrinol.* **2010**, *162*, 925–933. [CrossRef]
19. Bernardi, S.; Giudici, F.; Barbato, V.; Zanatta, L.; Grillo, A.; Fabris, B. Meta-Analysis on the Effect of Mild Primary Hyperparathyroidism and Parathyroidectomy Upon Arterial Stiffness. *J. Clin. Endocrinol. Metab.* **2021**, *106*, 1832–1843. [CrossRef]
20. McMahon, D.J.; Carrelli, A.; Palmeri, N.; Zhang, C.; DiTullio, M.; Silverberg, S.J.; Walker, M.D. Effect of Parathyroidectomy Upon Left Ventricular Mass in Primary Hyperparathyroidism: A Meta-Analysis. *J. Clin. Endocrinol. Metab.* **2015**, *100*, 4399–4407. [CrossRef]
21. Pamuk, N.; Akkan, T.; Dağdeviren, M.; Koca, A.O.; Beyan, E.; Ertuğrul, D.T.; Altay, M. Central and Peripheral Blood Pressures and Arterial Stiffness Increase in Hypoparathyroidism. *Arch. Endocrinol. Metab.* **2020**, *64*, 374–382. [CrossRef] [PubMed]
22. Underbjerg, L.; Sikjaer, T.; Rejnmark, L. Cardiovascular Findings in Patients with Nonsurgical Hypoparathyroidism and Pseudohypoparathyroidism: A Cohort Study. *Clin. Endocrinol.* **2019**, *90*, 592–600. [CrossRef] [PubMed]
23. Carrillo-Sepúlveda, M.A.; Ceravolo, G.S.; Fortes, Z.B.; Carvalho, M.H.; Tostes, R.C.; Laurindo, F.R.; Webb, R.C.; Barreto-Chaves, M.L.M. Thyroid Hormone Stimulates NO Production via Activation of the PI3K/Akt Pathway in Vascular Myocytes. *Cardiovasc. Res.* **2010**, *85*, 560–570. [CrossRef] [PubMed]
24. Moulakakis, K.G.; Sokolis, D.P.; Perrea, D.N.; Dosios, T.; Dontas, I.; Poulakou, M.V.; Dimitriou, C.A.; Sandris, G.; Karayannacos, P.E. The Mechanical Performance and Histomorphological Structure of the Descending Aorta in Hyperthyroidism. *Angiology* **2007**, *58*, 343–352. [CrossRef]
25. Klein, I.; Ojamaa, K. Thyroid Hormone and the Cardiovascular System. *N. Engl. J. Med.* **2001**, *344*, 501–509. [CrossRef]
26. Ojamaa, K.; Klemperer, J.D.; Klein, I. Acute Effects of Thyroid Hormone on Vascular Smooth Muscle. *Thyroid* **1996**, *6*, 505–512. [CrossRef]
27. Salvi, P.; Palombo, C.; Salvi, G.M.; Labat, C.; Parati, G.; Benetos, A. Left Ventricular Ejection Time, Not Heart Rate, Is an Independent Correlate of Aortic Pulse Wave Velocity. *J. Appl. Physiol.* **2013**, *115*, 1610–1617. [CrossRef]

88. Salvi, P.; Baldi, C.; Scalise, F.; Grillo, A.; Salvi, L.; Tan, I.; De Censi, L.; Sorropago, A.; Moretti, F.; Sorropago, G.; et al. Comparison between Invasive and Noninvasive Methods to Estimate Subendocardial Oxygen Supply and Demand Imbalance. *J. Am. Heart Assoc.* **2021**, *10*, e021207. [CrossRef]
89. Stabouli, S.; Papakatsika, S.; Kotsis, V. Hypothyroidism and Hypertension. *Expert Rev. Cardiovasc. Ther.* **2010**, *8*, 1559–1565 [CrossRef]
90. Duntas, L.H. Thyroid Disease and Lipids. *Thyroid* **2002**, *12*, 287–293. [CrossRef]
91. Wen, J.; Huang, Y.; Lu, Y.; Yuan, H. Associations of non-high-density lipoprotein cholesterol, triglycerides and the total cholesterol/HDL-c ratio with arterial stiffness independent of low-density lipoprotein cholesterol in a Chinese population *Hypertens. Res.* **2019**, *42*, 1223–1230. [CrossRef] [PubMed]
92. Kvetny, J.; Heldgaard, P.E.; Bladbjerg, E.M.; Gram, J. Subclinical Hypothyroidism Is Associated with a Low-Grade Inflammation, Increased Triglyceride Levels and Predicts Cardiovascular Disease in Males below 50 Years. *Clin. Endocrinol.* **2004**, *61*, 232–238 [CrossRef] [PubMed]
93. Taddei, S.; Caraccio, N.; Virdis, A.; Dardano, A.; Versari, D.; Ghiadoni, L.; Ferrannini, E.; Salvetti, A.; Monzani, F. Low-Grade Systemic Inflammation Causes Endothelial Dysfunction in Patients with Hashimoto's Thyroiditis. *J. Clin. Endocrinol. Metab.* **2006**, *91*, 5076–5082. [CrossRef] [PubMed]
94. Libby, P. Inflammation in Atherosclerosis. *Nature* **2002**, *420*, 868–874. [CrossRef] [PubMed]
95. Jain, S.; Khera, R.; Corrales–Medina, V.F.; Townsend, R.R.; Chirinos, J.A. Inflammation and Arterial Stiffness in Humans. *Atherosclerosis* **2014**, *237*, 381–390. [CrossRef] [PubMed]
96. Bernardi, S.; Grillo, A.; Antonello, R.M.; Cola, M.F.; Dobrinja, C.; Fabris, B.; Giudici, F. Meta-Analysis on the Association between Thyroid Hormone Disorders and Arterial Stiffness. *J. Endocr. Soc.* **2022**, *6*, bvac016. [CrossRef]
97. Hanson, A.S.; Linas, S.L. Parathyroid Hormone/adenylate Cyclase Coupling in Vascular Smooth Muscle Cells. *Hypertension* **1994**, *23*, 468–475. [CrossRef]
98. Rashid, G.; Bernheim, J.; Green, J.; Benchetrit, S. Parathyroid Hormone Stimulates the Endothelial Expression of Vascular Endothelial Growth Factor. *Eur. J. Clin. Investig.* **2008**, *38*, 798–803. [CrossRef]
99. Schlüter, K.D.; Piper, H.M. Cardiovascular Actions of Parathyroid Hormone and Parathyroid Hormone-Related Peptide. *Cardiovasc. Res.* **1998**, *37*, 34–41. [CrossRef]
100. Schiffl, H.; Sitter, T.; Lang, S.M. Noradrenergic Blood Pressure Dysregulation and Cytosolic Calcium in Primary Hyperparathyroidism. *Kidney Blood Press. Res.* **1997**, *20*, 290–296. [CrossRef]
101. Gennari, C.; Nami, R.; Gonnelli, S. Hypertension and Primary Hyperparathyroidism: The Role of Adrenergic and Renin-Angiotensin-Aldosterone Systems. *Miner. Electrolyte Metab.* **1995**, *21*, 77–81.
102. Park, B.; Lee, Y.J. Borderline high serum calcium levels are associated with arterial stiffness and 10-year cardiovascular disease risk determined by Framingham risk score. *J. Clin. Hypertens.* **2019**, *21*, 668–673. [CrossRef] [PubMed]
103. Wang, L.; Manson, J.E.; Sesso, H.D. Calcium intake and risk of cardiovascular disease: A review of prospective studies and randomized clinical trials. *Am. J. Cardiovasc. Drugs* **2012**, *12*, 105–116. [CrossRef] [PubMed]
104. Spronck, B.; Heusinkveld, M.H.G.; Vanmolkot, F.H.; Roodt, J.O.; Hermeling, E.; Delhaas, T.; Kroon, A.A.; Reesink, K.D. Pressure-Dependence of Arterial Stiffness: Potential Clinical Implications. *J. Hypertens.* **2015**, *33*, 330–338. [CrossRef]
105. Fliser, D.; Franek, E.; Fode, P.; Stefanski, A.; Schmitt, C.P.; Lyons, M.; Ritz, E. Subacute Infusion of Physiological Doses of Parathyroid Hormone Raises Blood Pressure in Humans. *Nephrol. Dial. Transplant.* **1997**, *12*, 933–938. [CrossRef]
106. Boutouyrie, P.; Chowienczyk, P.; Humphrey, J.D.; Mitchell, G.F. Arterial Stiffness and Cardiovascular Risk in Hypertension. *Circ. Res.* **2021**, *128*, 864–886. [CrossRef]

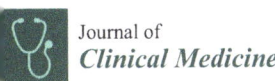

Article

The Impaired Elasticity of Large Arteries in Systemic Sclerosis Patients

Michele Colaci [1,2,*], Luca Zanoli [2,3], Alberto Lo Gullo [4], Domenico Sambataro [2], Gianluca Sambataro [2], Maria Letizia Aprile [1], Pietro Castellino [2,3] and Lorenzo Malatino [1,2]

1. Rheumatology Clinic, Internal Medicine Unit, AOE Cannizzaro, 95126 Catania, Italy; marialetizia_aprile@libero.it (M.L.A.); malatino@unict.it (L.M.)
2. Department of Clinical and Experimental Medicine, University of Catania, 95100 Catania, Italy; dott.zanoli@gmail.com (L.Z.); d.sambataro@hotmail.it (D.S.); dottorsambataro@gmail.com (G.S.); pcastell@unict.it (P.C.)
3. Internal Medicine Unit, Policlinico Rodolico—S. Marco, 95123 Catania, Italy
4. Rheumatology Unit, ARNAS Garibaldi, 95123 Catania, Italy; albertologullo@virgilio.it
* Correspondence: michele.colaci@unict.it

Abstract: (1) Background: Systemic sclerosis (SSc) is an autoimmune disease characterized by endothelial dysfunction and fibrosis of skin and visceral organs. In the last decade, attention has been focused on the macrovascular involvement of the disease. In particular, the observation of increased arterial stiffness represented an interesting aspect of the disease, as predictor of cardiovascular risk. (2) Methods: We recruited 60 SSc patients (52 ± 12 years old, 90% females) and 150 age/sex-matched healthy controls in order to evaluate both intima-media thickness of the right common carotid artery and arterial stiffness using the B-mode echography and the SphygmoCor system® tonometer. (3) Results: The carotid-femoral pulse wave velocity (PWV) was higher in SSc patients than in controls (8.6 ± 1.7 vs. 7.8 ± 1.5 m/s; $p < 0.001$), as was the carotid-radial PWV (7.8 ± 1.1 vs. 6.7 ± 1.4 m/s; $p < 0.001$). The intima-media thickness was higher in SSc than in controls (654 ± 108 vs. 602 ± 118 μm; $p = 0.004$). The other parameters measured at carotid (radial strain, Young's modulus, compliance and distensibility) all indicated that arterial stiffness in tension was more pronounced in SSc. Of interest, the direct correlation between PWV and age corresponded closely in SSc. Moreover, a significant difference between SSc and controls as regards the carotid parameters was evident in younger subjects. (4) Conclusions: SSc patients showed an increased arterial stiffness compared to healthy controls. In particular, an SSc-related pathologic effect was suggested by the more pronounced increase in PWV with age and lower values of carotid elasticity in younger SSc patients than in age-matched controls.

Keywords: pulse wave velocity; carotid distensibility; carotid strain; Young's elastic modulus; carotid compliance; systemic sclerosis; scleroderma; arterial stiffness

Citation: Colaci, M.; Zanoli, L.; Lo Gullo, A.; Sambataro, D.; Sambataro, G.; Aprile, M.L.; Castellino, P.; Malatino, L. The Impaired Elasticity of Large Arteries in Systemic Sclerosis Patients. *J. Clin. Med.* **2022**, *11*, 3256. https://doi.org/10.3390/jcm11123256

Academic Editor: Paolo Salvi

Received: 30 April 2022
Accepted: 6 June 2022
Published: 7 June 2022

Publisher's Note: MDPI stays neutral with regard to jurisdictional claims in published maps and institutional affiliations.

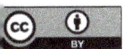

Copyright: © 2022 by the authors. Licensee MDPI, Basel, Switzerland. This article is an open access article distributed under the terms and conditions of the Creative Commons Attribution (CC BY) license (https://creativecommons.org/licenses/by/4.0/).

1. Introduction

Systemic sclerosis (SSc) is characterized by endothelial dysfunction and diffuse vasculopathy. Traditionally, the vascular involvement of SSc was considered mainly microvascular, leading to tissue ischemia. Raynaud's phenomenon, digital ulcers, as well as pulmonary arterial hypertension are typical SSc features that pathogenetically identify functional and structural alterations of microvasculature [1,2]. However, in the last decade, increasing evidence that large arteries are also affected was accumulated [3–5].

Arterial stiffness is a typical sign of arterial dysfunction, even in the absence of overt vascular abnormalities. The main pathogenetic feature is damage to elastin fibers of the aorta and its main branches, which are replaced by collagen overproduction [6]. Furthermore, the increase in vascular smooth-muscle cells and the infiltration of lymphocytes that secrete metalloproteinases and cytokines, such as transforming growth factor-ß, also contribute to arterial wall stiffening [6].

Arterial stiffness is well recognized as an independent cardiovascular risk factor; therefore, its assessment is clinically relevant [7–9]. The measurement of arterial stiffness may be easily performed by a simple, non-invasive evaluation of the pulse wave velocity (PWV). Several studies in the literature showed that SSc patients presented increased PWV if compared with healthy age/sex-matched controls, suggesting that the autoimmune disease is also responsible for macrovascular alterations [3,5,10–22]. Nonetheless, arterial stiffness is a well-recognized crossroad of different pathophysiological states, such as arterial hypertension, diabetes mellitus, smoking-related complications, and dyslipidemia [7–9,23]. In this study, we aimed to investigate the macrovascular involvement in SSc by measuring aortic stiffness together with the behavior of the so far unknown carotid elastic parameters, in order to identify additional alterations, if any, of carotid wall elasticity associated with SSc.

2. Materials and Methods

2.1. Patients

We recruited consecutive SSc patients classified according to the 2013 ACR/EULAR criteria [24] and referred to the Rheumatology Clinic of the Cannizzaro hospital or to the Rheumatology Unit of the ARNAS Garibaldi hospital, both in Catania, Italy. The SSc series was paired with a control group of the same ethnicity, matched for age and sex, randomly selected from a database including healthy outpatients referred to the clinic for cardiovascular diseases prevention, Internal Medicine Unit, Policlinico Rodolico—S.Marco, Catania, Italy.

SSc patients and controls affected by diseases associated with arterial stiffening, such as arterial hypertension, diabetes mellitus, chronic kidney disease, dyslipidemia, atherosclerotic diseases (i.e., myocardial infarction, stroke and peripheral arterial diseases), chronic heart failure and current or former smoking habits, permanent or paroxysmal atrial fibrillation, were excluded from this study.

Chronic vasoactive treatments were not interrupted for the study. However, in the case of prostanoid infusion therapy, the measurements of vascular parameters were performed at least 3 weeks after the last prostanoid administration.

All demographic, clinical, laboratory and instrumental characteristics of SSc patients had already been collected in their clinical records. These records included: clinical history, data from the physical examination, C-reactive protein, erythrocyte sedimentation rate, complete blood counts, indices of liver and renal function, autoantibody profiles, plasma NT-pro-BNP, spirometry, DLCO measurement, chest high-resolution computed tomography, ECG and echocardiography.

All patients gave their informed consent to the study, which was carried out in accordance with the ethical standards of the 1964 Helsinki Declaration and its later amendments and approved by the Ethics Committee of Catania 1 (protocol n. 403, 13 March 2017).

2.2. Methods

All participants were studied in a vascular clinic by the same trained operator (L.Z.) blinded to patients' clinical histories. Vascular evaluations were performed in a quiet room with a controlled temperature of $22 \pm 1\,°C$ between 9:00 and 11:00 a.m. The patients were fasting and refrained from caffeine, alcohol and exercise before the study for at least 12 h.

After 15 min of rest in a supine position, brachial blood pressure was measured three times, 2 min apart, using a validated oscillometric device (Spacelabs 90217 ambulatory blood pressure monitor: Issaquah, WA, USA) [25]. The mean value of three measurements was used in this study.

The study of right common carotid artery was performed as previously reported [26]. Longitudinal B-mode (60 Hz, 128 radiofrequency lines) and fast B-mode (600 Hz, 14 radiofrequency lines) images of the artery 2 cm below the carotid bulb were obtained using a high-precision echo tracking device (MyLab One; Esaote, Maastricht, The Netherlands) equipped with a high-resolution (13 MHz) linear-array transducer. The systolic and diastolic internal diameters (D_s and D_d) and the intima-media thickness (IMT) were measured at the right common carotid artery, according to Laurent et al. [27]. It is not excluded that IMT may be slightly different for measurements at the left side.

The right arm radial pulse wave profile was recorded by applanation tonometry (SphygmoCor system®, AtCor Medical, Sydney, Australia) after recalibration with brachial mean blood pressure (MBP) and diastolic blood pressure (DBP) in the contralateral arm and was used to calculate carotid pulse pressure (PP). Brachial MBP was calculated as brachial DBP + 1/3 × brachial PP.

The carotid PP was used for the calculation of carotid stiffness indexes [28].

The carotid-femoral and the carotid-radial PWV (cfPWV and crPWV, respectively) were measured with the SphygmoCor device, as previously reported [27], using the foot-to-foot velocity method, the intersecting tangent algorithm and the direct distance between the measurement sites [29]: cfPWV (m/s) = 0.8 × [carotid-femoral direct distance (m)/Δt]; crPWV (m/s) = 0.8 × [carotid-radial direct distance (m)/Δt]. The mean value of two consecutive recordings was used for this analysis. When the difference between the two measurements was $\geq$0.5 m/s, a third recording was performed, and the median value was used. The augmentation index (AIx%), an indirect measure of arterial stiffness, was calculated as the difference between the late systolic peak and the early systolic peak pressure, divided by the former.

The carotid distensibility, defined as the relative change in luminal area (ΔA) during systole for a given pressure change, was calculated as previously described [26], assuming the lumen to be circular and using the following equation: carotid distensibility = ΔA/A × carotid PP.

The carotid strain, defined as the relative change in the vessel diameter during systole, was calculated using the following equation: Strain = (Ds − Dd)/Dd, where Ds is the systolic internal diameter and Dd is the diastolic internal diameter.

The circumferential wall stress (CWS), which represents the tangential force that enlarges the vessel, was calculated as follows: CWS (kPa) = (mean BP × Dm)/2IMTm (where Dm and IMTm were the mean values of the internal diameter and the wall thickness during the cardiac cycle). The cross-sectional compliance coefficient (CC) represents the absolute change in lumen area during systole for a given pressure change and was calculated as follows: CC = stroke change in lumen area/local pulse pressure.

The incremental young elastic modulus (Einc), which represents the elastic properties of the material of the arterial wall (assuming that the vessel wall consists of a homogeneous material), was calculated as previously described [26], using the following equation: Einc = [3(1 + A/WCSA)]/DC, given that WCSA is the mean intima-media cross-sectional area.

2.3. Statistical Analysis

All continuous variables are presented as mean ± standard deviation (SD), after confirming their normal distribution by means of the Kolmogorov–Smirnov test; categorical variables are presented as a percentage value.

Clinical and hemodynamic variables were compared using analysis of variance (ANOVA) for continuous variables. Spearman linear regression analysis was performed to verify the existence of any significant correlation between two quantitative variables. p values < 0.05 were considered statistically significant.

The statistical analysis was performed using NCSS 2007 and PASS 11 software (Gerry Hintze, Kaysville, UT, USA).

3. Results

This cross-sectional study included 60 SSc patients and 150 age/sex-matched healthy controls. Table 1 shows demographic characteristics and findings obtained in this study.

Table 1. Data obtained in SSc patients and age/sex-matched healthy controls.

Parameter	SSc Patients $n = 60$	Controls $n = 150$	p-Values
Age, years	52 (12)	53 (13)	0.93
Females, %	90	86	0.62
BMI, Kg/m^2	24.4 (3.7)	25.0 (4.3)	0.40
SBP, mmHg	124 (19)	121 (18)	0.45
DBP, mmHg	70 (9)	71 (9)	0.62
MBP, mmHg	90 (12)	67 (11)	0.81
HR, b/m	68 (9)	67 (11)	0.46
cfPWV, m/s	8.6 (1.7)	7.8 (1.5)	**<0.001**
crPWV, m/s	7.8 (1.1)	6.7 (1.4)	**<0.001**
AIx%	33 (11)	29 (14)	0.06
Internal diameter, mm	5.78 (0.69)	5.69 (0.69)	0.39
Intima-media thickness, μm	654 (108)	602 (118)	**0.004**
Radial strain, %	5.28 (1.29)	6.14 (2.32)	**0.01**
Distensibility, KPa$^{-1} \times 10^{-3}$	20.3 (7.5)	26.4 (13.5)	**0.001**
Young's elastic modulus, KPa $\times 10^2$	517 (210)	436 (178)	**0.01**
Circumferential wall stress, KPa	54 (13)	58 (15)	0.07
CC, m$^2 \times$ KPa$^{-1} \times 10^{-7}$	6.72 (1.95)	7.98 (3.31)	**0.02**

Data are shown as mean (standard deviation). SSc = systemic sclerosis; BMI = body mass index; SBP = systolic blood pressure; DBP = diastolic blood pressure; MBP = mean blood pressure; HR = heart rate; cfPWV = carotid-femoral pulse wave velocity; crPWV = carotid-radial pulse wave velocity; AIx% = augmentation index; CC = cross-sectional compliance coefficient. The internal diameter was measured 2 cm below the bulb of the right common carotid artery. Significant p values have been reported in bold.

Fifty-six out of 60 (93.3%) SSc patients showed the limited skin subset, 27 patients (45%) presented digital ulcers in their clinical history, 32 (53.3%) interstitial lung disease and 3 (5%) pulmonary arterial hypertension (PAH). Furthermore, anti-centromere or anti-Scl70 autoantibodies were found in 35 (58.3%) and 22 (36.7%) SSc patients, respectively.

All patients were treated with calcium channel blockers for Raynaud's phenomenon. Moreover, 13 patients used endothelin-1 receptor antagonists for digital ulcer prevention or PAH, while 35 were treated with monthly infusion of prostanoids.

No significant difference between SSc patients and controls as regards the body mass index (BMI) was noted. The values for blood pressure confirmed that no patients with arterial hypertension were included.

The evaluation of the right common carotid artery showed an increase in IMT in SSc patients compared with controls, but a similar internal diameter. Moreover, stiffness of the arterial wall was significantly increased in SSc patients compared with controls (Table 1). In particular, PWV (measured both as carotid-femoral PWV and radial-femoral PWV) was clearly higher in SSc patients than in controls, indicating a diffuse vascular stiffening involving both elastic and muscular arteries in SSc patients.

Carotid-femoral PWV > 10 m/s was found in 13 out of 60 SSc patients and 11 out of 150 controls (21.7% vs. 7.3%; p = 0.003). These 13 SSc patients had a mean age of 63.9 (range 52–73) years, whereas the mean age of the entire SSc group was 52 ± 12 years (p = 0.0014). No other SSc characteristics distinguished this patient subgroup from the others.

Interestingly, PWV was directly and more closely correlated with age in SSc patients compared with healthy controls, with a steeper regression line, suggesting that SSc is responsible for an accelerated loss of elastic properties of large vessels (Figure 1).

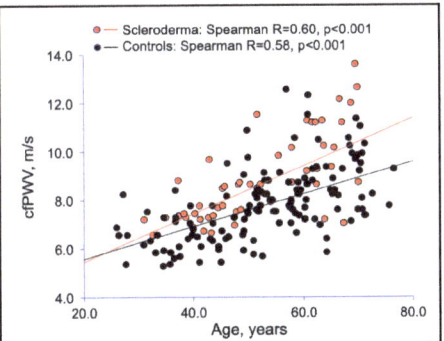

Figure 1. Correlations between carotid femoral PWV and age in SSc patients versus healthy controls.

Macrovascular stiffness was consistent with structural changes of the arterial wall, as shown by the higher IMT of the common carotid artery in SSc than in controls (Table 1, Figure 2), although a similar pattern of direct association between PWV and IMT was demonstrated in both SSc patients and healthy subjects (Figure 3).

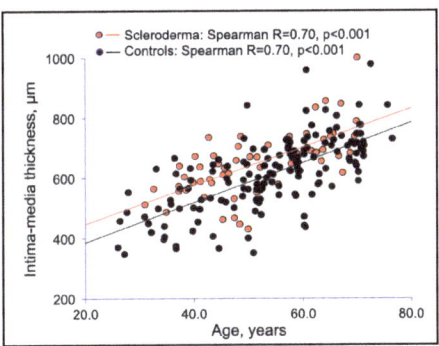

Figure 2. Correlations between IMT and age in SSc patients versus healthy controls.

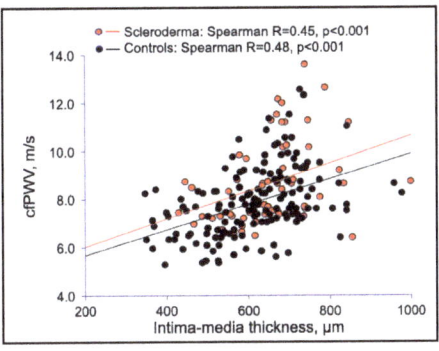

Figure 3. Correlations between carotid femoral PWV and IMT in SSc patients versus healthy controls.

An increased carotid elastic modulus index, along with reduced radial strain, compliance and distensibility, were also observed in SSc patients, compared with controls (Table 1). As shown in Figure 4, in younger SSc patients, carotid wall presented a reduction in its elasticity in comparison with healthy individuals. These findings suggest a direct effect of SSc on arterial wall, leading to a precocious arterial aging. In fact, carotid elastic changes (compliance, distensibility, and radial strain) in sclerodermic patients tends to be more different from controls in younger subjects and overlapping in the elderly (Figure 4).

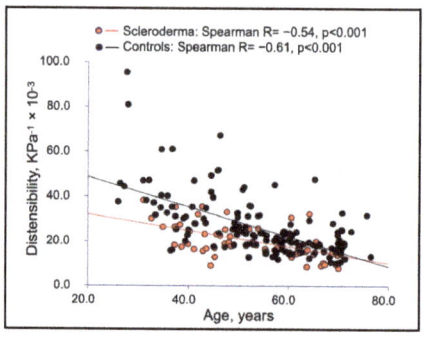
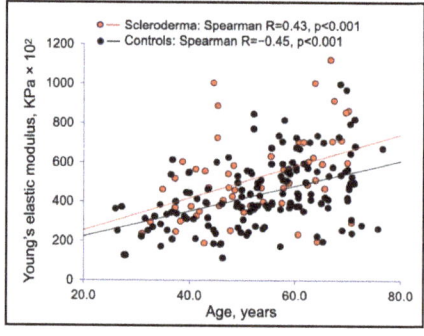
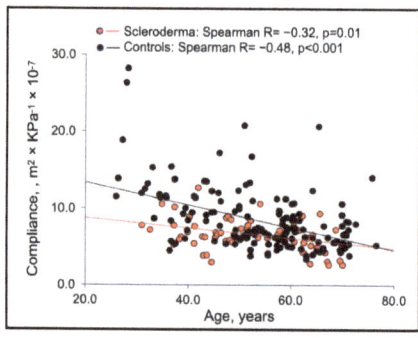
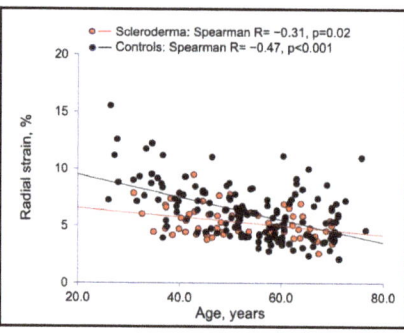

Figure 4. Carotid wall elasticity evaluation in SSc patients versus healthy controls.

Vasoactive therapies did not seem to influence our findings. Finally, except for SSc patients' age, no significant correlations between SSc characteristics and vascular parameters were found.

4. Discussion

In this study, we evaluated the arterial stiffness of large vessels in a group of SSc patients compared with healthy controls. PWV, an index of aortic stiffness, was higher in SSc patients than in controls, in accordance with the literature [3–6,10–22]. In particular, cfPWV was directly and more closely correlated with age in patients than in controls, and was positively associated with IMT. We also demonstrated that vascular stiffening involved both muscular and elastic arteries of SSc patients, as shown by the higher values for both crPWV and cfPWV (Table 1).

In a previous study [18], a cutoff of 9 m/s for cfPWV was considered in order to identify patients with a significant increase. At variance, in the present study, a cutoff of 10 m/s was considered, according to the ESC guidelines for arterial hypertension [30]. However, it would be more correct to consider the absolute values of PWV without choosing a cutoff, because no data are so far available on the clinical and prognostic significance of individual PWV values in rheumatic diseases.

Of note, the increase in carotid Young's elastic modulus and the reduction in radial strain, compliance and distensibility, provided for the first time in SSc evidence further corroborating the concept that a complex dysfunction of macrovascular arterial bed occurs in SSc patients. The carotid stiffening was particularly evident in younger SSc patients, thus emphasizing its association with SSc.

Vascular dysfunction of SSc involved both elastic (i.e., carotid artery and aorta) and muscular (i.e., brachial artery) arteries. Moreover, in SSc patients we found the coexistence of stiffening and thickening processes. The increase in the Young's elastic modulus suggested that alterations of the bioelastic material occur in the arterial wall in SSc. As a consequence of the stiffening process, the radial strain and the distensibility of the common carotid artery were reduced. Of interest, despite the increased common carotid artery IMT in SSc compared with control subjects, the internal diameter was comparable, thus suggesting that, in SSc patients, the thickening of large elastic arteries may proceed in parallel with the enlargement of the arterial wall. Further studies may be needed to confirm this hypothesis.

The increase in arterial stiffness in SSc is a crucial point in the assessment of the cardiovascular risk in SSc patients [5,10,12], providing additional predictive value above IMT measurement for the association with high risk of cardiovascular disease [31]. In our previous study [32] including female patients affected by SSc or diabetes mellitus, the incidence of established coronary artery disease was lower in SSc patients than in diabetics, but similar between the two groups when subjects older than 65 years were considered. This would mean that, when SSc patients grow older than 65 years, the SSc phenotype may become equivalent to that of diabetes.

Rheumatic diseases, such as rheumatoid arthritis (RA), were widely studied as independent risk factors for the increase in cardiovascular risk, due to the chronic inflammatory state [33–35]. In the literature, increased incidence of major adverse cardiovascular events was largely demonstrated for RA patients, in association with long disease duration and scarce disease control [33–35]. Moreover, it is well known that the chronic inflammatory state leads to endothelial activation/lesion and surface expression of adhesion molecules for migration of leukocytes [36]. The inflammatory infiltration of atherosclerotic plaques and progression of vascular injury through the inflammatory pathway may be considered as the *primum movens* of premature atherosclerosis in RA patients [33–36].

Differently from other rheumatic diseases, SSc is characterized by endothelial dysfunction even from its early phase [1,2]. Raynaud's phenomenon, or the onset of digital ulcers, may be considered a direct consequence of the imbalance between endothelium-derived relaxation and vasoconstrictive factors. Endothelial dysfunction is considered an early marker of atherosclerosis [37], so, therefore, we may assume that SSc could contribute *per se* to the development of accelerated atherosclerosis. Consistently, our findings (Figures 1 and 4) suggested that SSc could be involved in the pathogenetic chain of arterial stiffening. In this respect, in a previous study [38], we raised a suggestive hypothesis regarding aortic wall damage in SSc patients. In particular, we found a significant association between nailfold videocapillaroscopy abnormalities and aortic root dilation. These findings could lead us to hypothesize that a microvascular dysfunction of the aortic *vasa vasorum* may contribute to the early damage of the aortic wall. Then, fibrosis, due to collagen overproduction replacing elastin fibers, completes the aortic remodeling. The absence of histological studies on aortic wall from SSc patients, unfortunately, so far does not allow confirmation of this hypothesis

Overall, the presence of a macrovascular involvement in SSc is widely accepted, even though the large heterogeneity of the methodologies used in the literature has so far raised some inconsistencies [3]. However, the presence of SSc-specific endothelial dysfunction makes plausible the development of an SSc-related macrovascular alteration.

In clinical practice, SSc patients may be affected also by systemic hypertension, diabetes, and dyslipidemia or could be smokers. Therefore, the coexistence of several cardiovascular risk factors makes the identification of the intrinsic role of SSc more difficult. For this reason, in this study, we focused on SSc patients without other conditions known to be traditional cardiovascular risk factors.

In our study, we did not find correlations between arterial stiffness parameters and SSc patients' features, besides patients' age. It is probable that the relatively low number of cases included in our study (i.e., few cases with diffuse skin subset or PAH) did not allow us to find specific correlations found in previous studies [12,39]. Further larger cohort studies are needed to clarify this issue.

In conclusion, the evaluation of carotid elasticity, carried out for the first time in our study, could facilitate a better understanding of the specific characteristics of macrovascular abnormalities in patients with SSc.

This study, however, has limitations. In fact, some unknown or underestimated factors might have influenced our findings. For instance, many drugs used in SSc are vasoactive substances that could counteract the long-term evolution of arterial stiffness. Furthermore, immunosuppressive agents may inhibit leukocyte activities also in the arterial wall, thus influencing the natural progression of disease. Therefore, considering the high number of confounders influencing endothelial function and arterial alterations, protocols for the evaluation of cardiovascular risk in SSc should be designed within very large, multicenter, prospective studies.

Author Contributions: Conceptualization, M.C., L.Z., P.C. and L.M.; methodology, M.C. and L.Z.; formal analysis, L.Z.; investigation L.Z.; resources, A.L.G. and M.L.A.; data curation, D.S. and G.S.; writing—original draft preparation, M.C.; writing—review and editing, L.Z., D.S., G.S., P.C. and L.M.; supervision, P.C. and L.M. All authors have read and agreed to the published version of the manuscript.

Funding: This research received no external funding.

Institutional Review Board Statement: The study was conducted according to the guidelines of the Declaration of Helsinki and approved by the Ethics Committee of Catania 1 (protocol n. 403, 13 March 2017).

Informed Consent Statement: Informed consent was obtained from all subjects involved in the study.

Data Availability Statement: The data presented in this study are available on request from the corresponding author. The data are not publicly available due to privacy restrictions.

Acknowledgments: This study is part of the University Research plan 2016–2018, project #1A "Molecular and clinical-early instrumental markers in metabolic and chronic-degenerative pathologies" by Dept. of Clinical and Experimental Medicine.

Conflicts of Interest: The authors declare no conflict of interest.

References

1. Cutolo, M.; Soldano, S.; Smith, V. Pathophysiology of systemic sclerosis: Current understanding and new insights. *Expert Rev. Clin. Immunol.* **2019**, *15*, 753–764. [CrossRef] [PubMed]
2. Thoreau, B.; Chaigne, B.; Renaud, A.; Mouthon, L. Pathophysiology of systemic sclerosis. *Press. Med.* **2021**, *50*, 104087. [CrossRef]
3. Bertolino, J.; Scafi, M.; Benyamine, A.; Aissi, K.; Boufi, M.; Schleinitz, N.; Sarlon, G.; Rossi, P.; Granel, B. Atteintes macrovasculaires de la sclérodermie: État de la question en 2019 [Systemic sclerosis and macrovascular involvement: Status of the issue in 2019]. *J. Med. Vasc.* **2019**, *44*, 400–421. [CrossRef]
4. Psarras, A.; Soulaidopoulos, S.; Garyfallos, A.; Kitas, G.; Dimitroulas, T. A critical view on cardiovascular risk in systemic sclerosis. *Rheumatol. Int.* **2017**, *37*, 85–95. [CrossRef] [PubMed]
5. Meiszterics, Z.; Tímár, O.; Gaszner, B.; Faludi, R.; Kehl, D.; Czirják, L.; Szűcs, G.; Komócsi, A. Early morphologic and functional changes of atherosclerosis in systemic sclerosis-a systematic review and meta-analysis. *Rheumatology* **2016**, *55*, 2119–2130. [CrossRef]
6. Matucci-Cerinic, M.; Kahaleh, B.; Wigley, F.M. Review: Evidence that systemic sclerosis is a vascular disease. *Arthritis Rheum.* **2013**, *65*, 1953–1962. [CrossRef]
7. Chirinos, J.A.; Segers, P.; Hughes, T.; Townsend, R. Large-Artery Stiffness in Health and Disease: JACC State-of-the-Art Review. *J. Am. Coll. Cardiol.* **2019**, *74*, 1237–1263. [CrossRef]
8. Cavalcante, J.L.; Lima, J.A.; Redheuil, A.; Al-Mallah, M.H. Aortic stiffness: Current understanding and future directions. *J. Am. Coll. Cardiol.* **2011**, *57*, 1511–1522. [CrossRef] [PubMed]
9. Ohkuma, T.; Ninomiya, T.; Tomiyama, H.; Kario, K.; Hoshide, S.; Kita, Y.; Inoguchi, T.; Maeda, Y.; Kohara, K.; Tabara, Y.; et al. Brachial-Ankle Pulse Wave Velocity and the Risk Prediction of Cardiovascular Disease: An Individual Participant Data Meta-Analysis. *Hypertension* **2017**, *69*, 1045–1052. [CrossRef]
10. Pagkopoulou, E.; Soulaidopoulos, S.; Triantafyllidou, E.; Arvanitaki, A.; Katsiki, N.; Loutradis, C.; Karagiannis, A.; Doumas, M.; Garyfallos, A.; Kitas, G.D.; et al. Peripheral microcirculatory abnormalities are associated with cardiovascular risk in systemic sclerosis: A nailfold video capillaroscopy study. *Clin. Rheumatol.* **2021**, *40*, 4957–4968. [CrossRef]
11. Jud, P.; Meinitzer, A.; Strohmaier, H.; Schwantzer, G.; Foris, V.; Kovacs, G.; Avian, A.; Odler, B.; Moazedi-Fürst, F.; Brodmann, M.; et al. Evaluation of endothelial dysfunction and clinical events in patients with early-stage vasculopathy in limited systemic sclerosis. *Clin. Exp. Rheumatol.* **2021**, *39* (Suppl. 131), 57–65. [CrossRef]
12. Bartoloni, E.; Pucci, G.; Cannarile, F.; Battista, F.; Alunno, A.; Giuliani, M.; Cafaro, G.; Gerli, R.; Schillaci, G. Central Hemodynamics and Arterial Stiffness in Systemic Sclerosis. *Hypertension* **2016**, *68*, 1504–1511. [CrossRef] [PubMed]
13. Irzyk, K.; Bienias, P.; Rymarczyk, Z.; Bartoszewicz, Z.; Siwicka, M.; Bielecki, M.; Karpińska, A.; Dudzik-Niewiadomska, I.; Pruszczyk, P.; Ciurzyński, M. Assessment of systemic and pulmonary arterial remodelling in women with systemic sclerosis. *Scand. J. Rheumatol.* **2015**, *44*, 385–388. [CrossRef]
14. Ngian, G.S.; Sahhar, J.; Wicks, I.P.; Van Doornum, S. Arterial stiffness is increased in systemic sclerosis: A cross-sectional comparison with matched controls. *Clin. Exp. Rheumatol.* **2014**, *32* (Suppl. 86), S161–S166.
15. Uçar Elalmış, Ö.; Çiçekçioğlu, H.; Karagöz, A.; Ozbalkan Aşlar, Z.; Karaaslan, Y. Evaluation of aortic elastic properties in patients with systemic sclerosis. *Turk Kardiyol. Dern. Ars.* **2014**, *42*, 635–642. [CrossRef] [PubMed]
16. Sunbul, M.; Tigen, K.; Ozen, G.; Durmus, E.; Kivrak, T.; Cincin, A.; Kepez, A.; Atas, H.; Direskeneli, H.; Basaran, Y. Evaluation of arterial stiffness and hemodynamics by oscillometric method in patients with systemic sclerosis. *Wien. Klin. Wochenschr.* **2013**, *125*, 461–466. [CrossRef] [PubMed]
17. Turiel, M.; Gianturco, L.; Ricci, C.; Sarzi-Puttini, P.; Tomasoni, L.; Colonna, V.; Ferrario, P.; Epis, O.; Atzeni, F. Silent cardiovascular involvement in patients with diffuse systemic sclerosis: A controlled cross-sectional study. *Arthritis Care Res.* **2013**, *65*, 274–280. [CrossRef]
18. Colaci, M.; Giuggioli, D.; Manfredi, A.; Sebastiani, M.; Coppi, F.; Rossi, R.; Ferri, C. Aortic pulse wave velocity measurement in systemic sclerosis patients. *Reumatismo* **2012**, *64*, 360–367. [CrossRef]
19. Liu, J.; Zhang, Y.; Cao, T.S.; Duan, Y.Y.; Yuan, L.J.; Yang, Y.L.; Li, Y.; Yao, L. Preferential macrovasculopathy in systemic sclerosis detected by regional pulse wave velocity from wave intensity analysis: Comparisons of local and regional arterial stiffness parameters in cases and controls. *Arthritis Care Res.* **2011**, *63*, 579–587. [CrossRef]
20. Soltész, P.; Dér, H.; Kerekes, G.; Szodoray, P.; Szücs, G.; Dankó, K.; Shoenfeld, Y.; Szegedi, G.; Szekanecz, Z. A comparative study of arterial stiffness, flow-mediated vasodilation of the brachial artery, and the thickness of the carotid artery intima-media in patients with systemic autoimmune diseases. *Clin. Rheumatol.* **2009**, *28*, 655–662. [CrossRef] [PubMed]
21. Cypiene, A.; Laucevicius, A.; Venalis, A.; Dadoniene, J.; Ryliskyte, L.; Petrulioniene, Z.; Kovaite, M.; Gintautas, J. The impact of systemic sclerosis on arterial wall stiffness parameters and endothelial function. *Clin. Rheumatol.* **2008**, *27*, 1517–1522. [CrossRef]
22. Tímár, O.; Soltész, P.; Szamosi, S.; Dér, H.; Szántó, S.; Szekanecz, Z.; Szűcs, G. Increased arterial stiffness as the marker of vascular involvement in systemic sclerosis. *J. Rheumatol.* **2008**, *35*, 1329–1333.
23. Maloberti, A.; Vallerio, P.; Triglione, N.; Occhi, L.; Panzeri, F.; Bassi, I.; Pansera, F.; Piccinelli, E.; Peretti, A.; Garatti, L.; et al. Vascular Aging and Disease of the Large Vessels: Role of Inflammation. *High Blood Press. Cardiovasc. Prev.* **2019**, *26*, 175–182. [CrossRef]

24. Van den Hoogen, F.; Khanna, D.; Fransen, J.; Johnson, S.R.; Baron, M.; Tyndall, A.; Matucci-Cerinic, M.; Naden, R.P.; Medsger, T.A., Jr.; Carreira, P.E.; et al. 2013 classification criteria for systemic sclerosis: An American College of Rheumatology/European League against Rheumatism collaborative initiative. *Arthritis Rheum.* **2013**, *65*, 2737–2747. [CrossRef]
25. O'Brien, E.; Waeber, B.; Parati, G.; Staessen, J.; Myers, M.G. Blood pressure measuring devices: Recommendations of the European Society of Hypertension. *BMJ* **2001**, *322*, 531–536. [CrossRef]
26. Zanoli, L.; Empana, J.P.; Perier, M.C.; Alivon, M.; Ketthab, H.; Castellino, P.; Laude, D.; Thomas, F.; Pannier, B.; Laurent, S.; et al. Increased carotid stiffness and remodelling at early stages of chronic kidney disease. *J. Hypertens.* **2019**, *37*, 1176–1182. [CrossRef]
27. Laurent, S.; Cockcroft, J.; Van Bortel, L.; Boutouyrie, P.; Giannattasio, C.; Hayoz, D.; Pannier, B.; Vlachopoulos, C.; Wilkinson, I.; Struijker-Boudier, H. European Network for Non-invasive Investigation of Large Arteries. Expert consensus document on arterial stiffness: Methodological issues and clinical applications. *Eur. Heart J.* **2006**, *27*, 2588–2605. [CrossRef]
28. Zanoli, L.; Lentini, P.; Boutouyrie, P.; Fatuzzo, P.; Granata, A.; Corrao, S.; Gaudio, A.; Inserra, G.; Rapisarda, F.; Rastelli, S.; et al. Pulse wave velocity differs between ulcerative colitis and chronic kidney disease. *Eur. J. Int. Med.* **2018**, *47*, 36–42. [CrossRef]
29. Van Bortel, L.M.; Laurent, S.; Boutouyrie, P.; Chowienczyk, P.; Cruickshank, J.K.; De Backer, T.; Filipovsky, J.; Huybrechts, S.; Mattace-Raso, F.U.; Protogerou, A.D.; et al. Expert consensus document on the measurement of aortic stiffness in daily practice using carotid-femoral pulse wave velocity. *J. Hypertens.* **2012**, *30*, 445–448. [CrossRef]
30. Williams, B.; Mancia, G.; Spiering, W.; Agabiti Rosei, E.; Azizi, M.; Burnier, M.; Clement, D.L.; Coca, A.; de Simone, G.; Dominiczak, A.; et al. 2018 ESC/ESH Guidelines for the management of arterial hypertension. *Eur. Heart J.* **2018**, *39*, 3021–3104. [CrossRef]
31. Yoon, J.H.; Cho, I.J.; Chang, H.J.; Sung, J.M.; Lee, J.; Ryoo, H.; Shim, C.Y.; Hong, G.R.; Chung, N. The Value of Elastic Modulus Index as a Novel Surrogate Marker for Cardiovascular Risk Stratification by Dimensional Speckle-Tracking Carotid Ultrasonography. *J. Cardiovasc. Ultrasound* **2016**, *24*, 215–222. [CrossRef]
32. Colaci, M.; Giuggioli, D.; Spinella, A.; Vacchi, C.; Lumetti, F.; Mattioli, A.V.; Coppi, F.; Aiello, V.; Perticone, M.; Malatino, L.; et al. Established coronary artery disease in systemic sclerosis compared to type 2 diabetic female patients: A cross-sectional study. *Clin. Rheumatol.* **2019**, *38*, 1637–1642. [CrossRef]
33. Restivo, V.; Candiloro, S.; Daidone, M.; Norrito, R.; Cataldi, M.; Minutolo, G.; Caracci, F.; Fasano, S.; Ciccia, F.; Casuccio, A.; et al. Systematic review and meta-analysis of cardiovascular risk in rheumatological disease: Symptomatic and non-symptomatic events in rheumatoid arthritis and systemic lupus erythematosus. *Autoimmun. Rev.* **2022**, *21*, 102925. [CrossRef]
34. Rezuș, E.; Macovei, L.A.; Burlui, A.M.; Cardoneanu, A.; Rezuș, C. Ischemic Heart Disease and Rheumatoid Arthritis-Two Conditions, the Same Background. *Life* **2021**, *11*, 1042. [CrossRef]
35. Weber, B.; Liao, K.P.; DiCarli, M.; Blankstein, R. Cardiovascular disease prevention in individuals with underlying chronic inflammatory disease. *Curr. Opin. Cardiol.* **2021**, *36*, 549–555. [CrossRef]
36. Hong, J.; Maron, D.J.; Shirai, T.; Weyand, C.M. Accelerated atherosclerosis in patients with chronic inflammatory rheumatologic conditions. *Int. J. Clin. Rheumatol.* **2015**, *10*, 365–381. [CrossRef]
37. Mussbacher, M.; Schossleitner, K.; Kral-Pointner, J.B.; Salzmann, M.; Schrammel, A.; Schmid, J.A. More than Just a Monolayer: The Multifaceted Role of Endothelial Cells in the Pathophysiology of Atherosclerosis. *Curr. Atheroscler. Rep.* **2022**, *24*, 483–492. [CrossRef]
38. Colaci, M.; Dal Bosco, Y.; Schinocca, C.; Ronsivalle, G.; Guggino, G.; De Andres, I.; Russo, A.A.; Sambataro, D.; Sambataro, G.; Malatino, L. Aortic root dilation is associated with the reduction in capillary density observed at nailfold capillaroscopy in SSc patients. *Clin. Rheumatol.* **2021**, *40*, 1185–1189. [CrossRef]
39. Soulaidopoulos, S.; Pagkopoulou, E.; Katsiki, N.; Triantafyllidou, E.; Karagiannis, A.; Garyfallos, A.; Kitas, G.D.; Dimitroulas, T. Arterial stiffness correlates with progressive nailfold capillary microscopic changes in systemic sclerosis: Results from a cross-sectional study. *Arthritis Res. Ther.* **2019**, *21*, 253. [CrossRef]

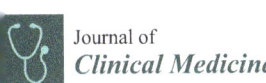

Review

The Gut Microbiota and Vascular Aging: A State-of-the-Art and Systematic Review of the Literature

Davide Agnoletti [1,2,*], Federica Piani [1,2], Arrigo F. G. Cicero [1,2] and Claudio Borghi [1,2]

1. Cardiovascular Internal Medicine, IRCCS Azienda Ospedaliero-Universitaria di Bologna, 40138 Bologna, Italy; federica.piani2@unibo.it (F.P.); arrigo.cicero@unibo.it (A.F.G.C.); claudio.borghi@unibo.it (C.B.)
2. Cardiovascular Internal Medicine, Medical and Surgical Sciences Department, University of Bologna, 40138 Bologna, Italy
* Correspondence: davide_agnoletti@hotmail.com

Abstract: The gut microbiota is a critical regulator of human physiology, deleterious changes to its composition and function (dysbiosis) have been linked to the development and progression of cardiovascular diseases. Vascular ageing (VA) is a process of progressive stiffening of the arterial tree associated with arterial wall remodeling, which can precede hypertension and organ damage, and is associated with cardiovascular risk. Arterial stiffness has become the preferred marker of VA. In our systematic review, we found an association between gut microbiota composition and arterial stiffness, with two patterns, in most animal and human studies: a direct correlation between arterial stiffness and abundances of bacteria associated with altered gut permeability and inflammation; an inverse relationship between arterial stiffness, microbiota diversity, and abundances of bacteria associated with most fit microbiota composition. Interventional studies were able to show a stable link between microbiota modification and arterial stiffness only in animals. None of the human interventional trials was able to demonstrate this relationship, and very few adjusted the analyses for determinants of arterial stiffness. We observed a lack of large randomized interventional trials in humans that test the role of gut microbiota modifications on arterial stiffness, and take into account BP and hemodynamic alterations.

Keywords: vascular ageing; arterial stiffness; central hemodynamics; pulse wave velocity; gut microbiota; gut microbiome; inflammation; oxidative stress

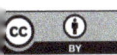

1. Introduction

For several decades, cardiovascular disease (CVD) has been the leading cause of death worldwide. CVD is mainly driven by high blood pressure (BP), which causes damage several target organs. However, there is some evidence that cardiovascular risk due to hypertension is not fully restored by antihypertensive treatment, leading to the concept of residual cardiovascular risk [1]. This is in line with the hypothesis that underlying factors drive both CVD and hypertension, and precede the clinical evidence of the disease, even before hypertension is established. Indeed, subclinical local and systemic inflammation could be one of the main drivers of target organ damage. One of the underlying factors contributing to increased cardiovascular risk is arteriosclerosis, a process of progressive stiffening of the arterial tree associated with arterial wall remodeling, which can precede hypertension and organ damage during the life course. This process has recently been mentioned as "vascular ageing" [2].

The main function of the arterial system is to dampen the pulsatility induced by the stroke volume during the systole.

This is of pivotal importance as organs with high flow and low resistance (e.g., the heart, brain, kidney) are prone to the side effects of increased pulsatility [3]. The large arteries, mainly the aorta, due to their elastic properties, contribute to preserving continuous and low pulsatile flow into target organs. The progressive stiffening of the arterial tree from the center to the periphery, together with the phenomenon of pressure wave reflection, maintains and even amplifies blood pressure in order to guarantee correct organ perfusion Eventually, the peripheral resistances preserve the target organ microcirculation from pulsatility. During the physiological process of ageing, the arterial tree becomes more and more stiff, due to a change in the elastin–collagen ratio and to the deterioration of the arterial extracellular matrix. This leads to increased pulsatility at the peripheral level, where target organs may be injured. Early vascular ageing (EVA) is an attempt to describe early vascular modifications, leading to a stiffer arterial tree as compared with the normal aging process, and conferring higher cardiovascular risk. Arterial stiffness has become the preferred marker of EVA and is easily estimated by the measurement of pulse wave velocity (PWV). The stiffness of an arterial segment can be estimated either "locally" (e.g., in the carotid artery by the doppler ultrasound technique, or in the ascending aorta by magnetic resonance) or "globally" (e.g., the entire aorta by the carotid-femoral PWV [cfPWV] by arterial tonometry). Aortic PWV has become the gold standard for the estimation of aortic stiffness and is an established marker of cardiovascular morbidity and mortality [4,5].

The gut microbiota has emerged as a critical regulator of human physiology, and deleterious changes of its composition and function, commonly referred to as dysbiosis, have been linked to the development and progression of numerous disorders, including cardiovascular diseases. In particular, both direct and indirect roles of gut microbiota have been described on blood pressure regulation and vascular inflammation and stiffening.

The human gastrointestinal tract harbors a vast array of microorganisms that significantly affect host nutrition, metabolic function, gut development, and maturation of the immune system and intestinal epithelial cells [6–8]. In the present review, we refer to "microbiota" as the composition of the whole gut bacterial microorganism. Overall, the microbiota comprises 5 major phyla and approximately more than 1000 species in the large intestine. The gut microbiota promotes digestion and food absorption for host energy production, whereas in the colon, complex carbohydrates are digested and subsequently fermented into short chain fatty acids (SCFAs) such as n-butyrate, acetate, and propionate. The resulting SCFAs seem to regulate neutrophil function and migration, reduce colonic mucosal permeability, inhibit inflammatory cytokines, and control the redox environment in the cell. From a physiological point of view, the main producers of SCFAs belong to the Firmicutes phylum, the single largest grouping of gut bacteria. The Clostridia class in the Firmicutes phylum includes diverse bacteria of medical, environmental, and biotechnological importance. In particular, butyrate and butyrate-producing microbes have been associated with gastrointestinal health in humans and various animal species, and in the human gut are predominately members of clostridial clusters IV (phylum Firmicutes, class Clostridia, genera: *Faecalibacterium, Oscillibacter, Ruminococcus, . . .*) and XIVa (phylum Firmicutes, class Clostridia, genera: *Coprococcus, Roseburia, Clostridum_g24, . . .*) [9]. *Clostridium* clusters XIVa and IV represent the gut's predominant bacteria, accounting for 10–40% of the total bacteria [10]. *Akkermansia muciniphila*, the only member of the Verrucomicrobia phylum, is one of the SCFA-producing bacteria and represents 3–5% of total faecal microbes. A large number of studies has shown that the abundance of *Akkermansia* in the gut is correlated with several health benefits in humans [11]. These beneficial effects are related to the ability of the bacterium of maintaining the mucus thickness and the integrity of the intestinal barrier, providing energy sources (SCFAs) for mucin-producing goblet cells [11]. Studies have shown a relationship between low *A. muciniphila* abundance and increased occurrence of inflammatory metabolic diseases, such as diabetes, obesity, and inflammatory bowel disease [12], which are associated with epithelial gut damage and high permeability.

In investigating gut microbiota characteristics, it is important to explore (i) α diversity: the microbial diversity at the smallest spatial scale (intra individual), assessed by the Shannon or Simplon index; (ii) ß diversity: the microbial diversity at the landscape scale (inter-individual diversity within the same population); (iii) Richness: the total number of species in the unit of study, measured as operational taxonomic units (Chao1 index); (iv)

Firmicutes:Bacteroidetes (F:B) ratio: an index of balance between the two most relevant bacterial families. Furthermore, a high-resolution analysis of the bacterial community down to the species level, and a functional profiling for the assessment of the most represented genes/metabolic pathways and their relative abundance is obtained by a metagenomics analysis, whereas metatranscriptomics is exploited to elucidate which microbial genes annotated in metagenomes are actually transcribed and to what extent. The abundance of health-promoting or detrimental microbiome-derived metabolites (e.g., lipidome and metabolome profile) is assessed by metabolomics analysis.

The mechanisms underlying the association between vascular ageing and the gut microbiota are presented in Figure 1.

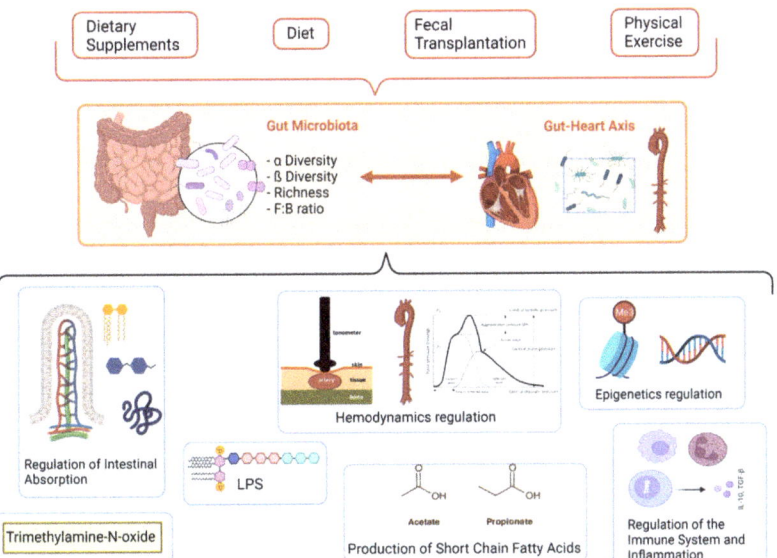

Figure 1. Schemes of the intercorrelation between environmental and biological mechanisms, gut microbiota, and vascular ageing.

2. State-of-the-Art Review

2.1. Microbiota and Hypertension

Data from literature indicate that fruit and vegetable intake is associated with both lower BP values and reduced cardiovascular mortality [13,14], despite a high fat intake [15]. Several micronutrients have been investigated as potential proactive means to achieve such results. Fibers interact with gut microbiota, stimulating growth of specific bacterial phyla, and fiber intake has been associated with lower cardiovascular and all-cause mortality [16].

Among the metabolites produced by the gut microbiota, alanine, n-methylnicotinate, hippurate, and formate have been associated with BP levels. While formate and hippurate are negatively correlated with BP, alanine (produced mainly under a carnivore diet) is associated with higher BP [17]. 4-hydroxyhippurate production by polyphenols microbial metabolism was associated with higher risk of developing hypertension at 10 years (1.17 [95%CL 1.08–1.28]) in a black normotensive population [18]. Subjects with prehypertension or stage 1 hypertension underwent a randomized crossover trial with three diet interventions: carbohydrate-rich, protein-rich, or mono-unsaturated fat-rich diet for 6 weeks each. Urinary metabolites were associated with blood pressure, in particular: proline-betaine (derived from carbohydrate, protein and fat-rich diets), 4-cresyl sulfate and phenylacetylglutamine (derived from the fat-rich diet), N-methyl-2-pyridone-5-carboxamide (derived from the carbohydrate-rich diet) were inversely associated with BP, while carnitine (derived from the protein-rich diet) and hippurate (derived from the carbohydrate-rich diet) were positively associated with BP levels [19]. These results show that different diet interventions, addressing macronutrient content, are associated with distinct hemodynamic effects.

From the available data, hypertension is associated with gut microbiota dysbiosis, characterized by an increased F:B ratio, as well as a drastic decrease in acetate-, butyrate-, and an accumulation of lactate-producing microbial populations. Treatment with an oral minocycline dose, which interferes with microbial growth, has been found to attenuate hypertension and produce beneficial effects on dysbiosis in a rat model [20]. Otherwise, primary alterations in the gut microbiota may elicit hypertension, as was highlighted by an animal study where hypertensive, stroke-prone rats (SHRSP) presented a dysbiotic gut. The main result was that, after transplantation of the SHRSP microbiota in normotensive rats, the authors observed a significant increase in systolic blood pressure (SBP) [21].

If the relationship between gut microbiota and hypertension is so far well described, it is not easy to understand by which pathophysiological mechanisms do the microbial environment and its metabolites regulate BP levels. One of the main characters in the scene is the group of SCFAs.

2.2. The Role of SCFAs

For more than two decades, SCFAs, mainly acetate, propionate and butyrate, have been found to be involved in dilatation in rat tail arteries and human colonic resistance arteries in a concentration-dependent way [22–24]. More recent findings suggest that propionate enhances renin release from juxta glomerular cells, and reduces BP levels in hypertensive mice, as well as in wild mice [25]. In a model of deoxycorticosterone acetate (DOCA)-salt mice, chronic acetate intake was associated with lower BP levels, together with reduced myocardial fibrosis and hypertrophy, and better cardiac function [26]. Interestingly, in the same study, the authors describe that fiber intake could modify the gut microbiota, increasing acetate-producing bacteria, and that fiber and acetate supplementation improved dysbiosis. The positive biological effects of fibers and acetate were ascribed to: (i) the downregulation of cardiac and renal genes for early-growth-response-protein-1 (Egr1), involved in myocardial hypertrophy, fibrosis, and inflammation; (ii) the downregulation of the renin–angiotensin system in the kidney [26].

Several metabolite-sensing G-protein-coupled receptors (GPCRs) have been found to bind with SCFAs, and are important for gut health and immune response regulation [27]. Impaired signaling of these receptors may occur due to excess fat or sugar intake, and could be involved in the deterioration of the intestinal barrier, with lipopolysaccharide (LPS) translocation and subsequent local and systemic inflammation (leaky gut syndrome, see paragraph 2.6) [27,28]. In addition, SCFAs could influence cellular gene expression, binding to diverse histone deacetylases. One of the most important GPCRs is the olfactory receptor 51E2 (named Olfr78 or OR51E2), which is found mainly in arterial smooth muscle cells, autonomic nerves, and in juxtaglomerular apparatus, and binds acetate and propionate, resulting in increased renin release. In Olfr78-/- mice, both BP and plasma renin levels were found to be lower than in wild mice. Indeed, a challenge of propionate in wild mice resulted in a dose-dependent BP lowering, while in Olfr78-/- mice, an accentuated BP-lowering effect was observed with a very low propionate dose, indicating that Olfr78 activation antagonizes the acute hypotensive effect of propionate. This suggests that propionate receptors other than Olfr78 regulate BP levels [25]. GPR41 is found in the vascular endothelium and mediates vasodilation through SCFA stimulation. GPR41-/- mice are not prone to the BP-lowering effect of propionate, and present both higher BP levels and arterial stiffness [29]. This realizes a complex schema where the same metabolite (propionate) can increase renin release, but can also exert a hypotensive effect, depending on the receptor it activates.

According to the data presented, it appears that a biological link exists between microbiota composition, the production of SCFAs, and blood pressure regulation. In particular, beside the effect of blood pressure, it is worth highlighting that SCFA production is almost constantly associated with a beneficial microbiota composition, and that higher butyrate levels are mostly associated with positive local and systemic effects. They include: improvement of colonocytes health; reduction of neutrophils migration; increased tight junction protein, and an anti-inflammatory effect.

2.3. Maternal Heritage and Genetic/Epigenetic Regulation

A study on mice fed with a high-fiber diet or acetate during pregnancy showed that acetate inhibited the histone deacetylaese-9, which resulted in the downregulation of atrial natriuretic peptide (ANP) in the offspring [30]. In another mouse model, mice fed with fiber or acetate presented an improved heart and kidney function, in particular through genetic regulation of fibrosis, fluid absorption, the renin angiotensin system, and inflammation pathways (e.g., by downregulation of transcription factor Egr1, IL-1, Rasal1, Cyp4a14, Cck) [26].

In offspring exposed in utero to maternal obesity, a mouse study found a specific methylation profile in the resistance of mesenteric arteries, which was associated with vascular remodeling and impaired vasodilation [31].

Overall, from the scarce information available, it seems that maternal characteristics and behavior influence offspring in terms of both inflammation pathways and hemodynamics.

2.4. Inflammation and Immune System in Hypertension

Hypertension is associated with immune activation. Increased numbers of central memory CD8+ T cells, activated CD8+ T cells producing Interferon-gamma (IFNγ) and tumor necrosis factor (TNF), and TH17 cells have been reported in patients with hypertension [32]. Monocytes from patients with essential hypertension are preactivated, producing greater amounts of IL-1β, TNF and IL-6 following ex vivo stimulation with angiotensin II or LPS than monocytes from healthy controls [33,34]. A major goal of hypertension treatment is the prevention of end-organ damage. A substantial portion of the vascular, renal, cardiac, and brain damage and dysfunction that accompanies hypertension is mediated by inflammation within these target organs. The innate and adaptive immune responses are critical to the development of hypertension and its consequences [35]. Adaptive immunity activation of both T-cells and B-cells is initiated early in the course of the disease and greatly contributes to important pathogenetic changes, through release of pro-inflammatory cytokines and antibodies [34].

While hypertension and aging are established factors contributing to arterial stiffness, the role of inflammation in the stiffening of the arteries is less well understood.

Arterial stiffness is associated with increased production of reactive oxygen species [36] and proinflammatory cytokines [37]. Furthermore, C-reactive protein itself may play an active role in mediating arterial stiffening, by inducing endothelial dysfunction. The increased vascular inflammation increases vascular fibrosis, smooth muscle cell proliferation, and impair endothelial-mediated vasodilation, which subsequently leads to increased arterial stiffness [38]. Oxidative stress appears to play a role in the pathogenesis of arterial stiffness, as oxidative injury may result in increased vascular inflammation and increased cellular proliferation, which may subsequently lead to impaired arterial elasticity [39].

Multiple studies have shown elevated indices of arterial stiffness in subjects with primary inflammatory disorders, and prospective studies (including 2 RCTs) have demonstrated a reduction in arterial stiffness following treatment with anti-TNF and other anti-inflammatory agents [40–44].

The gut microbiota is thought to modulate immune and inflammatory responses. Germ-free mice present lower levels of TH7 and Treg, and a higher TH2/TH1 ratio than wild mice, which is associated with hypertension development. Furthermore, GPCR are also localized in immunity cells, so that SCFAs are able to interact with and activate them [45]. From the evidence available so far, it is clear that: (i) Inflammatory dysregulation occurs during human hypertension, together with immune system activation; (ii) Vascular ageing, as estimated by arterial stiffness, is strictly influenced by inflammation and oxidative stress, and could precede the development of hypertension; (iii) The gut microbiota can regulate immunity cells and the inflammation response.

2.5. The Role of Trimethylamine-N-Oxide

The pivotal role of the gut microbiota in cardiovascular disease is highlighted by the data concerning trimethylamine-N-oxide (TMAO) and its link to both microbiota and atherosclerosis. TMAO is a molecule transformed from the metabolism of choline by the gut microbiota, starting from dietary phosphatidylcholine. The main sources of phosphatidylcholine are meat, eggs, and foods with a high cholesterol content. The final TMAO plasma concentration depends on diet, gut microbial composition, drugs, and the activity of the liver flavin monooxygenase [46,47].

Plasma TMAO concentration correlates with incidents of major adverse cardiovascular events in patients with acute coronary syndrome [48]. TMAO levels were also associated with ageing, systolic blood pressure, and cfPWV, independent of cardiovascular risk factors [49]. TMAO dietary supplementation increased arterial stiffness in both young and old mice, impaired aortic wall intrinsic mechanical stiffness, and increased aortic wall concentration of advanced glycation end-products [49]. Interestingly, in mice, TMAO infusion amplified the angiotensin II effect in increasing BP [17,50], but did not affect BP levels in normotensive rats, so that it is unclear whether TMAO is proatherogenic or a marker of atherosclerosis [50]. In any case, even if the results of an experimental study show an obligate role for intestinal microbiota in the generation of TMAO from the dietary lipid phosphatidylcholine [51], it is still not clear whether specific patterns of microbiota composition would be associated with different levels of TMAO production. This issue is highlighted by the results of a recent meta-analysis showing that supplementation with probiotic *Lactobacillus rhamnosus GG* was the most efficient in reducing the plasma TMAO level in both humans and animals [52].

2.6. The Role of Lipopolysaccharides

LPSs are found mainly in the gut lumen, as they form the outer membrane of gram-negative bacteria. In situations of increased permeability of the epithelial gut barrier, LPS transmigrates into the blood stream, and it binds to the toll-like receptor-4 by means of CD14 complex. This stimulation induces the release of several proinflammatory cytokines by the NF-kB pathway, with activation of the immune and inflammatory response [53].

Even if LPS enhances the atherosclerotic process and boosts the formation of unstable plaques, its link with hypertension is still debated.

Gut microbiota dysbiosis easily induces both an increase of lumen LPS and a deterioration of the gut epithelial barrier with amplification of tight junction permeability, resulting in the transmigration of LPS; this phenomenon is called the "leaky gut syndrome", and is one of the promoters of systemic inflammation driven by the gut microbiota.

2.7. The Role of Salt

As shown above, different dietary patterns, including a diverse composition of fiber, fructose, and fat, modulate the gut microbiota with various effects on inflammation, the immune system, and BP levels. In this domain, dietary sodium intake has emerged as an important player for its interaction not only with BP levels, but also with gut microbiota, inflammation, and the immune system [54,55].

Sodium and water absorption are regulated by the sodium–proton exchanger 3 (NHE3), which is found both in the gastrointestinal tract and the renal proximal tubule [56]. In a model of spontaneously hypertensive rats, the inhibition of NHE3 resulted in increased fecal content of sodium and water, decreased urinary sodium excretion, and lower BP levels [57]. NHE3-ko mice presented altered gut microbiota, with a beneficial decrease of the F:B ratio [58], but NHE3 deficiency was also found to induce irritable bowel syndrome, with gut dysbiosis [59], making the results difficult to interpret. High salt intake alters gut microbiota, inducing low microbial diversity [60] and the depletion of *Lactobacillus* spp., which is restored after normalization of the sodium dietary content [61]. Moreover, supplementing *Lactobacillus* reduced BP levels and TH-17 cell activation in mice fed with a high-salt diet [61]. Salt intake also affects the Clostridial order, with a reduction of several genera, and an increase in Christensenellaceae, Corynebacteriaceae, Lachnospiraceae, Ruminococcaceae and *Oscillospira*, with exacerbation of colitis [60,62]. It is worth noting that the biological result of the modifications of the genera abundances in the gut is not always predictable, as it depends also on bacterial species-to-species interaction and on activation of specific genes. Indeed, mice fed with a high-salt diet show a higher abundance of *Roseburia*, a butyrate-producing species [60], but lower butyrate production, perhaps due to the loss of interaction with *Lactobacillus* spp., which is depleted [62].

High salt intake can increase several proinflammatory cytokines, such as interleukin (IL)-6 and IL-23 [63], and may activate TH-17 cells with production of IL-17 and IL-22 [55,61], which are associated with the development of hypertension [64]. Interestingly, as shown before, these activation mechanisms are likely mediated by the gut microbiota [45,65].

From the data presented here, it emerges that salt intake is associated with several biological mechanisms related to disbiosis and inflammatory pathways.

2.8. Microbiota and Exercise

A relatively recent observational study comparing the fecal bacterial profile of elite male rugby players with non-athlete healthy subjects [66] showed significant differences between the two groups; in particular, athletes had lower levels of Bacteroidetes and greater amounts of Firmicutes than the controls. After analyzing the gut microbiota composition of the participants of the American Gut Project, it was concluded that increasing exercise frequency from never to daily causes greater diversity among the Firmicutes phylum (including *Faecalibacterium prausnitzii* and species from the genus *Oscillospira*, *Lachnospira*, and *Coprococcus*), which contributes to a healthier gut environment. In the limited studies available in animal models, exercise in rats was associated with higher Bacteroidetes and lower Firmicutes in fecal matter, whereas the cecal microbiota following 6 weeks of exercise activity presented a greater abundance of selected Firmicutes species and a lower abundance of *Bacteroides/Prevotella* genera. Similarly, at the phyla level, exercise reduced Bacteroidetes, while it increased Firmicutes, Proteobacteria, and Actinobacteria in mice. Even if data on bacterial genera are lacking, this microbiota composition could represent a beneficial adaptation to exercise. Rats that participated in voluntary running exercise had increased colonic butyrate concentrations compared to sedentary rats, due to higher levels of butyrate-producing bacteria from the Firmicutes phylum (SM7/11 and T2-87) in their cecum. Hsu et al. investigated the influence that intestinal microbiota has on endurance swimming time in specific pathogen-free (SPF), germ-free (GF), and *Bacteroides fragilis* (BF) gnotobiotic mice. They found that the antioxidant capacity was deeply different in the three mice models, as serum levels of glutathione peroxidase (GPx) and catalase (CAT), two major antioxidants able to convert hydrogen peroxide into water, were greater in SPF than GF mice. Additionally, serum superoxide dismutase (SOD) activity, pivotal for the clearance of superoxyde radicals, was lower in BF than SPF and GF mice. The authors found that endurance swimming time was longer for SPF and BF mice than GF mice, suggesting that the gut microbiota composition is crucial for exercise performance, and could also be linked to the activity of antioxidant enzyme systems. The types and amount of SCFAs produced by gut microorganisms are determined by the composition of the gut microbiota and the metabolic interactions between microbial species, but also by the amount, type, and balance of the main dietary macro- and micronutrients [67].

Exercise training seems to have a role in gut microbiota composition and function, and the bacterial patterns may evolve during exercise, potentially providing beneficial adaptation to physical stress. At the same time, the gut microbiota composition itself may influence the exercise performance.

2.9. Nutrition and Stiffness

The relationship between dietary components and arterial stiffness has been investigated in limited and heterogeneous studies that seem to indicate a beneficial effect of certain nutrients on vascular ageing.

Higher anthocyanin and flavone, cocoa intake, as well as phytoestrogens such as isoflavones and lignans, are associated with lower arterial stiffness [68].

Dietary polyphenols have been investigated in several small heterogeneous studies. Cocoa and chocolate, rich in flavonoids and proanthocyanidins, seem to reduce BP levels and cardiovascular risk, with an improvement in measures of vascular health (arterial stiffness and endothelial function), possibly due to the activation of nitric oxide (NO) synthase, and to other antioxidant/anti-inflammatory properties [69,70]. The European Food Safety Authority approved a health claim about the effectiveness of cocoa polyphenols on arterial elasticity, indicating an ideal assumption of 200 mg of cocoa flavanols daily, consumed as 2.5 g high-flavanol cocoa powder, or 10 gr high-flavanol dark chocolate [71]. Although anti-inflammatory and antioxidant effects have been associated with berry and grape juice consumption, there are no sufficient data to establish their relationship with arterial stiffness. On the other hand, the importance of isoflavone (a soy metabolite) in reducing arterial stiffness and BP levels has been highlighted [72].

Curcumin capsule supplementation has shown to reduce PWV in diabetic patients in a randomized trial [73].

3. Systematic Review

3.1. Aim

This systematic review aims to investigate (i) the interdependence between gut microbiota composition and central hemodynamics, and (ii) whether modifications to gut microbiota translate into different vascular aging profiles.

3.2. Methods

3.2.1. Eligibility Criteria

This systematic review is based on population, intervention, comparator, outcome, and setting criteria. Participants: humans or animals included in both observational and interventional studies. Interventions: we considered every kind of intervention (dietary, antibiotics, fecal transplant, dietary supplements, etc.). Comparators: we included any kind of comparator. Outcomes: primary outcomes: (i) modification in PWV; (ii) modification in gut microbiota composition (alpha- and beta-diversity, genera abundances); secondary outcome: relationship between changes in PWV and gut microbiota composition. Study designs: observational, experimental, and interventional trials in humans and animals are included. No restrictions were imposed on language or date of publication. Exclusion criteria: studies without information about either microbiota or arterial stiffness were excluded; editorials, study protocols, reviews, commentary, and letters were also excluded.

3.2.2. Information Sources and Search

The following databases from inception to February 2022 were searched: PubMed/MEDLINE, Scopus, Web of Science. The main electronic search strategy was designed for PubMed/MEDLINE and was adapted as appropriate for each of the other databases.

D.A. and F.P. screened titles, abstracts, and full texts of articles identified in this search, and extracted the data for eligible studies; discrepancies were resolved by consensus.

3.3. Results

The systematic search led to the identification of 24 articles from three databases, of which 12 were based on animal studies and 12 on humans. A flowchart of the final selection of items is shown in Figure 2. Main characteristics of the selected articles are summarized in Table 1.

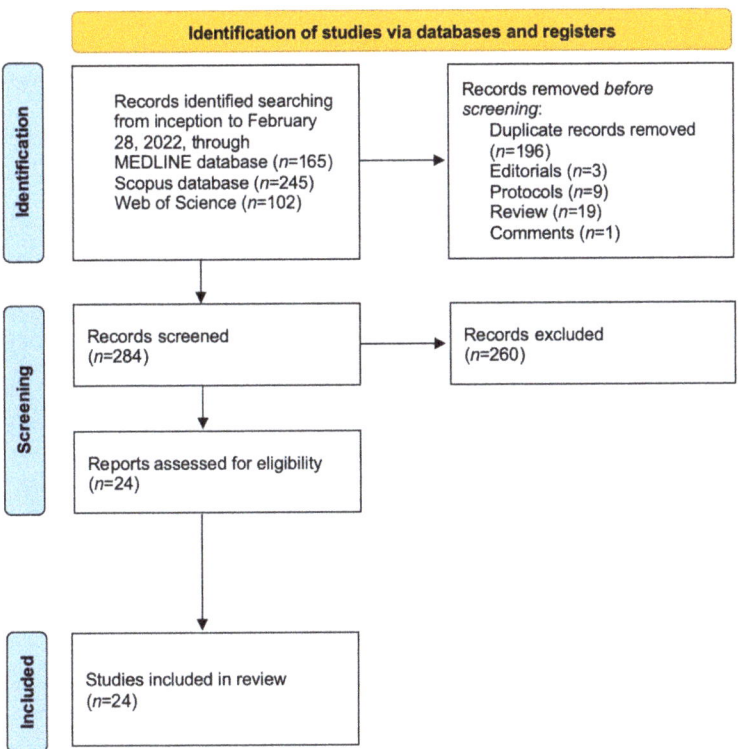

Figure 2. Flow diagram of the Systematic Review.

3.4. Discussion

3.4.1. Animal Studies

Among twelve studies based on animal models, four studies tested diet supplementation with soy [74], dapaglifozin [75], indole-3-propionic acid [76], and hesperidin [77]. Three studies focused on fecal transplantation [78–80], and two on antibiotic treatment [81,82]. Other studies investigated the SCFA receptor [29] and germ-free mice [83]. Only three studies reported data on BP levels [29,49,77]. Nine studies analyzed arterial stiffness by recording PWV by aortic doppler (see Table 1).

Table 1. Characteristics of animal studies.

Authors	n	Marker of VA	Intervention	Duration	Effect on Vascular Ageing	Mechanisms Linked to Microbiota
Guirro, M., 2020 [77]	48	Neuraminidase circulating levels	Hesperidin treatment; two diets for 9 wk (n = 24): standard diet and cafeteria (CAF) diet	9 weeks of diet + 8 weeks of hesperidin	CAF feeding resulted in increased endothelial dysfunction, arterial stiffness, and inflammation. Hesperidin supplementation reduced SBP and markers of arterial stiffness in CAF-fed rats	Urinary metabolites of hesperidin were positively correlated with Bacteroidaceae family.
Liu, H., 2020 [78]	35	PWV at the left common carotid artery	Gavage with feces from either healthy donors (controls) or myocardial infarction patients (CAD) + high fat diet	12 weeks	Mice treated with CAD feces had higher vascular stiffness than controls (Controls: 2.75 ± 0.29 m/s vs. CAD: 3.59 ± 0.27 m/s; $p = 0.043$). No BP data.	In mice treated with CAD feces: increased LPS and pro-inflammatory cytokines; increased activated TH17 cells; reduced Treg cells.

Table 1. Cont.

Authors	n	Marker of VA	Intervention	Duration	Effect on Vascular Ageing	Mechanisms Linked to Microbiota
Battson, M.L., 2019 [79]	40	Aortic PWV (doppler)	Fecal transplantation, 10 controls and 10 obese mice received healthy microbiota, and 10 and 10 received obese microbiota	8 weeks	Control mice receiving microbiota of obese subjects had higher PWV. *Akkermansia* abundance inversely related to PWV. No BP data.	Obese mice had reduced *Clostridia* and *Oscillospira*. Control mice and obese mice receiving microbiota of obese subjects had higher level of *Bacteroides* sp. Control mice receiving microbiota of obese subjects had reduced level of *Akkermansia*.
Natarajan, N., 2016 [29]	10	Aortic stiffness (PWV by doppler and ex vivo)	Gpr41 KO group vs Grp41 WT group	3 and 6 months	At 6 months PWV was significantly higher in KO mice vs WT mice, with similar compliance in ex vivo analysis, suggesting functional vascular alteration. KO mice presented isolated systolic hypertension at baseline	Gpr41 (SCFA receptor) localizes in the vascular endothelium. Vascular endothelium is essential for SCFA-mediated vasodilation to occur, as vasodilation is absent in endothelium-denuded vessels ex vivo.
Edwards, J.M., 2020 [83]	12	Resistance arteries stiffness (ex vivo)	Ex vivo evaluation of vascular stiffness		Resistance arteries from male GF mice present increased vascular stiffness. No changes in vascular stiffness in arteries from female mice. No BP data.	Microbiota influenced the vasoconstriction response.
Cross, T.W.L., 2017 [74]	40	Aortic PWV (doppler)	Ovariectomy vs sham surgery; soy-rich vs soy-free diet	28 weeks	PWV was lowered with soy feeding but was not affected by ovariectomy. No BP data.	Soy-rich diet modified intestinal microbiota composition (lower F:B ratio).
Battson, M.L., 2018 [81]	36	Aortic PWV (doppler)	Standard diet (SD) (n 12) or Western diet (WD) (n 24) for 5 months, then WD mice were randomized to receive broad-spectrum antibiotic cocktail (WD + Abx) or placebo (n 12/group) for 2 months	7 months	PWV progressively increased in WD mice during the 7-month intervention. In WD + Abx, PWV was completely normalized to SD levels. No BP data.	WD had increased Firmicutes and decreased Bacteroidetes and Actinobacteria. Abundance of numerous bacterial taxa were altered by diet; in particular, *Bifidobacterium* spp. were significantly more abundant in SD animals compared with WD.
Brunt, V.E., 2019 [82]	73	Aortic PWV (doppler); ex vivo intrinsic mechanical stiffness	Cocktail of broad-spectrum, poorly absorbed antibiotics in drinking water vs placebo. 4 groups: young controls (YC); young antibiotics (YA); old controls (OC); old antibiotics (OA).	3–4 weeks	At baseline, PWV was higher in OC and OA vs YC ($p < 0.01$). PWV increased in YC but not in YA during intervention. In OA, PWV was reduced at the end of the intervention. Antibiotic treatment in old mice was associated with a partial improvement back towards young levels ($p = 0.047$ vs. OC). Aortic elastin protein expression was lower in OC vs. YC ($p = 0.02$), but was restored in OA. No BP modifications were registered.	Ageing was associated with greater alpha diversity. Old mice demonstrated several bacterial markers of gut dysbiosis and/or inflammation. Three-fold age-related increase in circulating plasma TMAO levels. In both young and old mice, antibiotic treatment suppressed TMAO levels.

Table 1. Cont.

Authors	n	Marker of VA	Intervention	Duration	Effect on Vascular Ageing	Mechanisms Linked to Microbiota
Lee, D.M., 2018 [75]	47	Aortic PWV (doppler); ex vivo	(1) standard diet; (2) standard diet + dapagliflozin (60 mg dapagliflozin/kg diet). Controls ($n = 11$); Controls + dapa ($n = 12$); Diabetics (Db) ($n = 12$); Db + dapa ($n = 12$).	8 weeks	Dapagliflozin treatment improved both endothelium-dependent dilatation (EDD) and Endothelium-independent dilation (EID) in Db mice. PWV was negatively and EID-EDD positively correlated with *Akkermansia* abundance. PWV was positively correlated with Firmicutes and F:B ratio. No BP data.	Significantly reduced richness and diversity in the Db + dapa group compared to controls. Bacteroidetes and Proteobacteria were influenced by dapagliflozin treatment in Db + dapa. Db + dapa had a significantly lower F:B ratio than the other treatment groups. *Oscillospira* was significantly reduced in the Db + dapa compared to all other groups
Lee, D.M., 2020 [76]	48	Aortic PWV (doppler)	Standard (SD) vs Western diet (WD). Indole-3-propionic acid (IPA) vs placebo. (1) SD + placebo, (2) WD +placebo, (3) SD + IPA, (4) WD + IPA. ($n = 12$ mice/group).	5 months	IPA supplementation did not affect PWV in WD, but impaired PWV in SD. *Bifidobacterium* reduction by WD was related to PWV. No BP data.	WD feeding decreased *Bifidobacterium*. Reduced abundance of *Bifidobacterium* was observed in SD + IPA.
Trikha, S.R.J., 2021 [80]	10	Aortic PWV (doppler)	2 age-matched male and 2 female (1 of each lean [LM], and 1 obese [OBM]) microbiota donors to form cohorts 1 and 2 of inoculated mice.		PWV was increased in OBM mice vs. GF mice. In cohort 2, OBM mice displayed a marked increase in PWV vs. LM mice. No BP data.	Mouse microbiota profiles clustered according to their transplant donor groups. Taxa appear to be driving this separation, *Bacteroides ovatus* and *Parabacteroides diastonis* were consistently associated with LM mice.

VA stands for Vascular ageing; SBP, systolic blood pressure; PWV, pulse wave velocity; LPS, lipopolysaccharides; Gpr, G-protein coupled receptor; SCFA, short-chain fatty acid; GF, germ-free; F:B, Firmicutes/Bacteroidetes ratio; TMAO, trimethylamine-N-oxide.

Supplementation studies. In all studies, independent of the type of supplement, the modifications of gut microbiota were associated with parallel modification to arterial stiffness. In particular, it seems that the changes of the gut microbiota linked to a better configuration are correlated with lower arterial stiffness. (i) In rats selectively bred for low running capacity, soy supplementation significantly improved their blood lipid profile, adipose tissue inflammation, and aortic stiffness; it shifted the cecal microbiota toward a lower F:B ratio. Soy-fed rats had lower mRNA expression of CD11c (inflammatory macrophage marker) and of the proinflammatory cytokine IL-6 [74]. (ii) Diabetic mice presented higher cfPWV than controls. Supplementation with dapagliflozin was associated with reduced microbiota diversity and richness, but failed to improve arterial stiffness in the study by Lee DM. Interestingly, arterial stiffness was negatively associated with *Akkermansia* abundance and positively with F:B ratio [75]. (iii) The supplementation with indole-3-propionic acid (a microbial metabolite of the essential aromatic amino acid, tryptophan) did not improve cfPWV in mice fed a western diet, and even worsened cfPWV in control mice, which also presented a reduced abundance of *Bifidobacterium* [76]. (iv) Supplementation with hesperidin resulted in higher urinary excretions of hippurate and other polyphenols metabolites. As most polyphenols are metabolized by gut microbiota before being absorbed, in this study, urinary metabolites of hesperidin were positively correlated with a microbial family, the Bacteroidaceae (phylum Bacteroidetes). From the vascular point of view, hesperidin supplementation was able to reduce both the circulating levels of neuraminidase (a biological marker of arterial stiffness [84]) and the systolic BP [77].

These results show a biological effect of polyphenols on vascular ageing, and indicate gut microbiota modification as the potential mechanism of the effect.

Fecal transplantation. Arterial stiffness was associated with gut microbiota modifications induced by fecal transplantation. In particular, PWV was positively associated with Clostridium genus, which contains most of the deleterious *Clostridium* species (e.g., *C. botulinum, C. perfringens, C. difficile*), and with gut permeability and obese microbiota, whereas it was negatively associated with Akkermansia abundance. (i) Local carotid stiffness was investigated in mice fed with a high-fat diet and gavaged with gut microbiota of either healthy donors ("Con" group) or patients with myocardial infarction ("CAD" group). The characteristics of the gut microbiota from CAD patients were transmissible and associated with low fermentation and high inflammation, and with increased abundance of *Clostridium symbiosum* (Clostridium genus) and Eggerthella genus. CAD mice also presented a higher carotid stiffness than the Con group of about 1 m/s [78]. (ii) An interesting study from Battson M et al. investigated fecal transplantation in four groups: control mice fed with either normal microbiota (Con + Con) or microbiota from obese mice (Con + Ob); and obese mice fed with either normal microbiota (Ob + Con) or obese (Ob + Ob) microbiota. Higher PWV was observed after obese microbiota gavage in control mice, together with altered gut permeability and SCFA content. Importantly, Akkermansia abundance was strongly inversely related to PWV with r = −0.8 ($p < 0.0001$) [79]. (iii) In another experimental study, the microbiota from either lean (LM) or obese (OBM) patients was used to feed two cohorts of mice: one from male and one from female patients. Aortic stiffness was higher in OBM than germ-free mice, and in cohort 2, it was also higher in OBM than LM mice. Mouse microbiota profiles clustered according to their transplant donor groups, possibly explaining the difference in arterial stiffness [80].

Antibiotic treatment. In both studies that we found, antibiotic treatment induced deep changes in gut microbiota composition, which were associated with parallel changes in arterial stiffness. (i) The role of antibiotic treatment was investigated in mice fed with a western diet for 5 months. During the study, mice presented a progressive increase in aortic PWV, which was completely reversed by 2-month antibiotic supplementation. The western diet increased the F:B ratio and Ruminococcus abundance; it reduced the abundance of Bifidobacterium, and increased inflammatory markers like LPS-binding protein, IL-6, plasminogen activator inhibitor-1, which were normalized after the antibiotic treatment. Four groups were analyzed: old control mice (OC), old mice fed with antibiotic supplementation (OA), young control mice (YC); young mice with antibiotics (YA). Old mice presented several markers of dysbiosis and inflammation, with higher levels of TMAO and PWV. During the intervention, PWV increased in young mice without antibiotic supplementation only. In old mice, antibiotic treatment was associated with: (i) partial PWV improvement ($p = 0.047$ vs. OC); (ii) increased aortic elastin expression; (iii) suppressed TMAO levels [81]. (ii) In one study from Brunt V et al., 35 young and 38 old mice were treated with antibiotic supplement for 3 to 4 weeks. After the supplementation, most of major phyla were suppressed. The intervention restored arterial stiffness in old mice to normal levels, and normalized oxidative stress and inflammation [82].

The role of SCFA receptor Gpr41 in vascular function was investigated in Gpr41-KO mice. Gpr41 was found in the vascular endothelium, which was necessary for SCFA-mediated vasodilation. At baseline, Gpr41-/- mice presented isolated systolic hypertension, but with no differences in plasma renin concentration between WT and KO mice. At 6mo, Gpr41-/- mice showed accelerated vascular ageing with higher PWV than wild mice. Of note, ex vivo analysis at 6mo showed no difference in tensile vessel properties. The disparity between higher PWV and unchanged structural vessel properties indicates that functional alterations may occur before structural modifications exist [29].

The gut microbiota influences the resistance properties of arteries, with increased stiffness in male germ-free mice with respect to either wild or female germ-free mice [83].

All these experimental animal studies consistently show a strict correlation between modification of gut microbiota and arterial stiffness. Moreover, some of them highlight the role of inflammation as a mediator between the gut microbiota and arterial stiffness.

3.4.2. Human Studies

Among studies on humans (see Table 2), we found five cross-sectional and seven intervention studies. Ten studies present information on BP, and six employed cfPWV as a measure of arterial stiffness. Three studies did not directly evaluate modification in microbiota.

Cross-sectional studies. In this study setting, a correlation between gut microbiota modifications and arterial stiffness parameters was consistently found across the included studies. In particular, the abundance of beneficial bacteria (mainly butyrate producers) is constantly associated with lower arterial stiffness. (i) Menni et al. investigated more than 600 women from the TwinsUK registry, and measured tonometric carotid-femoral PWV and microbiota composition. They found that gut microbiome diversity was significantly inversely associated with arterial stiffness. PWV was also negatively associated with the abundance of Ruminococcaceae family bacteria, which are beneficial butyrate-producing bacteria linked to lower endotoxemia [85]. (ii) In 10 hemodialysis patients, Firmicutes and Bacteroidetes phyla were the most abundant. Faecalibacterium spp. (butyrate producer from the Oscillospiraceae family, class Clostridia, phylum Firmicutes) were positively associated with total carbohydrate intake ($\rho = 0.636$; $p = 0.048$) and negatively associated with cfPWV ($\rho = -0.867$, $p = 0.001$). Lipopolysaccharide-Binding Protein, a marker of bacterial translocation through the intestinal barrier and endotoxemia, was negatively associated with butyrate-producing bacteria [86]. This result supports the association between the favorable microbiota composition and vascular ageing, through a reduction of the systemic inflammation derived from leaky gut syndrome. (iii) In sixty-nine subjects not treated for hypertension who underwent an ambulatory BP monitoring, an ambulatory arterial stiffness index (AASI) was obtained. AASI is calculated from the regression line between 24 h systolic and diastolic BP values, and is believed to be a marker of arterial stiffness. Although no definite evidence exists on its accuracy, at least it seems able to predict cardiovascular events. No association was found between microbiota diversity indexes and AASI. AASI was associated with lower abundance of Lactobacillus spp. and higher abundance of several deleterious species from the genus Clostridium [87]. (iv) In children with chronic kidney disease with different categories of estimated glomerular filtration rate (G1: eGFR $\geq$ 90 mL/min/1.73 m^2, 9.5 years-old; G2-G3: eGFR 30–89, 13.7 ys), carotid-PWV was correlated to the severity of the disease. Although various beneficial bacteria (Lactobacillus, Bifidobacterium, Akkermansia) were not influenced by the severity of the disease, genus Lactobacillus abundance was negatively correlated with PWV [88].

Supplement intervention. Three studies investigated the effect of supplementation on gut microbiota and arterial stiffness, without any significant result. Only one study found a significant effect on arterial stiffness reduction associated with a specific microbiota pattern, but the effect was only marginal. (i) A total of sixty-six healthy men were enrolled in a randomized, double-blind placebo-controlled trial where two forms of aronia supplementation were compared to a placebo after 12-week treatment: a (poly)phenol-rich aronia extract, and an aronia fruit powder. No effect on aortic stiffness was registered. Gut microbial diversity was very high and did not show significant variation among the treatment groups after aronia intake; the aronia extract group presented an increased abundance of genus Anaerostipes (butyrate producer, family Lachnospiraceae, class Clostridia) [89]. (ii) A relatively young uncontrolled hypertensive sample was randomized to receive garlic (n 23) supplementation or a placebo (n 26) for 12 weeks. Tonometric cfPWV presented a trend for reduction in the garlic group (from 12.8 to 12.1 m/s), but with no statistical difference versus the placebo. Of note, SBP was reduced in garlic versus the placebo arm, with a mean difference of 10 mmHg. The garlic group presented an increase in Lactobacillus and Clostridium spp, without deeper characterization of the bacterial species [90]. (iii) A total of twelve young men were studied after consumption of 2 eggs/day for 2 weeks in a non-randomized trial. Brachial-ankle PWV and endothelial function improved, with no effect on BP, inflammation, oxidative stress, or TMAO. Microbiota was not modified, but a reduction of tryptophan degradation was observed [91].

Exercise intervention. Both the following studies found a significant relationship between the gut microbiota and arterial stiffness surrogates. In particular, the second study, focused on a very intense exercise training program, found a significant microbiota modification after the training, associated with improvement of the augmentation index (an indirect index of arterial stiffness, which is associated both with vascular peripheral resistances and with the phenomenon of the pulse wave reflection). Unfortunately, the trial was not randomized and the augmentation index is not only related with arterial stiffness, but also to the peripheral resistances and heart rate. This mines the interpretation of the results. (i) A crossover trial with 5 wks of exercise training and 5 wks of washout period found a significant positive correlation between Clostridium difficile and arterial stiffness in 33 men, measured by the cardio-ankle vascular index (CAVI), ($r = 0.306$, $p = 0.016$) and SBP, but with no exercise effect. Microbiota diversity was not affected by exercise, but the relative abundances of Oscillospira and Clostridium difficile were increased and decreased by exercise, respectively [92]. Considering that Oscillospira species (family Oscillospiraceae, class Clostridia) are associated with leanness and may have anti-inflammatory properties [93], the results of this study support the beneficial role of exercise training in microbiota composition. (ii) In a non-randomized interventional trial, 24 obese adolescents underwent a 6-wk program of endurance/strength training for 5 h/day and 6 d/wk, together with caloric restriction. The subendocardial viability ratio, an index of the workload of the left ventricle depending on ventricle-vascular coupling, and the augmentation index were improved by the program, with no significant change in BP. Microbiota diversity increased, together with the abundance of the Christensenellaceae family, which is inversely related to the host body mass index [94].

Studies without direct microbiota measures. Three studies present results on arterial stiffness modification in relation to either comorbidities or supplementation design, assuming an indirect role of gut microbiota. (i) In the paper by Ponziani et al., 39 patients with suspected small intestinal bacterial overgrowth (SIBO) were included. Vitamin-K2 status was measured, and Vitamin-K2 intake and carotid PWV were obtained. In patients with confirmed SIBO ($n = 12$), despite similar dietary vitamin-K2 intake, measured vitamin-K2 status was markedly reduced versus the no-SIBO group ($p = 0.02$), suggesting an altered vitamin-K2 production by intestinal bacteria. Median PWV was significantly higher in the SIBO group than the no-SIBO group (10.25 m/s vs. 7.68 m/s; $p = 0.002$). Furthermore, in both groups, vitamin-K2 status was significantly correlated with carotid PWV ($R2 = 0.29$, $p < 0.001$) [95]. This study supports the role of gut dysbiosis in vascular ageing. (ii) In a randomized trial, 15 patients received 1-month cocoa extract with 130 mg epicatechin and 560 mg procyanidins (group D1-10), 15 patients received 20 mg epicatechin and 540 procyanidins (group D2-10), and were compared with the placebo ($n = 15$). Of note, both epicatechin and procyanidins are catabolized by gut microbes in the colon. CfPWV was reduced in the D1-10 group by about 1 m/s versus the placebo and by 0.8 m/s versus D2-10 group. SBP was also reduced in D1-10 versus the control and D2-10 groups. In this study, the reduction of SBP could explain the observed variation in PWV. The impact of cocoa flavonols on vascular health was mainly linked to epicatechin, and is mediated by epicatechin metabolites, which in turn depends on gut microbiota metabolism [96]. (iii) One study focused on the effect of equol, a microbial-derived metabolite of the isoflavone daidzein. Equol is produced by gut microbiota after soy intake in almost one-third of the Western population. Acute soy supplementation slightly reduced cfPWV only in equol producers (-0.2 m/s) at 24 h, with no change in BP [97].

Even if a direct association with microbiota composition and function has not been addressed, the three studies presented here show a significant correlation between vascular ageing and the metabolites of gut microbiota. This confirms the role of gut microbiota in modulating human systemic biological pathways.

Antibiotics in humans. In contrast to what has been shown in animal studies, this paragraph aims to warn the reader not to consider antibiotic treatment beneficial for cardiovascular health in humans. Indeed, the role of antibiotics in humans is not fully established. Studies investigating the role of antibiotics in microbiota and the effect on cardiovascular risk are lacking. According to the literature, it appears that antibiotics impact the gut microbiota, reducing bacterial diversity and changing relative abundances [98]. They were also found to enhance pathways linked to increased atherosclerosis [99]. Long-term use of antibiotics in late adulthood has been associated with all-cause and cardiovascular mortality [100]. Macrolide antibiotic consumption is associated with increased risk for sudden cardiac death or ventricular tachyarrhythmias and cardiovascular death, but not increased all-cause mortality [101]. Furthermore, no association with long-term cardiovascular risk (ranging from >30 days to >3 years) was noted in observational studies or randomized controlled trials on treatment with macrolides [102]. A significant association was found between fluoroquinolone use and an increased risk for arrhythmia and cardiovascular mortality [103]. Antibiotic exposure in infancy was associated with a slightly increased risk of childhood overweight and obesity [104]. The pooled colorectal cancer risk was increased among individuals who ever used antibiotics, particularly for broad-spectrum antibiotics [105]. The pooled breast cancer risk was modestly increased among individuals who ever used antibiotics [106].

Limitations. This study presents several limitations. Firstly, due to the small number of studies and great heterogenicity among them, it was not possible to make a meta-analysis of the results. Second, the quality of most of the studies was questionable, due either to sample size, or to the assessment of microbiota or arterial stiffness. Third, for the reason just mentioned, it was not possible to entirely follow the PRISMA statement for systematic review.

3.5. Conclusions

From the available literature, we found an association between gut microbiota composition and arterial stiffness. We identified two association patterns, consistently present in most animal and human studies: (i) a direct correlation between arterial stiffness and abundances of bacteria associated with altered gut permeability and inflammation (mainly from the *Clostridium* genus), as well as with biological markers of inflammation; (ii) an inverse relationship between arterial stiffness, microbiota diversity, and abundances of bacteria associated with most fit microbiota composition (butyrate producers, *Akkermansia, Bifidobacterium, Ruminococcaceae, Faecalibacterium, Lactobacillus*).

While in animal studies most of the interventions were able to show a stable link between microbiota modification and arterial stiffness, in humans that was not the case. In particular, none of the identified interventional trials was able to demonstrate this relationship. However, most strikingly, nearly half of human studies measured BP, and very few adjusted the vascular analyses for BP variation, which is a major determinant of arterial stiffness.

The main finding of this review is the lack of large randomized interventional trials in humans that test the role of gut microbiota modifications on arterial stiffness, and take into account BP and hemodynamic alterations.

Table 2. Characteristics of human studies.

Authors	n	Marker of VA	Intervention	Duration	Effect on Vascular Ageing	Mechanisms Linked to Microbiota
Rodriguez-Mateos, A., 2018 [96]	45	cfPWV	DP1-10 group: cocoa extract with 690 mg (130 mg epicatechin; 560 mg DP2-10 procyanidins). DP2-10 group: cocoa extract with 560 mg (20 mg epicatechin; 540 mg DP2-10 procyanidins). Controls.	1 month	DP1-10 group: decrease in PWV at 1 mo of -1.0 m/s (95% CI: -1.6, -0.4 m/s) compared with the control and of -0.8 m/s (95% CI: -1.4, -0.2 m/s) compared with DP2-10. Decrease in SBP at 1 month in both treatment groups.	Epicatechin is absorbed via the colon after catabolism by the microbiota; Pro-cyanidins are also subject to microbiome-mediated catabolism.
Istas, G., 2019 [89]	66	cfPWV; AIx	Aronia whole fruit capsule: 12 mg (poly)phenols; aronia extract capsule: 116 mg (poly)phenols.	Acute: 0–2 h Chronic: 0–12 weeks	No significant difference in PWV and BP.	The aronia extract group: higher abundance of *Anaerostipes*; the aronia whole fruit group: increases in *Bacteroides*.
Taniguchi, H., 2018 [92]	33	CAVI	Exercise program ($n = 16$) and control period ($n = 17$).	10 weeks	Changes in *Clostridium Difficile* were positively correlated both with CAVI (r 0.31, p 0.02; no effect of exercise) and with SBP	Diversity and composition of microbiota were not affected by exercise; exercise increased the relative abundance of *Oscillospira* and decreased the abundance of *C. Difficile*.
Menni, C., 2018 [85]	617	cfPWV	Observational study in female twins.	N/a	Carotid-femoral PWV is inversely correlated with gut microbiome diversity and with the abundance of specific microbes in the gut (Ruminococcaceae family bacteria). Analysis was adjusted for MAP.	N/a
Biruete, A., 2019 [86]	10	cfPWV	Observational study in hemodialysis patients.	N/a	*Faecalibacterium* spp. (with anti-inflammatory properties), was negatively associated with aortic PWV. F:B ratio was positively associated with SBP.	N/a
Ponziani, F.R., 2017 [95]	39	Carotid PWV	Patients with small intestinal bacterial overgrowth (SIBO).	N/a	PWV was increased in the SIBO group compared to the no-SIBO group (10.25 m/s vs 7.68 m/s; p = 0.002). dp-ucMGP levels (marker of low vitamin-K2 status) correlated with PWV in whole population. No BP data.	Dietary vitamin-K2 intake does not correlate with vitamin-K2 status (measured by dp-ucMGP serum levels). The gut microbiota is crucial for overcoming dietary vitamin-K2 insufficiencies.
Ried, K., 2018 [90]	49	cfPWV (tonometry)	Kyolic Aged Garlic Extract vs placebo.	12 weeks	No significant differences in PWV between groups and intra-group before and after treatment. Garlic reduced SBP.	Increase of *Lactobacillus* and *Clostridia* species in the garlic group. *Faecalibacterium prausnitzii* markedly increased in the placebo group.
Hazim, S., 2016 [97]	28	cfPWV	Soy isoflavones acute supplementation.	3 days	Acute soy intakes modified cfPWV only in equol producer subjects at 24 h; equol concentrations were significantly correlated with changes in cfPWV. No changes in BP.	N/a

Table 2. Cont.

Authors	n	Marker of VA	Intervention	Duration	Effect on Vascular Ageing	Mechanisms Linked to Microbiota
Huang, J., 2020 [94]	24	AIx75; SEVR	Obese individuals underwent exercise: endurance/strength training 5 h/day, 6 days/week; diet: calorie-restricted.	6 weeks	Significant increase of SEVR; reduction of AIx. No changes in BP.	Increase in intestinal microbial diversity; abundance of *Lactobacillales*, *Bacilli*, *Streptococcaceae*, and *Veillonella* were significantly reduced. *Christensenellaceae* were significantly enhanced; changes in *Cronobacter*, *Lachnospiraceae* UCG-003, and *Helicobacter* were all positively or negatively associated with the changes in SEVR, AIx75.
Dinakis, E., 2021 [87]	69	AASI	Observational study.		No associations were found between alpha diversity and AASI; no significant clustering patterns of AASI; Small but positive correlation between plasma butyrate levels and AASI. No BP data.	AASI was associated with lower abundance of *Lactobacillus* spp. and higher abundance of several species from the genus *Clostridium*.
Liu, X., 2022 [91]	12	baPWV/FMD	2 eggs/day in healthy young men.	2 weeks	Egg consumption improved baPWV and FMD. No effect on inflammation and oxidative stress. No changes in BP.	No change in taxonomy, alpha and beta diversity; reduced tryptophan degradation.
Hsu, C.N., 2018 [88]	86	carotid-PWV (echo-tracking)	Observational study on children and adolescents with chronic kidney disease (CKD).	N/a	Carotid-PWV was elevated in children with CKD and eGFR category G2–G3 compared to those with eGFR category G1. 65% of children and adolescents with CKD G1–G3 had BP abnormalities on ABPM.	CKD children with an abnormal ABPM profile had lower abundance of the genus *Prevotella*; the abundances of genera *Bifidobacterium* and *Lactobacillus* were correlated with urinary TMAO level.

VA stands for Vascular ageing; SBP, systolic blood pressure; cfPWV, carotid-femoral pulse wave velocity; CAVI, cardio-ankle vascular index; MAP, mean arterial pressure; AIx75, augmentation index corrected for heart rate at 75 bpm; SEVR, sub-endocardial viability ratio; AASI, ambulatory arterial stiffness index; baPWV, brachial-ankle pulse wave velocity; FMD, flow-mediated dilation; eGFR, estimated glomerular filtration rate; eGFR categories: G1 $\geq$ 90 mL/min/1.73 m^2, G2 50–89, G3 30–59; ABPM, ambulatory blood pressure measurement; TMAO, trimethylamine-N-oxide.

Author Contributions: Conceptualization, D.A., F.P., A.F.G.C., C.B.; methodology, D.A., F.P., A.F.G.C.; validation, D.A., F.P., A.F.G.C., C.B.; writing—original draft preparation, D.A.; writing—review and editing, F.P., A.F.G.C., C.B.; supervision, C.B. All authors have read and agreed to the published version of the manuscript.

Funding: This research received no external funding.

Institutional Review Board Statement: Not applicable.

Informed Consent Statement: Not applicable.

Data Availability Statement: No new data were created or analyzed in this study. Data sharing is not applicable to this article.

Acknowledgments: We thank Professor Patrizia Brigidi, from the Department of Clinical and Surgical Sciences, University of Bologna, for kind support in manuscript conceptualization and revision.

Conflicts of Interest: A.F.G.C. is consultant to Roelmi and Viatris. C.B. is on the scientific board of Servier International and Menarini International. D.A. and F.P. declare they have no financial interest.

References

1. Blacher, J.; Evans, A.; Arveiler, D.; Amouyel, P.; Ferrières, J.; Bingham, A.; Yarnell, J.; Haas, B.; Montaye, M.; Ruidavets, J.-B.; et al. Residual cardiovascular risk in treated hypertension and hyperlipidaemia: The PRIME Study. *J. Hum. Hypertens.* **2010**, *24*, 19–26. [CrossRef] [PubMed]
2. Nilsson, P.M. Early Vascular Aging in Hypertension. *Front. Cardiovasc. Med.* **2020**, *7*, 1–5. [CrossRef] [PubMed]
3. Lakatta, E.G.; Wang, M.; Najjar, S.S. Arterial Aging and Subclinical Arterial Disease are Fundamentally Intertwined at Macroscopic and Molecular Levels. *Med. Clin. N. Am.* **2009**, *93*, 583–604. [CrossRef] [PubMed]
4. Ben-Shlomo, Y.; Spears, M.; Boustred, C.; May, M.; Anderson, S.G.; Benjamin, E.J.; Boutouyrie, P.; Cameron, J.; Chen, C.-H.; Cruickshank, J.K.; et al. Aortic Pulse Wave Velocity Improves Cardiovascular Event Prediction. *J. Am. Coll. Cardiol.* **2014**, *63*, 636–646. [CrossRef]
5. Mitchell, G.F.; Hwang, S.-J.; Vasan, R.S.; Larson, M.G.; Pencina, M.J.; Hamburg, N.M.; Vita, J.A.; Levy, D.; Benjamin, E.J. Arterial stiffness and cardiovascular events the Framingham Heart Study. *Circulation* **2010**, *121*, 505–511. [CrossRef]
6. Lozupone, C.; Faust, K.; Raes, J.; Faith, J.J.; Frank, D.N.; Zaneveld, J.; Gordon, J.I.; Knight, R. Identifying genomic and metabolic features that can underlie early successional and opportunistic lifestyles of human gut symbionts. *Genome Res.* **2012**, *22*, 1974–1984. [CrossRef]
7. Zhernakova, A.; Kurilshikov, A.; Bonder, M.J.; Tigchelaar, E.F.; Schirmer, M.; Vatanen, T.; Mujagic, Z.; Vila, A.V.; Falony, G.; Vieira-Silva, S.; et al. Population-based metagenomics analysis reveals markers for gut microbiome composition and diversity. *Science* **2016**, *352*, 565–569. [CrossRef]
8. Gilbert, J.A.; Blaser, M.J.; Caporaso, J.G.; Jansson, J.K.; Lynch, S.V.; Knight, R. Current understanding of the human microbiome. *Nat. Med.* **2018**, *24*, 392–400. [CrossRef]
9. Levine, U.Y.; Looft, T.; Allen, H.K.; Stanton, T.B. Butyrate-producing bacteria, including mucin degraders, from the swine intestinal tract. *Appl. Environ. Microbiol.* **2013**, *79*, 3879–3881. [CrossRef]
10. Nagano, Y.; Itoh, K.; Honda, K. The induction of Treg cells by gut-indigenous Clostridium. *Curr. Opin. Immunol.* **2012**, *24*, 392–397. [CrossRef]
11. Ghaffari, S.; Abbasi, A.; Somi, M.H.; Moaddab, S.Y.; Nikniaz, L.; Kafil, H.S.; Ebrahimzadeh Leylabadlo, H. Akkermansia muciniphila: From its critical role in human health to strategies for promoting its abundance in human gut microbiome. *Crit. Rev. Food Sci. Nutr.* **2022**, 1–21. [CrossRef] [PubMed]
12. Ouyang, J.; Lin, J.; Isnard, S.; Fombuena, B.; Peng, X.; Marette, A.; Routy, B.; Messaoudene, M.; Chen, Y.; Routy, J.-P. The Bacterium Akkermansia muciniphila: A Sentinel for Gut Permeability and Its Relevance to HIV-Related Inflammation. *Front. Immunol.* **2020**, *11*, 645. [CrossRef] [PubMed]
13. Wang, X.; Ouyang, Y.; Liu, J.; Zhu, M.; Zhao, G.; Bao, W.; Hu, F.B. Fruit and vegetable consumption and mortality from all causes, cardiovascular disease, and cancer: Systematic review and dose-response meta-analysis of prospective cohort studies. *BMJ* **2014**, *349*, g4490. [CrossRef] [PubMed]
14. Miura, K.; Greenland, P.; Stamler, J.; Liu, K.; Daviglus, M.L.; Nakagawa, H. Relation of vegetable, fruit, and meat intake to 7-year blood pressure change in middle-aged men: The Chicago Western Electric Study. *Am. J. Epidemiol.* **2004**, *159*, 572–580. [CrossRef]
15. Alonso, A.; de la Fuente, C.; Martín-Arnau, A.M.; de Irala, J.; Martínez, J.A.; Martínez-González, M.A. Fruit and vegetable consumption is inversely associated with blood pressure in a Mediterranean population with a high vegetable-fat intake: The Seguimiento Universidad de Navarra (SUN) Study. *Br. J. Nutr.* **2004**, *92*, 311–319. [CrossRef]
16. Park, Y.; Subar, A.F.; Hollenbeck, A.; Schatzkin, A. Dietary fiber intake and mortality in the NIH-AARP diet and health study. *Arch. Intern. Med.* **2011**, *171*, 1061–1068. [CrossRef]
17. Tzoulaki, I.; Iliou, A.; Mikros, E.; Elliott, P. An Overview of Metabolic Phenotyping in Blood Pressure Research. *Curr. Hypertens. Rep.* **2018**, *20*, 78. [CrossRef]
18. Zheng, Y.; Yu, B.; Alexander, D.; Mosley, T.H.; Heiss, G.; Nettleton, J.A.; Boerwinkle, E. Metabolomics and Incident Hypertension Among Blacks. *Hypertension* **2013**, *62*, 398–403. [CrossRef]
19. Loo, R.L.; Zou, X.; Appel, L.J.; Nicholson, J.K.; Holmes, E. Characterization of metabolic responses to healthy diets and association with blood pressure: Application to the Optimal Macronutrient Intake Trial for Heart Health (OmniHeart), a randomized controlled study. *Am. J. Clin. Nutr.* **2018**, *107*, 323–334. [CrossRef]
20. Yang, T.; Santisteban, M.M.; Rodriguez, V.; Li, E.; Ahmari, N.; Carvajal, J.M.; Zadeh, M.; Gong, M.; Qi, Y.; Zubcevic, J.; et al. Gut Dysbiosis is Linked to Hypertension. *Hypertension* **2015**, *65*, 1331–1340. [CrossRef]
21. Adnan, S.; Nelson, J.W.; Ajami, N.J.; Venna, V.R.; Petrosino, J.F.; Bryan, R.M.J.; Durgan, D.J. Alterations in the gut microbiota can elicit hypertension in rats. *Physiol. Genom.* **2017**, *49*, 96–104. [CrossRef] [PubMed]
22. Daugirdas, J.T.; Nawab, Z.M.; Klok, M. Acetate relaxation of isolated vascular smooth muscle. *Kidney Int.* **1987**, *32*, 39–46. [CrossRef] [PubMed]
23. Nutting, C.W.; Islam, S.; Daugirdas, J.T. Vasorelaxant effects of short chain fatty acid salts in rat caudal artery. *Am. J. Physiol. Circ. Physiol.* **1991**, *261*, H561–H567. [CrossRef] [PubMed]
24. Mortensen, F.V.; Nielsen, H.; Mulvany, M.J.; Hessov, I. Short chain fatty acids dilate isolated human colonic resistance arteries. *Gut* **1990**, *31*, 1391–1394. [CrossRef]

25. Pluznick, J.L.; Protzko, R.J.; Gevorgyan, H.; Peterlin, Z.; Sipos, A.; Han, J.; Brunet, I.; Wan, L.X.; Rey, F.; Wang, T.; et al. Olfactory receptor responding to gut microbiotaderived signals plays a role in renin secretion and blood pressure regulation. *Proc. Natl. Acad. Sci. USA* **2013**, *110*, 4410–4415. [CrossRef]
26. Marques, F.Z.; Nelson, E.; Chu, P.-Y.Y.; Horlock, D.; Fiedler, A.; Ziemann, M.; Tan, J.K.; Kuruppu, S.; Rajapakse, N.W.; El-Osta, A.; et al. High-fiber diet and acetate supplementation change the gut microbiota and prevent the development of hypertension and heart failure in hypertensive mice. *Circulation* **2017**, *135*, 964–977. [CrossRef]
27. Tan, J.K.; McKenzie, C.; Mariño, E.; Macia, L.; Mackay, C.R. Metabolite-Sensing G Protein–Coupled Receptors—Facilitators of Diet-Related Immune Regulation. *Annu. Rev. Immunol.* **2017**, *35*, 371–402. [CrossRef]
28. Macia, L.; Tan, J.; Vieira, A.T.; Leach, K.; Stanley, D.; Luong, S.; Maruya, M.; Ian McKenzie, C.; Hijikata, A.; Wong, C.; et al. Metabolite-sensing receptors GPR43 and GPR109A facilitate dietary fibre-induced gut homeostasis through regulation of the inflammasome. *Nat. Commun.* **2015**, *6*, 6734. [CrossRef]
29. Natarajan, N.; Hori, D.; Flavahan, S.; Steppan, J.; Flavahan, N.A.; Berkowitz, D.E.; Pluznick, J.L. Microbial short chain fatty acid metabolites lower blood pressure via endothelial G protein-coupled receptor 41. *Physiol. Genom.* **2016**, *48*, 826–834. [CrossRef]
30. Thorburn, A.N.; McKenzie, C.I.; Shen, S.; Stanley, D.; MacIa, L.; Mason, L.J.; Roberts, L.K.; Wong, C.H.Y.; Shim, R.; Robert, R.; et al. Evidence that asthma is a developmental origin disease influenced by maternal diet and bacterial metabolites. *Nat. Commun.* **2015**, *6*, 7320. [CrossRef]
31. Payen, C.; Guillot, A.; Paillat, L.; Fothi, A.; Dib, A.; Bourreau, J.; Schmitt, F.; Loufrani, L.; Aranyi, T.; Henrion, D.; et al. Pathophysiological adaptations of resistance arteries in rat offspring exposed in utero to maternal obesity is associated with sex-specific epigenetic alterations. *Int. J. Obes.* **2021**, *45*, 1074–1085. [CrossRef] [PubMed]
32. Itani, H.A.; McMaster, W.G.; Saleh, M.A.; Nazarewicz, R.R.; Mikolajczyk, T.P.; Kaszuba, A.M.; Konior, A.; Prejbisz, A.; Januszewicz, A.; Norlander, A.E.; et al. Activation of Human T Cells in Hypertension. *Hypertension* **2016**, *68*, 123–132. [CrossRef] [PubMed]
33. Dörffel, Y.; Lätsch, C.; Stuhlmüller, B.; Schreiber, S.; Scholze, S.; Burmester, G.R.; Scholze, J. Preactivated Peripheral Blood Monocytes in Patients With Essential Hypertension. *Hypertension* **1999**, *34*, 113–117. [CrossRef] [PubMed]
34. Mikolajczyk, T.P.; Guzik, T.J. Adaptive Immunity in Hypertension. *Curr. Hypertens. Rep.* **2019**, *21*, 68. [CrossRef]
35. Norlander, A.E.; Madhur, M.S.; Harrison, D.G. Correction: The immunology of hypertension. *J. Exp. Med.* **2018**, *215*, 719. [CrossRef]
36. Csiszar, A.; Ungvari, Z.; Edwards, J.G.; Kaminski, P.; Wolin, M.S.; Koller, A.; Kaley, G. Aging-Induced Phenotypic Changes and Oxidative Stress Impair Coronary Arteriolar Function. *Circ. Res.* **2002**, *90*, 1159–1166. Available online: http://www.ncbi.nlm.nih.gov/pubmed/12065318 (accessed on 14 July 2013). [CrossRef]
37. Wang, M.; Zhang, J.; Jiang, L.-Q.Q.; Spinetti, G.; Pintus, G.; Monticone, R.; Kolodgie, F.D.; Virmani, R.; Lakatta, E.G. Proinflammatory profile within the grossly normal aged human aortic wall. *Hypertension* **2007**, *50*, 219–227. [CrossRef]
38. Boos, C.J.; Lip, G.Y.H. Elevated high-sensitive C-reactive protein, large arterial stiffness and atherosclerosis: A relationship between inflammation and hypertension? *J. Hum. Hypertens.* **2005**, *19*, 511–513. [CrossRef]
39. Patel, R.S.; Al Mheid, I.; Morris, A.A.; Ahmed, Y.; Kavtaradze, N.; Ali, S.; Dabhadkar, K.; Brigham, K.; Hooper, W.C.; Alexander, R.W.; et al. Oxidative stress is associated with impaired arterial elasticity. *Atherosclerosis* **2011**, *218*, 90–95. [CrossRef]
40. Jain, S.; Khera, R.; Corrales-Medina, V.F.; Townsend, R.R.; Chirinos, J.A. Inflammation and arterial stiffness in humans. *Atherosclerosis* **2014**, *237*, 381–390. [CrossRef]
41. Wykretowicz, A.; Guzik, P.; Kąsinowski, R.; Krauze, T.; Bartkowiak, G.; Dziarmaga, M.; Wysocki, H. Augmentation index, pulse pressure amplification and superoxide anion production in patients with coronary artery disease. *Int. J. Cardiol.* **2005**, *99*, 289–294. [CrossRef] [PubMed]
42. Yasmin; McEniery, C.M.; Wallace, S.; Mackenzie, I.S.; Cockcroft, J.R.; Wilkinson, I.B. C-reactive protein is associated with arterial stiffness in apparently healthy individuals. *Arterioscler. Thromb. Vasc. Biol.* **2004**, *24*, 969–974. [CrossRef] [PubMed]
43. Schillaci, G.; Bartoloni, E.; Pucci, G.; Pirro, M.; Settimi, L.; Alunno, A.; Gerli, R.; Mannarino, E. Aortic stiffness is increased in polymyalgia rheumatica and improves after steroid treatment. *Ann. Rheum. Dis.* **2012**, *71*, 1151–1156. [CrossRef]
44. Mäki-Petäjä, K.M.; Hall, F.C.; Booth, A.D.; Wallace, S.M.L.; Yasmin; Bearcroft, P.W.P.; Harish, S.; Furlong, A.; McEniery, C.M.; Brown, J.; et al. Rheumatoid arthritis is associated with increased aortic pulse-wave velocity, which is reduced by anti-tumor necrosis factor-alpha therapy. *Circulation* **2006**, *114*, 1185–1192. [CrossRef] [PubMed]
45. Marques, F.Z.; Mackay, C.R.; Kaye, D.M. Beyond gut feelings: How the gut microbiota regulates blood pressure. *Nat. Rev. Cardiol.* **2018**, *15*, 20–32. [CrossRef]
46. Janeiro, M.; Ramírez, M.; Milagro, F.; Martínez, J.; Solas, M. Implication of Trimethylamine N-Oxide (TMAO) in Disease: Potential Biomarker or New Therapeutic Target. *Nutrients* **2018**, *10*, 1398. [CrossRef]
47. Louca, P.; Menni, C.; Padmanabhan, S. Genomic Determinants of Hypertension with a Focus on Metabolomics and the Gut Microbiome. *Am. J. Hypertens.* **2020**, *33*, 473–481. [CrossRef]
48. Li, X.S.; Obeid, S.; Klingenberg, R.; Gencer, B.; Mach, F.; Räber, L.; Windecker, S.; Rodondi, N.; Nanchen, D.; Muller, O.; et al. Gut microbiota-dependent trimethylamine N-oxide in acute coronary syndromes: A prognostic marker for incident cardiovascular events beyond traditional risk factors. *Eur. Heart J.* **2017**, *38*, ehw582. [CrossRef]
49. Brunt, V.E.; Casso, A.G.; Gioscia-Ryan, R.A.; Sapinsley, Z.J.; Ziemba, B.P.; Clayton, Z.S.; Bazzoni, A.E.; VanDongen, N.S.; Richey, J.J.; Hutton, D.A.; et al. Gut Microbiome-Derived Metabolite Trimethylamine N-Oxide Induces Aortic Stiffening and Increases Systolic Blood Pressure With Aging in Mice and Humans. *Hypertension* **2021**, *78*, 499–511. [CrossRef]

50. Ufnal, M.; Jazwiec, R.; Dadlez, M.; Drapala, A.; Sikora, M.; Skrzypecki, J. Trimethylamine-N-Oxide: A Carnitine-Derived Metabolite That Prolongs the Hypertensive Effect of Angiotensin II in Rats. *Can. J. Cardiol.* **2014**, *30*, 1700–1705. [CrossRef]
51. Wang, Z.; Klipfell, E.; Bennett, B.J.; Koeth, R.; Levison, B.S.; Dugar, B.; Feldstein, A.E.; Britt, E.B.; Fu, X.; Chung, Y.-M.; et al. Gut flora metabolism of phosphatidylcholine promotes cardiovascular disease. *Nature* **2011**, *472*, 57–63. [CrossRef] [PubMed]
52. Cantero, M.A.; Guedes, M.R.A.; Fernandes, R.; Lollo, P.C.B. Trimethylamine N-oxide reduction is related to probiotic strain specificity: A systematic review. *Nutr. Res.* **2022**, *104*, 29–35. [CrossRef] [PubMed]
53. Raetz, C.R.H.; Whitfield, C. Lipopolysaccharide Endotoxins. *Annu. Rev. Biochem.* **2002**, *71*, 635–700. [CrossRef]
54. Smiljanec, K.; Lennon, S.L. Sodium, hypertension, and the gut: Does the gut microbiota go salty? *Am. J. Physiol.-Hear. Circ. Physiol.* **2019**, *317*, H1173–H1182. [CrossRef] [PubMed]
55. Kleinewietfeld, M.; Manzel, A.; Titze, J.; Kvakan, H.; Yosef, N.; Linker, R.A.; Muller, D.N.; Hafler, D.A. Sodium chloride drives autoimmune disease by the induction of pathogenic TH17 cells. *Nature* **2013**, *496*, 518–522. [CrossRef] [PubMed]
56. He, P.; Yun, C.C. Mechanisms of the Regulation of the Intestinal Na+/H+ Exchanger NHE3. *J. Biomed. Biotechnol.* **2010**, *2010*, 238080. [CrossRef]
57. Linz, D.; Wirth, K.; Linz, W.; Heuer, H.O.O.; Frick, W.; Hofmeister, A.; Heinelt, U.; Arndt, P.; Schwahn, U.; Böhm, M.; et al. Antihypertensive and Laxative Effects by Pharmacological Inhibition of Sodium-Proton-Exchanger Subtype 3–Mediated Sodium Absorption in the Gut. *Hypertension* **2012**, *60*, 1560–1567. [CrossRef] [PubMed]
58. Engevik, M.A.; Aihara, E.; Montrose, M.H.; Shull, G.E.; Hassett, D.J.; Worrell, R.T. Loss of NHE3 alters gut microbiota composition and influences Bacteroides thetaiotaomicron growth. *Am. J. Physiol. Liver Physiol.* **2013**, *305*, G697–G711. [CrossRef]
59. Laubitz, D.; Harrison, C.A.; Midura-Kiela, M.T.; Ramalingam, R.; Larmonier, C.B.; Chase, J.H.; Caporaso, J.G.; Besselsen, D.G.; Ghishan, F.K.; Kiela, P.R. Reduced Epithelial Na+/H+ Exchange Drives Gut Microbial Dysbiosis and Promotes Inflammatory Response in T Cell-Mediated Murine Colitis. *PLoS ONE* **2016**, *11*, e0152044. [CrossRef]
60. Wang, C.; Huang, Z.; Yu, K.; Ding, R.; Ye, K.; Dai, C.; Xu, X.; Zhou, G.; Li, C. High-Salt Diet Has a Certain Impact on Protein Digestion and Gut Microbiota: A Sequencing and Proteome Combined Study. *Front. Microbiol.* **2017**, *8*, 1838. [CrossRef]
61. Wilck, N.; Matus, M.G.; Kearney, S.M.; Olesen, S.W.; Forslund, K.; Bartolomaeus, H.; Haase, S.; Mähler, A.; Balogh, A.; Markó, L.; et al. Salt-responsive gut commensal modulates TH17 axis and disease. *Nature* **2017**, *551*, 585–589. [CrossRef] [PubMed]
62. Miranda, P.M.; De Palma, G.; Serkis, V.; Lu, J.; Louis-Auguste, M.P.; McCarville, J.L.; Verdu, E.F.; Collins, S.M.; Bercik, P. High salt diet exacerbates colitis in mice by decreasing Lactobacillus levels and butyrate production. *Microbiome* **2018**, *6*, 57. [CrossRef]
63. Yi, B.; Titze, J.; Rykova, M.; Feuerecker, M.; Vassilieva, G.; Nichiporuk, I.; Schelling, G.; Morukov, B.; Choukèr, A. Effects of dietary salt levels on monocytic cells and immune responses in healthy human subjects: A longitudinal study. *Transl. Res.* **2015**, *166*, 103–110. [CrossRef] [PubMed]
64. Madhur, M.S.; Lob, H.E.; McCann, L.A.; Iwakura, Y.; Blinder, Y.; Guzik, T.J.; Harrison, D.G. Interleukin 17 Promotes Angiotensin II–Induced Hypertension and Vascular Dysfunction. *Hypertension* **2010**, *55*, 500–507. [CrossRef]
65. Ivanov, I.I.; Atarashi, K.; Manel, N.; Brodie, E.L.; Shima, T.; Karaoz, U.; Wei, D.; Goldfarb, K.C.; Santee, C.A.; Lynch, S.V.; et al. Induction of Intestinal Th17 Cells by Segmented Filamentous Bacteria. *Cell* **2009**, *139*, 485–498. [CrossRef] [PubMed]
66. Clarke, S.F.; Murphy, E.F.; O'Sullivan, O.; Lucey, A.J.; Humphreys, M.; Hogan, A.; Hayes, P.; O'Reilly, M.; Jeffery, I.B.; Wood-Martin, R.; et al. Exercise and associated dietary extremes impact on gut microbial diversity. *Gut* **2014**, *63*, 1913–1920. [CrossRef]
67. Mach, N.; Fuster-Botella, D. Endurance exercise and gut microbiota: A review. *J. Sport Health Sci.* **2017**, *6*, 179–197. [CrossRef]
68. De Bruyne, T.; Steenput, B.; Roth, L.; De Meyer, G.R.Y.; Dos Santos, C.N.; Valentová, K.; Dambrova, M.; Hermans, N. Dietary polyphenols targeting arterial stiffness: Interplay of contributing mechanisms and gut microbiome-related Metabolism. *Nutrients* **2019**, *11*, 578. [CrossRef]
69. Ludovici, V.; Barthelmes, J.; Nägele, M.P.; Enseleit, F.; Ferri, C.; Flammer, A.J.; Ruschitzka, F.; Sudano, I. Cocoa, Blood Pressure, and Vascular Function. *Front. Nutr.* **2017**, *4*, 36. [CrossRef]
70. Vlachopoulos, C.; Alexopoulos, N.; Stefanadis, C. Effects of nutrition on arterial rigidity and reflected waves. *Sang Thromb. Vaiss.* **2007**, *19*, 479–486. [CrossRef]
71. EFSA Panel on Dietetic Products, Nutrition and Allergies (NDA). Scientific Opinion on the substantiation of a health claim related to cocoa flavanols and maintenance of normal endothelium-dependent vasodilation pursuant to Article 13(5) of Regulation (EC) No 1924/2006. *EFSA J.* **2012**, *10*, 2809. [CrossRef]
72. Richter, C.K.; Skulas-Ray, A.C.; Fleming, J.A.; Link, C.J.; Mukherjea, R.; Krul, E.S.; Kris-Etherton, P.M. Effects of isoflavone-containing soya protein on ex vivo cholesterol efflux, vascular function and blood markers of CVD risk in adults with moderately elevated blood pressure: A dose-response randomised controlled trial. *Br. J. Nutr.* **2017**, *117*, 1403–1413. [CrossRef] [PubMed]
73. Chuengsamarn, S.; Rattanamongkolgul, S.; Phonrat, B.; Tungtrongchitr, R.; Jirawatnotai, S. Reduction of atherogenic risk in patients with type 2 diabetes by curcuminoid extract: A randomized controlled trial. *J. Nutr. Biochem.* **2014**, *25*, 144–150. [CrossRef] [PubMed]
74. Cross, T.W.L.; Zidon, T.M.; Welly, R.J.; Park, Y.M.; Britton, S.L.; Koch, L.G.; Rottinghaus, G.E.; De Godoy, M.R.C.; Padilla, J.; Swanson, K.S.; et al. Soy improves cardiometabolic health and cecal microbiota in female low-fit rats. *Sci. Rep.* **2017**, *7*, 9261. [CrossRef]
75. Lee, D.M.; Battson, M.L.; Jarrell, D.K.; Hou, S.; Ecton, K.E.; Weir, T.L.; Gentile, C.L. SGLT2 inhibition via dapagliflozin improves generalized vascular dysfunction and alters the gut microbiota in type 2 diabetic mice. *Cardiovasc. Diabetol.* **2018**, *17*, 62. [CrossRef]

26. Lee, D.M.; Ecton, K.E.; Trikha, S.R.J.; Wrigley, S.D.; Thomas, K.N.; Battson, M.L.; Wei, Y.; Johnson, S.A.; Weir, T.L.; Gentile, C.L. Microbial metabolite indole-3-propionic acid supplementation does not protect mice from the cardiometabolic consequences of a Western diet. *Am. J. Physiol. - Gastrointest. Liver Physiol.* **2020**, *319*, G51–G62. [CrossRef]
27. Guirro, M.; Gual-Grau, A.; Gibert-Ramos, A.; Alcaide-Hidalgo, J.M.; Canela, N.; Arola, L.; Mayneris-Perxachs, J. Metabolomics elucidates dose-dependent molecular beneficial effects of hesperidin supplementation in rats fed an obesogenic diet. *Antioxidants* **2020**, *9*, 79. [CrossRef]
28. Liu, H.; Tian, R.; Wang, H.; Feng, S.; Li, H.; Xiao, Y.; Luan, X.; Zhang, Z.; Shi, N.; Niu, H.; et al. Gut microbiota from coronary artery disease patients contributes to vascular dysfunction in mice by regulating bile acid metabolism and immune activation. *J. Transl. Med.* **2020**, *18*, 382. [CrossRef]
29. Battson, M.L.; Lee, D.M.; Li Puma, L.C.; Ecton, K.E.; Thomas, K.N.; Febvre, H.P.; Chicco, A.J.; Weir, T.L.; Gentile, C.L. Gut microbiota regulates cardiac ischemic tolerance and aortic stiffness in obesity. *Am. J. Physiol. Circ. Physiol.* **2019**, *317*, 1210–1220. [CrossRef]
30. Trikha, S.R.J.; Lee, D.M.; Ecton, K.E.; Wrigley, S.D.; Vazquez, A.R.; Litwin, N.S.; Thomas, K.N.; Wei, Y.; Battson, M.L.; Johnson, S.A.; et al. Transplantation of an obesity-associated human gut microbiota to mice induces vascular dysfunction and glucose intolerance. *Gut Microbes* **2021**, *13*, 1940791. [CrossRef]
31. Battson, M.L.; Lee, D.M.; Jarrell, D.K.; Hou, S.; Ecton, K.E.; Weir, T.L.; Gentile, C.L. Suppression of gut dysbiosis reverses Western diet-induced vascular dysfunction. *Am. J. Physiol. Endocrinol. Metab.* **2018**, *314*, E468–E477. [CrossRef] [PubMed]
32. Brunt, V.E.; Gioscia-Ryan, R.A.; Richey, J.J.; Zigler, M.C.; Cuevas, L.M.; Gonzalez, A.; Vázquez-Baeza, Y.; Battson, M.L.; Smithson, A.T.; Gilley, A.D.; et al. Suppression of the gut microbiome ameliorates age-related arterial dysfunction and oxidative stress in mice. *J. Physiol.* **2019**, *597*, 2361–2378. [CrossRef] [PubMed]
33. Edwards, J.M.; Roy, S.; Tomcho, J.C.; Schreckenberger, Z.J.; Chakraborty, S.; Bearss, N.R.; Saha, P.; McCarthy, C.G.; Vijay-Kumar, M.; Joe, B.; et al. Microbiota are critical for vascular physiology: Germ-free status weakens contractility and induces sex-specific vascular remodeling in mice. *Vascul. Pharmacol.* **2020**, *125–126*, 106633. [CrossRef] [PubMed]
34. Foote, C.A.; Castorena-Gonzalez, J.A.; Ramirez-Perez, F.I.; Jia, G.; Hill, M.A.; Reyes-Aldasoro, C.C.; Sowers, J.R.; Martinez-Lemus, L.A. Arterial Stiffening in Western Diet-Fed Mice Is Associated with Increased Vascular Elastin, Transforming Growth Factor-β, and Plasma Neuraminidase. *Front. Physiol.* **2016**, *7*, 285. [CrossRef]
35. Menni, C.; Lin, C.; Cecelja, M.; Mangino, M.; Matey-Hernandez, M.L.; Keehn, L.; Mohney, R.P.; Steves, C.J.; Spector, T.D.; Kuo, C.-F.; et al. Gut microbial diversity is associated with lower arterial stiffness in women. *Eur. Heart J.* **2018**, *39*, 2390–2397. [CrossRef]
36. Biruete, A.; Allen, J.M.; Kistler, B.M.; Jeong, J.H.; Fitschen, P.J.; Swanson, K.S.; Wilund, K.R. Gut Microbiota and Cardiometabolic Risk Factors in Hemodialysis Patients. *Top. Clin. Nutr.* **2019**, *34*, 153–160. [CrossRef] [PubMed]
37. Dinakis, E.; Nakai, M.; Gill, P.A.; Yiallourou, S.; Sata, Y.; Muir, J.; Carrington, M.; Head, G.A.; Kaye, D.M.; Marques, F.Z. The Gut Microbiota and Their Metabolites in Human Arterial Stiffness. *Heart Lung Circ.* **2021**, *30*, 1716–1725. [CrossRef]
38. Hsu, C.-N.; Lu, P.-C.; Lo, M.-H.; Lin, I.-C.; Chang-Chien, G.-P.; Lin, S.; Tain, Y.-L. Gut Microbiota-Dependent Trimethylamine N-Oxide Pathway Associated with Cardiovascular Risk in Children with Early-Stage Chronic Kidney Disease. *Int. J. Mol. Sci.* **2018**, *19*, 3699. [CrossRef]
39. Istas, G.; Wood, E.; Le Sayec, M.; Rawlings, C.; Yoon, J.; Dandavate, V.; Cera, D.; Rampelli, S.; Costabile, A.; Fromentin, E.; et al. Effects of aronia berry (poly)phenols on vascular function and gut microbiota: A double-blind randomized controlled trial in adult men. *Am. J. Clin. Nutr.* **2019**, *110*, 316–329. [CrossRef]
40. Ried, K.; Travica, N.; Sali, A. The Effect of Kyolic Aged Garlic Extract on Gut Microbiota, Inflammation, and Cardiovascular Markers in Hypertensives: The GarGIC Trial. *Front. Nutr.* **2018**, *5*, 122. [CrossRef]
41. Liu, X.; Shao, Y.; Sun, J.; Tu, J.; Wang, Z.; Tao, J.; Chen, J. Egg consumption improves vascular and gut microbiota function without increasing inflammatory, metabolic, and oxidative stress markers. *FOOD Sci. Nutr.* **2022**, *10*, 295–304. [CrossRef]
42. Taniguchi, H.; Tanisawa, K.; Sun, X.; Kubo, T.; Hoshino, Y.; Hosokawa, M.; Takeyama, H.; Higuchi, M. Effects of short-term endurance exercise on gut microbiota in elderly men. *Physiol. Rep.* **2018**, *6*, e13935. [CrossRef] [PubMed]
43. Konikoff, T.; Gophna, U. Oscillospira: A Central, Enigmatic Component of the Human Gut Microbiota. *Trends Microbiol.* **2016**, *24*, 523–524. [CrossRef] [PubMed]
44. Huang, J.; Liao, J.; Fang, Y.; Deng, H.; Yin, H.; Shen, B.; Hu, M. Six-Week Exercise Training With Dietary Restriction Improves Central Hemodynamics Associated With Altered Gut Microbiota in Adolescents With Obesity. *Front. Endocrinol. (Lausanne).* **2020**, *11*, 569085. [CrossRef]
45. Ponziani, F.R.; Pompili, M.; Di Stasio, E.; Zocco, M.A.; Gasbarrini, A.; Flore, R. Subclinical atherosclerosis is linked to small intestinal bacterial overgrowth via vitamin K2-dependent mechanisms. *World J. Gastroenterol.* **2017**, *23*, 1241–1249. [CrossRef] [PubMed]
46. Rodriguez-Mateos, A.; Weber, T.; Skene, S.S.; Ottaviani, J.I.; Crozier, A.; Kelm, M.; Schroeter, H.; Heiss, C. Assessing the respective contributions of dietary flavanol monomers and procyanidins in mediating cardiovascular effects in humans: Randomized, controlled, double-masked intervention trial. *Am. J. Clin. Nutr.* **2018**, *108*, 1229–1237. [CrossRef]
47. Hazim, S.; Curtis, P.J.; Schär, M.Y.; Ostertag, L.M.; Kay, C.D.; Minihane, A.M.; Cassidy, A. Acute benefits of the microbial-derived isoflavone metabolite equol on arterial stiffness in men prospectively recruited according to equol producer phenotype: A double-blind randomized controlled trial. *Am. J. Clin. Nutr.* **2016**, *103*, 694–702. [CrossRef]

98. Elvers, K.T.; Wilson, V.J.; Hammond, A.; Duncan, L.; Huntley, A.L.; Hay, A.D.; van der Werf, E.T. Antibiotic-induced changes in the human gut microbiota for the most commonly prescribed antibiotics in primary care in the UK: A systematic review. *BMJ Open* **2020**, *10*, e035677. [CrossRef]
99. Kappel, B.A.; De Angelis, L.; Heiser, M.; Ballanti, M.; Stoehr, R.; Goettsch, C.; Mavilio, M.; Artati, A.; Paoluzi, O.A. Adamski, J.; et al. Cross-omics analysis revealed gut microbiome-related metabolic pathways underlying atherosclerosis development after antibiotics treatment. *Mol. Metab.* **2020**, *36*, 100976. [CrossRef]
100. Heianza, Y.; Ma, W.; Li, X.; Cao, Y.; Chan, A.T.; Rimm, E.B.; Hu, F.B.; Rexrode, K.M.; Manson, J.E.; Qi, L. Duration and Life-Stage of Antibiotic Use and Risks of All-Cause and Cause-Specific Mortality: Prospective Cohort Study. *Circ. Res.* **2020**, *126*, 364–373. [CrossRef]
101. Cheng, Y.-J.; Nie, X.-Y.; Chen, X.-M.; Lin, X.-X.; Tang, K.; Zeng, W.-T.; Mei, W.-Y.; Liu, L.-J.; Long, M.; Yao, F.-J.; et al. The Role of Macrolide Antibiotics in Increasing Cardiovascular Risk. *J. Am. Coll. Cardiol.* **2015**, *66*, 2173–2184. [CrossRef]
102. Wong, A.Y.S.; Chan, E.W.; Anand, S.; Worsley, A.J.; Wong, I.C.K. Managing Cardiovascular Risk of Macrolides: Systematic Review and Meta-Analysis. *Drug Saf.* **2017**, *40*, 663–677. [CrossRef] [PubMed]
103. Gorelik, E.; Masarwa, R.; Perlman, A.; Rotshild, V.; Abbasi, M.; Muszkat, M.; Matok, I. Fluoroquinolones and Cardiovascular Risk: A Systematic Review, Meta-analysis and Network Meta-analysis. *Drug Saf.* **2019**, *42*, 529–538. [CrossRef] [PubMed]
104. Rasmussen, S.H.; Shrestha, S.; Bjerregaard, L.G.; Ängquist, L.H.; Baker, J.L.; Jess, T.; Allin, K.H. Antibiotic exposure in early life and childhood overweight and obesity: A systematic review and meta-analysis. *Diabetes. Obes. Metab.* **2018**, *20*, 1508–1514. [CrossRef] [PubMed]
105. Simin, J.; Fornes, R.; Liu, Q.; Olsen, R.S.; Callens, S.; Engstrand, L.; Brusselaers, N. Antibiotic use and risk of colorectal cancer: A systematic review and dose-response meta-analysis. *Br. J. Cancer* **2020**, *123*, 1825–1832. [CrossRef] [PubMed]
106. Simin, J.; Tamimi, R.M.; Engstrand, L.; Callens, S.; Brusselaers, N. Antibiotic use and the risk of breast cancer: A systematic review and dose-response meta-analysis. *Pharmacol. Res.* **2020**, *160*, 105072. [CrossRef]

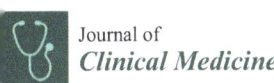

Article

Haemodynamic Adaptive Mechanisms at High Altitude: Comparison between European Lowlanders and Nepalese Highlanders

Paolo Salvi [1,*], Andrea Grillo [2], Sylvie Gautier [3], Luca Montaguti [4], Fausto Brunacci [4], Francesca Severi [4], Lucia Salvi [5], Enzo Pretolani [4], Gianfranco Parati [1,6,†] and Athanase Benetos [3,7,†]

1. Department of Cardiology, Istituto Auxologico Italiano, IRCCS, 20149 Milan, Italy; gianfranco.parati@unimib.it
2. Medicina Clinica, Azienda Sanitaria Universitaria Giuliano Isontina, 34149 Trieste, Italy; andr.grillo@gmail.com
3. CHRU-Nancy, Pôle "Maladies du Vieillissement, Gérontologie et Soins Palliatifs", Université de Lorraine, 54000 Nancy, France; s.gautier@chru-nancy.fr (S.G.); a.benetos@chru-nancy.fr (A.B.)
4. Department of Internal Medicine, 'M. Bufalini' Hospital, AUSL Romagna, 47521 Cesena, Italy; luca.montaguti@auslromagna.it (L.M.); fausto.brunacci@libero.it (F.B.); francescaseveri777@gmail.com (F.S.); psalvi.md@libero.it (E.P.)
5. Medicina II Cardiovascolare, AUSL-IRCCS di Reggio Emilia, 42123 Reggio Emilia, Italy; lsalvi.md@gmail.com
6. Department of Medicine and Surgery, University of Milano-Bicocca, 20126 Milan, Italy
7. INSERM, Université de Lorraine, DCAC u1116, 54000 Nancy, France
* Correspondence: psalvi.md@gmail.com
† These authors contributed equally to this work.

Abstract: Background: Exposure to high altitudes determines several adaptive mechanisms affecting in a complex way the whole cardiovascular, respiratory, endocrine systems because of the hypobaric hypoxic condition. The aim of our study was to evaluate the circulatory adaptive mechanisms at high altitudes, during a scientific expedition in the Himalayas. Methods: Arterial distensibility was assessed measuring carotid-radial and carotid-femoral pulse wave velocity. Tests were carried out at several altitudes, from 1350 to 5050 m above sea level, on 8 lowlander European researchers and 11 highlander Nepalese porters. Results: In Europeans, systolic blood pressure and pulse pressure increased slightly but significantly with altitude ($p < 0.05$ and $p < 0.001$, respectively). Norepinephrine showed a significant increase after the lowlanders had spent some time at high altitude ($p < 0.001$). With increasing altitude, a progressive increase in carotid-radial and carotid-femoral pulse wave velocity values was observed in lowlanders, showing a particularly significant increase ($p < 0.001$) after staying at high altitude (carotid-radial pulse wave velocity, median value (interquartile range) from 9.2 (7.9–10.0) to 11.2 (10.9–11.8) m/s and carotid-femoral pulse wave velocity from 8.5 (7.9–9.0) to 11.3 (10.9–11.8) m/s). At high altitudes (3400 and 5050 m above sea level), no significant differences were observed between highlanders and lowlanders in hemodynamic parameters (blood pressure, carotid-radial and carotid-femoral pulse wave velocity). Conclusions: The progressive arterial stiffening with altitude observed in European lowlanders could explain the increase in systolic and pulse pressure values observed at high altitudes in this ethnic group. Further studies are needed to evaluate the role of aortic stiffening in the pathogenesis of acute mountain sickness.

Keywords: altitude; altitude sickness; aortic stiffness; aortic distensibility; atrial natriuretic factor; blood pressure; pulse wave velocity; vascular stiffness

1. Introduction

Exposure to high altitudes determines several adaptive mechanisms which affect in a complex way the whole cardiovascular, respiratory, and endocrine systems because of the hypobaric hypoxic condition. Altitude may lead to detrimental effects on health, the most common of which is Acute Mountain Sickness (AMS). This condition is favoured by rapid ascent, exercise, cold, and individual predisposition [1,2] and is characterized by a clinical syndrome which may result in pulmonary and cerebral oedema, which are potentially lethal events [3,4]. The interrelation of several haemodynamic factors contributes to the development of pulmonary oedema. With the scope to evaluate the role of cardiovascular alterations in the pathogenesis of high-altitude pulmonary oedema, several studies have been conducted on humans to study the pulmonary and cardiac adaptations to high altitudes [5]. The adrenergic system activation is particularly important for the control of the cardiac function and of the vascular tone in the first phases of high altitudes adaptation [6]. In men, this activation seems to be particularly evident during a sub maximal physical stress [7] and could be responsible for the increased values of the basal renin plasmatic activity observed in these individuals [8]. Further studies have also demonstrated a modification in the number and functions of beta-adrenergic receptors in highlanders [9]. In the critical conditions of high altitudes, some human populations, such as Nepalese highlanders, have developed some phenotypic traits influenced by hypoxia, namely, a broader chest, larger lung capacity, and increase haemoglobin concentration [10–12]. The biological response of healthy lowlanders exposed to high altitude may therefore differ from that of native highlanders.

Despite the large number of studies conducted on humans to study the pulmonary and cardiac adaptations to altitude, the adaptive mechanisms of the large elastic arteries at very high altitude are not yet clearly understood. Given the difficulty and complexity of performing clinical research in extreme hypoxic-hypobaric conditions, a very small number of studies evaluated a possible process of aortic stiffening induced by exposure at very high altitudes. Lewis et al. [13] assessed arterial viscoelastic properties on 12 healthy lowlanders and 12 highlanders at very high altitude. In this study aortic distensibility, estimated by carotid-femoral pulse wave velocity (PWV), was measured in lowlanders at sea level, upon arrival at 5050 m above sea level (a.s.l.), and after 12–14 days of acclimatization, while highlanders completed only one session at 5050 m a.s.l. Compared with lowlanders at sea level, highlanders showed a higher aortic PWV; however, once lowlanders were exposed to high altitude, these between group differences were not present. However, the small number of people involved in the study and the absence of assessments at intermediate altitudes require further studies to confirm these results. On the other hand, acute ascent at an altitude of 4559 m a.s.l. (HIGHCARE Alps Study, Capanna Regina Margherita, Monte Rosa, Italy) did not show a significant change in aortic PWV in a group of 22 healthy volunteers [14].

The large arteries play an important role in blood pressure and peripheral flux regulation. It is well known that large arteries physiologically have not only a conduit function but also a buffering function, and owing to their distensibility, they are able to decrease the pulsatile systolic output of the left ventricle. Therefore, the large arteries have a regulation role, redeeming the pulsatility of the systolic ejection and transforming the regime of the cardiac pump from discontinuous to continuous. This buffering function results from the viscoelastic properties of the arterial wall, which depend on the arterial structure and tone. Structure is determined by the three arterial wall components: elastin, collagen, and smooth muscle cells. On the other hand, the arterial tone is mainly modulated by the autonomic nervous system's activity and by other vasoactive systems (adrenergic system, renin-angiotensin system, vasopressin, etc.) [15]. The functional and structural conditions of the arteries determine their ability to buffer the systolic wave and influence systemic blood pressure values [16].

The aim of our research was to study the changes in blood pressure and haemodynamic parameters during the ascent and staying at high altitudes, in two groups of European lowlanders and Nepalese highlanders.

2. Materials and Methods

This study was performed during the scientific expedition in the Himalayas "Circulatory adaptive mechanisms at high altitudes", inside the research project Everest-K2 of the Italian National Research Council (CNR). Our scientific expedition involved a group of white European lowlander researchers, who lived permanently almost at sea level, and a group of Nepalese highlanders, of Rai ethnicity, born and residing in the Khumbu valley between 3400 and 4930 m a.s.l., on average at 4007 ± 583 m a.s.l. The presence of chronic disease involving habitual therapy was considered an exclusion criterion from the study. No chronic treatments were taken by the study participants, and no drugs were taken during the high-altitude ascension.

The lowlanders, coming from Europe (Milan and Paris), after a 3-day stay in Kathmandu (Nepal, 1350 m a.s.l.), were taken by air transport to Lukla airport (2840 m a.s.l.). Nepalese highlander porters were enrolled at Lukla airport. Enrolment was random, linked to the needs of the scientific expedition (transport of scientific instruments and personal baggage of the researchers). After staying overnight in the nearby village of Phakding (2500 m a.s.l.), the group of lowlanders and highlanders trekked the next day to the village of Namche Bazaar (3400 m a.s.l.), where they stayed two full days for ac-climatization. From Namche Bazaar, the two groups of lowlanders and highlanders hiked together for 3 days to Lobuche (5050 m a.s.l.) on the Nepalese side of Everest at the "Pyramid International Laboratory" of the Italian National Research Council (CNR).

Data were collected at Kathmandu and Namche Bazaar in hotel rooms and at Lobuche in the Pyramid International Laboratory. Barometric pressure was recorded by a microclimatic station at the time of each study. Ambient temperature was similarly recorded and kept constant throughout the study. Examinations were performed in the morning after at least 18 h of physical rest and after a stay of at least 1 h in a room with a constant temperature of $19 \pm 1\ °C$.

2.1. Protocol of the Study

Participants were studied at different altitudes.
For the Europeans, measurements were performed (Figure 1):

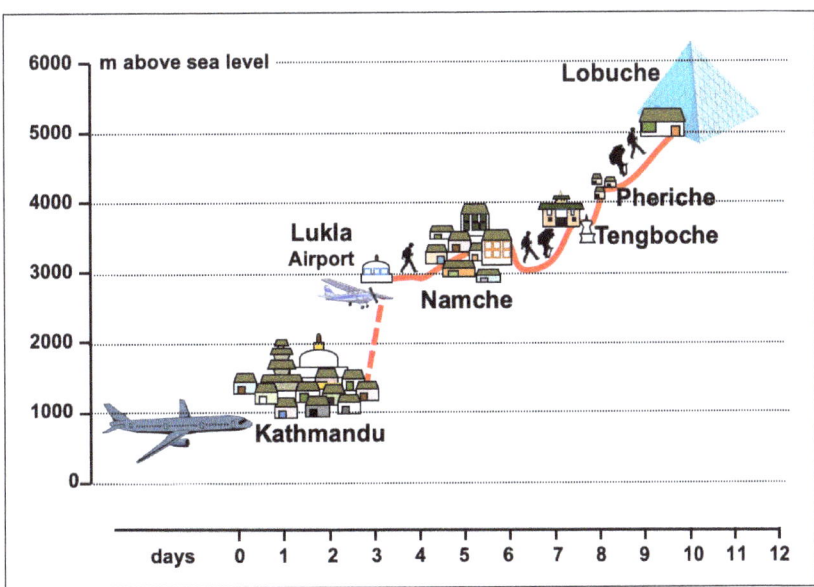

Figure 1. Timing, altimetry, and steps of the scientific expedition.

- In Italy, at sea level (only clinical and blood parameters);
- On the second day of permanence in Kathmandu, at 1350 m a.s.l.;
- On the second day of permanence in Namche Bazar, at 3400 m a.s.l.;
- On the second day of permanence in Lobuche, at 5050 m. a.s.l.;
- On the eighth day of stay in this high altitude laboratory.

For Nepalese participants, the same measurements were performed the same day as for the Europeans at 3400 m a.s.l. and the second day after their arrival in Lobuche.

2.2. Arterial Stiffness Assessment

The viscoelastic properties of large arteries were estimated by measuring PWV. Currently, carotid-femoral PWV (cf-PWV) is considered the most reliable non-invasive method for assessing aortic stiffness, while carotid-radial PWV (cr-PWV) reflects the stiffness of the muscular arteries in the upper limb [17]. A Millar Mikro-Tip Pulse Transducer SPT-301B tonometer (Millar Instruments, Inc., Houston, TX, USA) [16,18,19] integrated into a Cardioline Delta 3 electrocardiograph (Remco SpA, San Pedrino di Vignate, Italy) was used to record pulse pressure curves. PWV was measured by recording pressure wave curves in the carotid and peripheral arteries (femoral or radial) in rapid succession. PWV was defined as 80% of the distance between measurement sites [20] divided by the time delay between the distal (femoral or radial) pulse wave and the proximal (carotid) pulse wave, using the ECG trace as a reference. This method was previously described in detail [21,22].

2.3. Blood Pressure Measurement

Blood pressure measurements were carried out by means of mercury sphygmomanometer and a validated oscillometric system (Dinamap, model 1846 SX, Critikon, Tampa, FL, USA). Blood pressure with the latter device was acquired every 2 min in the left arm, during the tonometric recording.

2.4. Oxygen Saturation

Arterial oxygen saturation was measured by means of a Kontron Pulse Oximeter 7845 (Kontron, S&T group, Linz, Austria) with finger clip sensor.

2.5. Biochemical Dosages

The radioenzymatic assay was performed for the dopamine, epinephrine, and norepinephrine assays and the radioimmunoassay for the determination of the atrial natriuretic factor. These dosages were performed only at 1350 m a.s.l., at 5050 m a.s.l., and after stay at 5050 m a.s.l.

2.6. Statistical Analysis

Results are expressed as median and interquartile range. Normal distribution of variables was assessed by Shapiro–Wilk test. Differences between two groups (Europeans and Nepalese) for all variables were evaluated with Student's t-test for unpaired data or with independent samples Mann–Whitney U test for variables not normally distributed. Levene's test was used to assess equality of variances. Statistical analysis of parameter's alterations with altitude was calculated using Friedman's test and the subsequent two tailed Wilcoxon test for non-parametric paired data. Multivariate analysis using logistic regression models adjusted for age and body mass index were performed to assess differences in parameters between the European and Nepalese groups. Statistical analysis was performed by using the Statistical Package for the Social Sciences (SPSS for Windows, Release 20.0; SPSS, Chicago, IL, USA). A p value less than 0.05 was considered as significant.

3. Results

3.1. Population

All 8 European participants in the scientific expedition (6 men and 2 women) and 11 male Nepalese porters belonging to the Rai ethnic group agreed to participate in the study. Table 1 shows how highlander Nepalese were significantly shorter and leaner than European lowlanders.

Table 1. Main anthropometric characteristics of participants.

Parameter	Lowlanders	Highlanders	p-Value
Sex, f/m	2/6	0/11	
Age, years	35.0 (1.5–37.7)	25.0 (23.0–33.0)	0.004
Height, cm	176.0 (167.0–178.7)	158.0 (155.0–166.0)	<0.001
Weight, Kg	76.5 (70.5–82.2)	51.0 (49.0–54.0)	<0.001
BMI, Kg/m^2	25.0 (23.9–27.5)	20.6 (18.5–21.5)	<0.001
BSA, m^2	1.93 (1.81–2.01)	1.50 (1.47–1.56)	<0.001

Data are shown as median (interquartile range). Significance is expressed by the p-value. BMI, body mass index; BSA, body surface area; f, females; m, males.

Among the eight Europeans participating in this expedition, six reported headaches after 4000 m a.s.l. Three had moderate dyspnoea at rest, and one experienced vomiting at 5000 m a.s.l. Finally, upon arrival at Lobuche, one person in the lowlander group presented with signs of moderate cerebral oedema (ataxia, headache, dizziness, vomiting), which rapidly regressed after oxygen and corticoid therapy. None of the highlander porters reported any symptoms.

3.2. Blood Pressure and Large Arteries Parameters

Table 2 shows the clinical and haemodynamic parameters changes with altitude in the lowlander European volunteers and in the Nepalese porters.

Table 2. Clinical and haemodynamic parameters changes with altitude in lowlander European volunteers (n = 8) and in highlander Nepalese porters (n = 11).

Parameters	European Lowlanders				
	Sea Level	1350 m a.s.l.	3400 m a.s.l.	5050 m a.s.l.	5050 m a.s.l. after 8 Days of Stay
SaO$_2$, %	96.0 (95.2–97.0)	95.9 (95.4–97.0)	92.6 (89.0–94.5)	80.5 (77.0–84.0) **	83.5 (77.8–89.5) **
Respiratory Rate, breaths/m	10.5 (10.0–11.0)	10.0 (10.0–10.7)	12.0 (11.2–13.7)	14.0 (12.2–15.0) *	14.0 (12.3–15.0) *
Heart Rate, beat/m	62.6 (62.0–69.3)	67.2 (59.8–74.9)	71.2 (54.8–86.7)	78.3 (74.6–82.4)	76.5 (63.8–83.7)
Systolic BP, mmHg	109.2 (107.7–115.2)	112.7 (109.1–116.4)	118.5 (112.2–120.9)	119.2 (114.5–122.2)	121.0 (111.5–133.0) *
Diastolic BP, mmHg	71.3 (68.0–79.5)	66.7 (62.6–71.3)	68.0 (64.7–77.1)	70.5 (66.2–75.6)	70.5 (63.1–80.2)
Mean BP, mmHg	84.0 (81.2–93.7)	81.6 (78.6–87.1)	84.8 (81.4–91.8)	87.2 (82.5–90.0)	87.3 (79.7–97.3)
Pulse Pressure, mmHg	39.3 (32.3–44.0)	45.3 (44.3–47.7) *	46.8 (42.3–49.1) *	48.0 (46.0–51.7) **	50.7 (46.0–55.1) **
Carotid-femoral PWV, m/s	8.47 (7.87–9.00)	8.97 (7.82–9.78)	9.75 (9.13–10.11) *	8.90 (8.63–10.09) *	11.27 (9.82–12.96) **
Carotid-radial PWV, m/s	9.21 (7.90–10.06)	9.76 (8.00–10.01)	9.58 (8.43–10.01)	9.83 (9.07–10.19)	11.17 (10.90–11.76) **
Parameters	Nepalese Highlanders				
			3400 m a.s.l.	5050 m a.s.l.	
SaO$_2$, %			94.0 (92.4–95.5)	85.0 (83.0–91.0) **,†	
Respiratory Rate, breaths/m			11.0 (11.0–12.0)	12.0 (12.0–13.0) †	
Heart Rate, beat/m			62.7 (57.0–69.7)	64.3 (60.7–79.0)	
Systolic BP, mmHg			115.0 (109.7–118.7)	118.3 (102.7–121.3)	
Diastolic BP, mmHg			70.0 (66.7–76.0)	72.3 (70.7–78.7)	
Mean BP, mmHg			85.1 (80.8–90.2)	88.7 (81.6–92.4)	
Pulse Pressure, mmHg			42.7 (40.0–45.3)	42.7 (36.0–46.7) †	
Carotid-femoral PWV, m/s			8.65 (7.73–9.97)	9.09 (8.59–11.17)	
Carotid-radial PWV, m/s			9.59 (8.54–11.64)	10.42 (8.92–12.21)	

Data are shown as median (interquartile range). Significance is expressed by the p-value. *, p < 0.05; **, p < 0.001; versus basal condition (sea level for lowlanders and 3400 m a.s.l. for highlanders). †, p < 0.05; highlanders versus lowlanders at the same altitude (unadjusted data). BP, blood pressure; PWV, pulse wave velocity; SaO$_2$, arterial oxygen saturation.

In the European group, systolic blood pressure and pulse pressure increased slightly but significantly with altitude (Figure 2), reaching the highest levels eight days after the arrival at 5050 m (p < 0.05). Diastolic blood pressure and mean blood pressure did not show significant changes with altitude. In the Nepalese participants, blood pressure values did not change between 3500 and 5050 m.

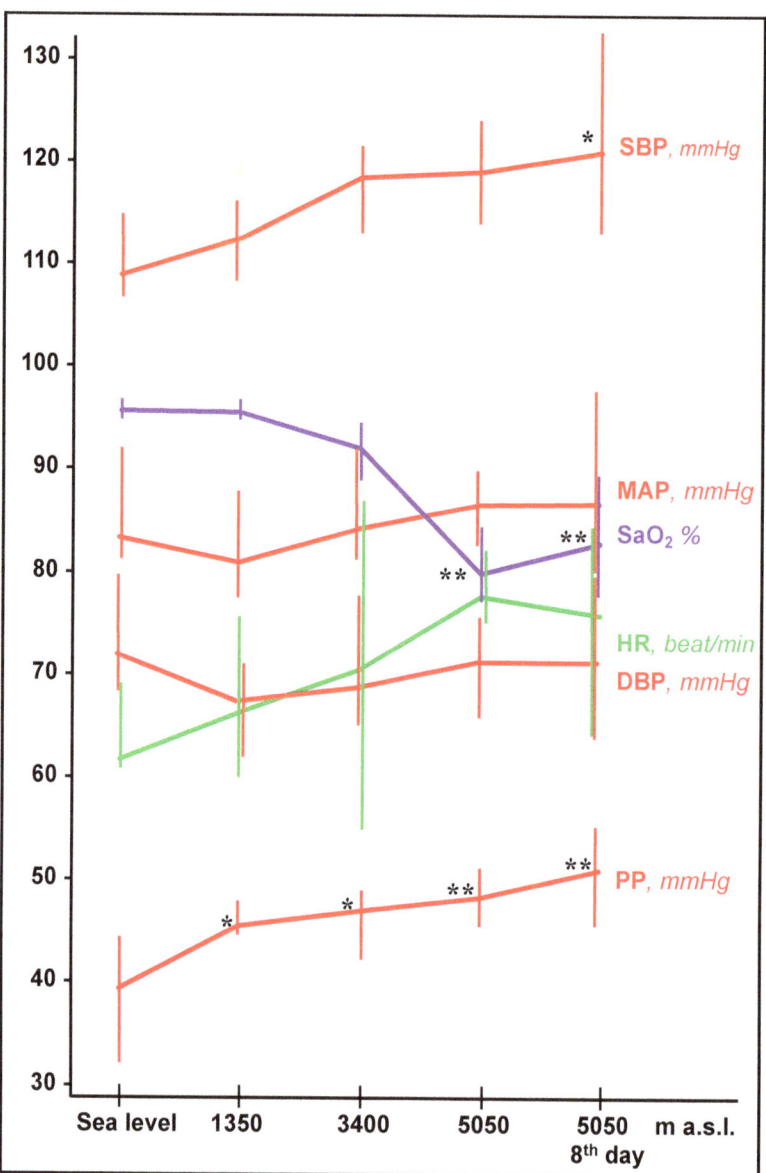

Figure 2. Heart rate (HR, green line), arterial oxygen saturation (SaO$_2$, violet line), and blood pressure (red lines) changes with altitude in 8 lowlander European volunteers. Data are shown as median and interquartile range. Significance is expressed by the *p*-value: *, $p < 0.05$; **, $p < 0.001$ versus sea level values. a.s.l., above sea level; DBP, diastolic blood pressure; MAP, mean arterial pressure; PP, pulse pressure (= SBP − DBP); SBP, systolic blood pressure.

Carotid-femoral and carotid-radial PWV increased in Europeans with altitude (Figures 3 and 4) showing the highest significant values ($p < 0.001$) on the eighth day in Lobuche (carotid-femoral: from 8.5 (7.9–9.0) to 11.3 (10.9–11.8) m/s, carotid-radial: from

9.2 (7.9–10.0) to 11.2 (10.9–11.8) m/s. As for systolic blood pressure in the Nepalese, no changes in PWV were observed with altitude.

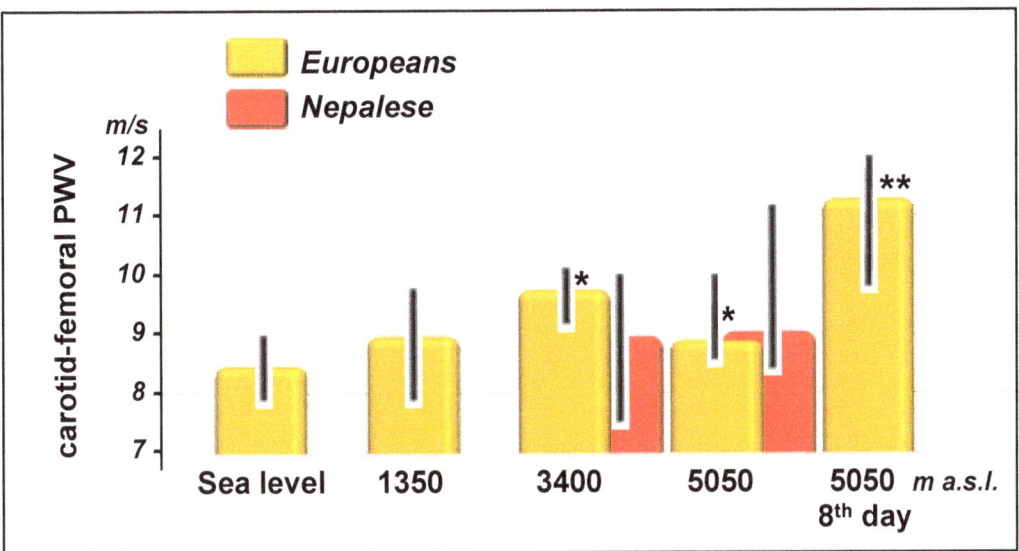

Figure 3. Changes in carotid-femoral pulse wave velocity (PWV) during the ascent and stay at very high altitudes in Europeans and Nepalese. Data are shown as median and interquartile range. Significance versus basal condition (sea level for lowlanders and 3400 m a.s.l. for highlanders) is expressed by the p-value: *, $p < 0.05$; **, $p < 0.001$.

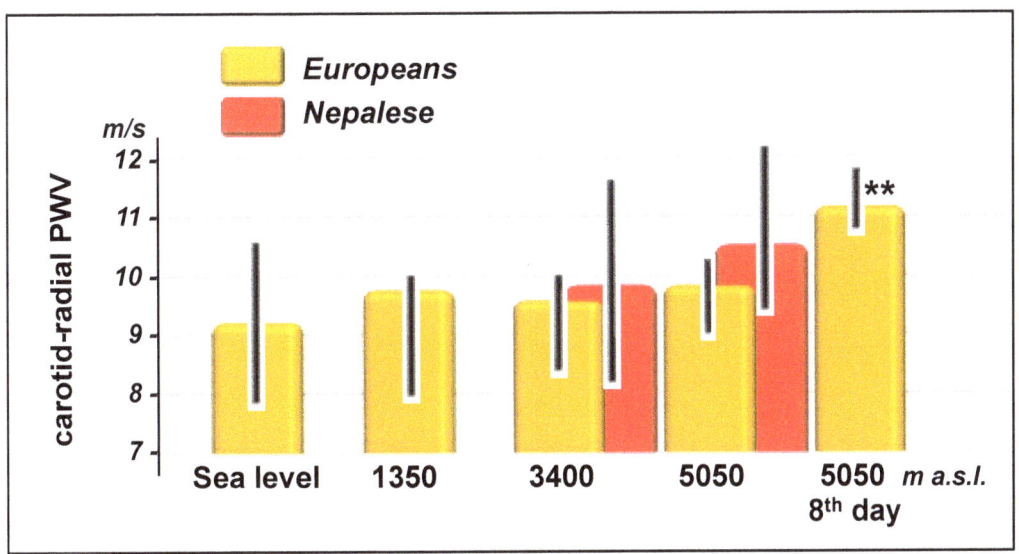

Figure 4. Changes in carotid-radial pulse wave velocity (PWV) during the ascent and stay at very high altitudes in Europeans and Nepalese. Data are shown as median and interquartile range. Significance versus basal condition (sea level for lowlanders and 3400 m a.s.l. for highlanders) is expressed by the p-value: **, $p < 0.001$.

A constant elevation of norepinephrine was observed in lowlanders at high altitude (5050 m a.s.l.), especially on the eighth day compared to the values recorded at 1350 m a.s.l. ($p < 0.05$): from median (interquartile range) 18 (9–45) pg/mL at 1350 m a.s.l. to 186 (158–222) pg/mL at 5050 m a.s.l., to 350 (193–833) pg/mL after 8 days of stay at 5050 m a.s.l. Nepalese people had higher levels of norepinephrine than the Europeans at the same altitude (428 (326–572) pg/mL at 5050 m a.s.l., $p < 0.05$). Epinephrine, dopamine, and atrial natriuretic factor tended to increase with altitude in lowlanders, without reaching statistical significance (Figure 5). No significant differences were found in the dosages of these molecules between lowlanders and highlanders at 5050 m a.s.l.

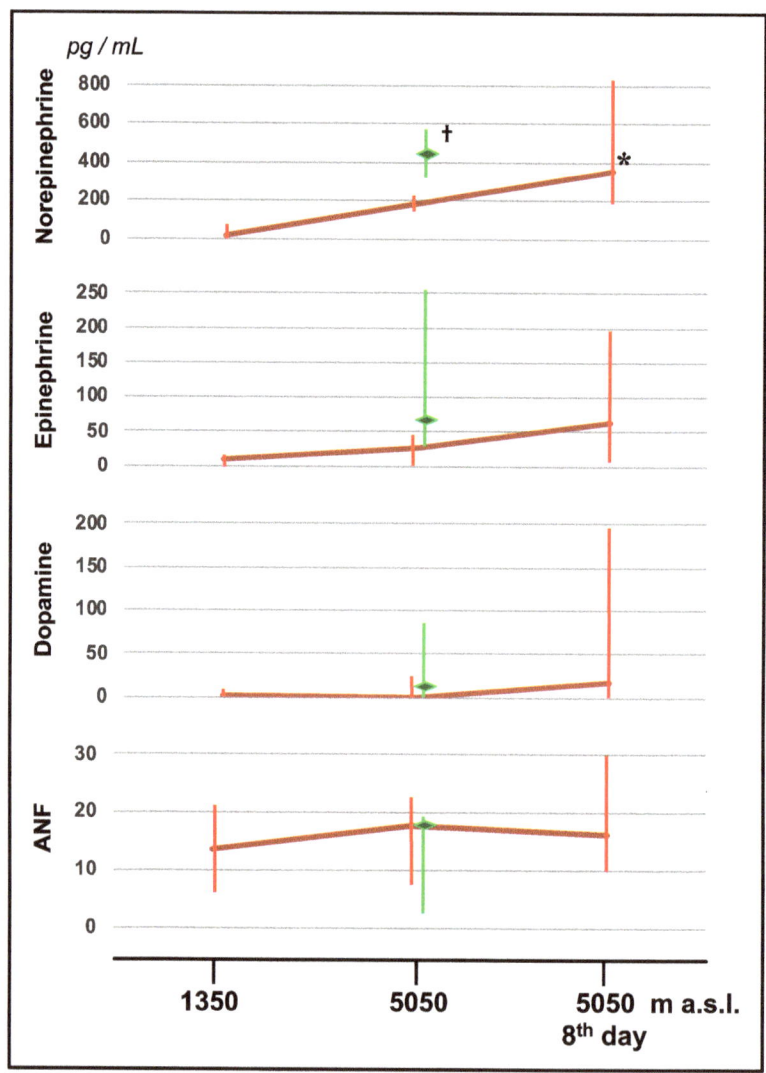

Figure 5. Changes in norepinephrine, epinephrine, dopamine, and atrial natriuretic factor values in lowlanders (red lines) with altitude. Data recorded in highlanders at 5050 m a.s.l. are shown as green lines. Data are shown as median and interquartile range. a.s.l., above sea level. Significance is expressed by the p-value: *, $p < 0.05$ versus values at 1350 m a.s.l.; †, $p < 0.05$ highlanders versus lowlanders.

4. Discussion

Our study provides three main findings. One, in healthy lowlander volunteers, acute exposure to high altitude causes a significant increase in arterial stiffness, as documented by the increase in PWV. Two, this process of stiffening of the large arteries not only affects the aorta but also involves the large muscular arteries of the upper limbs. Three, PWV values (both carotid-femoral and carotid-radial) recorded in Nepalese highlanders were similar to those recorded in European lowlanders at the same altitude. These changes remained significant after adjusting for mean arterial pressure and heart rate changes with altitude.

The viscoelastic properties of the aorta and of the large elastic arteries are guaranteed by an adequate ratio between elastic and collagen fibres of the arterial wall, as well as by a balance between these fibres, the extracellular matrix, and the smooth muscle cells. While changes in arterial wall structure may be evoked as an adaptation phenomenon for Nepalese highlanders, on the other hand, it is difficult to hypothesize that structural changes in the arterial wall can occur in the relatively short time of high-altitude ascension. A further element that makes PWV change at high altitude unlikely to be due to structural changes in the arterial wall comes from the results of the HIGHCARE Study. In agreement with results of our study, the HIGHCARE study showed, after an increase in PWV values at high altitudes, a rapid return of the PWV to baseline after returning to Europe at sea level [23].

We can therefore hypothesize, at least in lowlanders, a prevalent role played by functional factors in the changes in arterial distensibility at high altitudes. The role of functional factors affecting arterial mechanical properties is complex, and their changes are transitory. The main functional factors determining changes in vascular distensibility include left ventricular systolic ejection function, heart rate, arterial smooth muscle, and mean arterial pressure [16]. The sympathetic nervous system is considered to be one of the major elements affecting arterial functional properties. The activation of the sympathetic nervous system increases heart rate, ventricular contractility, and modulates the activity of the smooth muscle cell of the arterial wall, inducing peripheral vasoconstriction, increase in peripheral vascular resistance, and, therefore, a rise in mean arterial pressure. Additionally, increased peripheral vascular resistance can modify the amplitude and distribution of reflected pressure waves, increasing aortic systolic blood pressure as well as pulse pressure.

As already emerged in the HIGHCARE Study [23,24], and as shown by other research at high altitude [25,26], we confirm that exposure to high-altitude hypoxia is accompanied by a significant increase in plasma norepinephrine proportional to the altitude reached. This sympathetic activation is accentuated during the stay at high altitude. The adrenergic system activation is particularly important for the control of cardiac function and vascular tone in the first phases of adaptation to high altitude [6,24]. A modification of the number and functions of beta-adrenergic receptors in subjects who live at a high altitudes has been clearly shown [9]. Indeed, elevated epinephrine values at high altitudes were also found in our study, even in highlander porters.

The trend of the norepinephrine increase curve is associated with a corresponding significant increase in PWV. The stiffening of the aorta at high altitudes, documented by the increase in cf-PWV, may justify the increase in systolic blood pressure and pulse pressure recorded at high altitudes. The PWV values which were registered in the native people are similar to those registered in the Europeans at the same altitude; therefore, it may be inferred that the modifications which were observed in the Europeans are chronically present in the natives.

Muscular arteries should be much more sensitive to the activity of the sympathetic nervous system than the aorta and elastic arteries. We would therefore have expected a greater increase in cr-PWV compared to cf-PWV at high altitudes. Therefore, the weaker increase in carotid-radial PWV with altitude suggests that other factors besides sympathetic activation may influence the aortic stiffening. Among other factors that can contribute to increased aortic stiffness at high altitudes, we can consider haemoconcentration with consequent increase in blood viscosity [27], oxidative stress [28,29], interstitial oedema of the arterial wall [30], and endothelial dysfunction [31,32]. Previous studies have shown a link between altitude-induced increases in pulmonary artery pressure and increases in plasma and urinary tract endothelin-1 levels [33], suggesting that acute exposure to high altitude may impair both endothelial and vascular smooth muscle cell function. At present all these etiopathogenetic hypotheses are mainly based on speculative considerations, and further experimental studies are necessary to define the mechanisms underlying the increase in arterial stiffness related to hypobaric-hypoxia.

According to our knowledge, only the study developed by Lewis et al. compared aortic PWV values in lowlanders and highlanders at the same altitude, above 5000 m a.s.l., and provided evidence of impaired vascular function in highlanders versus lowlanders at sea level, as indicated by significantly higher central PWV values [13]. These observed changes in vascular function and central PWV in the Nepalese natives were remarkably comparable to those of European lowlanders at 5050 m a.s.l., suggesting that these changes may not depend on time spent at high altitudes. Contrary to what was evidenced in our study and in Lewis's study, Bruno et al. found no differences in aortic PWV values when comparing a cohort of 95 Nepalese living permanently in three rural villages at 2600, 3800, and 3800 m a.s.l. with a group of 64 Caucasian Italian volunteers, matched for age, sex, mean arterial pressure, and body mass index [34]. The discrepancy between the results of these studies could be attributed to a selection bias in the lowlander control group of the latter study. Further studies are needed to clarify this issue.

The main limitation of our study was the relatively small number of enrolled individuals. However, the limit conditions in which the researchers worked must be taken into account. Materials were carried on back by Nepalese porters and yaks (therefore, the weight was limited to small amounts), the energy supply was scarce. In Namche, the electric power was available only for few hours a day and sometimes it was unsteady.

5. Conclusions

These data demonstrate how altitude determines important and significant haemodynamic changes. The stiffening of the aorta at high altitudes, documented by the increase in cf-PWV, could justify the increase in systolic blood pressure and pulse pressure recorded at high altitudes [23,35]. Further studies are needed to evaluate the role of aortic stiffening in the pathogenesis of high-altitude pulmonary oedema and of the cardiac hypertrophy-dilation, which is often observed in people exposed to prolonged stays at high altitudes and in highlanders affected by chronic mountain sickness.

Author Contributions: Conceptualization, E.P., P.S. and A.B.; methodology, P.S., A.G., S.G., E.P., F.B. and F.S.; data analysis, P.S., A.G., L.S. and L.M.; formal analysis, G.P. and A.B.; investigation, P.S., L.M., F.B., F.S., S.G. and A.B.; writing—original draft preparation, P.S., A.G., L.S. and A.B; writing—review and editing, G.P. and A.B.; supervision, A.G., S.G., L.M., E.P. and A.B. All authors have read and agreed to the published version of the manuscript.

Funding: This research was partially supported by the Italian Ministry of Health. This research was funded by ICOT Impianti srl, Forlí, Italy, with the collaboration of Zeneca Italia s.p.a. supporting the Italian group, and Laboratoires Knoll France supporting the French group.

Institutional Review Board Statement: The study was conducted in accordance with the Declaration of Helsinki and approved by the Ethics Committee of Azienda Unità Sanitaria Locale di Cesena for studies involving humans (protocol n. 1993060801).

Informed Consent Statement: Informed consent was obtained from all participants at the study.

Data Availability Statement: The data presented in this study are available upon reasonable request from the corresponding author. The data are not publicly available due to privacy concerns.

Acknowledgments: This study was organized, coordinated, and led by Enzo Pretolani, within the research project Everest-K2 of the Italian National Research Council (CNR). Logistic support in Nepal was given by Mountain Equipe s.r.l., Bergamo, Italy. Special thanks to the engineer Giuseppe Lio, who oversaw the development of the device used in this study to assess pulse wave velocity.

Conflicts of Interest: The authors declare no conflict of interest.

References

1. Hackett, P.H.; Rennie, D. Avoiding mountain sickness. *Lancet* **1978**, *2*, 938. [CrossRef]
2. Selland, M.A.; Stelzner, T.J.; Stevens, T.; Mazzeo, R.S.; McCullough, R.E.; Reeves, J.T. Pulmonary function and hypoxic ventilatory response in subjects susceptible to high-altitude pulmonary edema. *Chest* **1993**, *103*, 111–116. [CrossRef] [PubMed]
3. Grocott, M.; Montgomery, H.; Vercueil, A. High-altitude physiology and pathophysiology: Implications and relevance for intensive care medicine. *Crit. Care* **2007**, *11*, 203. [CrossRef] [PubMed]
4. Hackett, P.H.; Rennie, D.; Levine, H.D. The incidence, importance, and prophylaxis of acute mountain sickness. *Lancet* **1976**, *2*, 1149–1155. [CrossRef]
5. Heistad, D.D.; Abboud, F.M.; Dickinson, W. Richards Lecture: Circulatory adjustments to hypoxia. *Circulation* **1980**, *61*, 463–470. [CrossRef]
6. Richalet, J.P.; Kacimi, R.; Antezana, A.M. The control of cardiac chronotropic function in hypobaric hypoxia. *Int. J. Sports Med.* **1992**, *13* (Suppl. 1), S22–S24. [CrossRef]
7. Rowell, L.B.; Blackmon, J.R.; Kenny, M.A.; Escourrou, P. Splanchnic vasomotor and metabolic adjustments to hypoxia and exercise in humans. *Am. J. Physiol.* **1984**, *247*, H251–H258. [CrossRef]
8. Milledge, J.S.; Catley, D.M.; Blume, F.D.; West, J.B. Renin, angiotensin-converting enzyme, and aldosterone in humans on Mount Everest. *J. Appl. Physiol. Respir. Environ. Exerc. Physiol.* **1983**, *55*, 1109–1112. [CrossRef]
9. Aldashev, A.A.; Borbugulov, U.M.; Davletov, B.A.; Mirrakhimov, M.M. Human adrenoceptor system response to the development of high altitude pulmonary arterial hypertension. *J. Mol. Cell. Cardiol.* **1989**, *21* (Suppl. 1), 175–179. [CrossRef]
10. Moore, L.G. Human Genetic Adaptation to High Altitudes: Current Status and Future Prospects. *Quat. Int.* **2017**, *461*, 4–13. [CrossRef]
11. Brutsaert, T.D.; Soria, R.; Caceres, E.; Spielvogel, H.; Haas, J.D. Effect of developmental and ancestral high altitude exposure on chest morphology and pulmonary function in Andean and European/North American natives. *Am. J. Hum. Biol.* **1999**, *11*, 383–395. [CrossRef]
12. Beall, C.M.; Brittenham, G.M.; Strohl, K.P.; Blangero, J.; Williams-Blangero, S.; Goldstein, M.C.; Decker, M.J.; Vargas, E.; Villena, M.; Soria, R.; et al. Hemoglobin concentration of high-altitude Tibetans and Bolivian Aymara. *Am. J. Phys. Anthropol.* **1998**, *106*, 385–400. [CrossRef]
13. Lewis, N.C.; Bailey, D.M.; Dumanoir, G.R.; Messinger, L.; Lucas, S.J.; Cotter, J.D.; Donnelly, J.; McEneny, J.; Young, I.S.; Stembridge, M.; et al. Conduit artery structure and function in lowlanders and native highlanders: Relationships with oxidative stress and role of sympathoexcitation. *J. Physiol.* **2014**, *592*, 1009–1024. [CrossRef] [PubMed]
14. Parati, G.; Revera, M.; Giuliano, A.; Faini, A.; Bilo, G.; Gregorini, F.; Lisi, E.; Salerno, S.; Lombardi, C.; Ramos Becerra, C.G.; et al. Effects of acetazolamide on central blood pressure, peripheral blood pressure, and arterial distensibility at acute high altitude exposure. *Eur. Heart J.* **2013**, *34*, 759–766. [CrossRef] [PubMed]
15. Bollinger, A.; Hoffmann, U.; Franzeck, U.K. Evaluation of flux motion in man by the laser Doppler technique. *Blood Vessels* **1991**, *28* (Suppl. 1), 21–26. [CrossRef] [PubMed]
16. Salvi, P. *Pulse Waves. How Vascular Hemodynamics Affects Blood Pressure*, 2nd ed.; Springer Nature: Heidelberg, Germany, 2017.
17. Townsend, R.R.; Wilkinson, I.B.; Schiffrin, E.L.; Avolio, A.P.; Chirinos, J.A.; Cockcroft, J.R.; Heffernan, K.S.; Lakatta, E.G.; McEniery, C.M.; Mitchell, G.F.; et al. Recommendations for Improving and Standardizing Vascular Research on Arterial Stiffness: A Scientific Statement from the American Heart Association. *Hypertension* **2015**, *66*, 698–722. [CrossRef]
18. Nichols, W.; O'Rourke, M.; Vlachopoulos, C. *McDonald's Blood Flow in Arteries. Theoretical, Experimental and Clinical Principles*, 6th ed.; Oxford University Press: New York, NY, USA, 2011.
19. Kelly, R.; Hayward, C.; Ganis, J.; Daley, J.; Avolio, A.; O'Rourke, M. Non-invasive registration of the arterial pressure pulse waveform using highfidelity applanation tonometry. *J. Vasc. Med. Biol.* **1989**, *1*, 142–149.
20. Reference Values for Arterial Stiffness Collaboration. Determinants of pulse wave velocity in healthy people and in the presence of cardiovascular risk factors: 'Establishing normal and reference values'. *Eur. Heart J.* **2010**, *31*, 2338–2350. [CrossRef]
21. Salvi, P.; Lio, G.; Labat, C.; Ricci, E.; Pannier, B.; Benetos, A. Validation of a new non-invasive portable tonometer for determining arterial pressure wave and pulse wave velocity: The PulsePen device. *J. Hypertens.* **2004**, *22*, 2285–2293. [CrossRef]
22. Salvi, P.; Scalise, F.; Rovina, M.; Moretti, F.; Salvi, L.; Grillo, A.; Gao, L.; Baldi, C.; Faini, A.; Furlanis, G.; et al. Noninvasive Estimation of Aortic Stiffness Through Different Approaches. *Hypertension* **2019**, *74*, 117–129. [CrossRef]
23. Revera, M.; Salvi, P.; Faini, A.; Giuliano, A.; Gregorini, F.; Bilo, G.; Lombardi, C.; Mancia, G.; Agostoni, P.; Parati, G.; et al. Renin-Angiotensin-Aldosterone System Is Not Involved in the Arterial Stiffening Induced by Acute and Prolonged Exposure to High Altitude. *Hypertension* **2017**, *70*, 75–84. [CrossRef]
24. Parati, G.; Bilo, G.; Faini, A.; Bilo, B.; Revera, M.; Giuliano, A.; Lombardi, C.; Caldara, G.; Gregorini, F.; Styczkiewicz, K.; et al. Changes in 24 h ambulatory blood pressure and effects of angiotensin II receptor blockade during acute and prolonged high-altitude exposure: A randomized clinical trial. *Eur. Heart J.* **2014**, *35*, 3113–3122. [CrossRef]
25. Bernardi, L. Heart rate and cardiovascular variability at high altitude. *Annu Int Conf IEEE Eng Med Biol Soc.* **2007**, *2007*, 6679–6681. [CrossRef] [PubMed]

26. Bernardi, L.; Passino, C.; Spadacini, G.; Calciati, A.; Robergs, R.; Greene, R.; Martignoni, E.; Anand, I.; Appenzeller, O. Cardiovascular autonomic modulation and activity of carotid baroreceptors at altitude. *Clin. Sci.* **1998**, *95*, 565–573. [CrossRef]
27. Reinhart, W.H.; Kayser, B.; Singh, A.; Waber, U.; Oelz, O.; Bartsch, P. Blood rheology in acute mountain sickness and high-altitude pulmonary edema. *J. Appl. Physiol.* **1991**, *71*, 934–938. [CrossRef]
28. Patel, R.S.; Al Mheid, I.; Morris, A.A.; Ahmed, Y.; Kavtaradze, N.; Ali, S.; Dabhadkar, K.; Brigham, K.; Hooper, W.C.; Alexander, R.W.; et al. Oxidative stress is associated with impaired arterial elasticity. *Atherosclerosis* **2012**, *218*, 90–95. [CrossRef] [PubMed]
29. Noma, K.; Goto, C.; Nishioka, K.; Jitsuiki, D.; Umemura, T.; Ueda, K.; Kimura, M.; Nakagawa, K.; Oshima, T.; Chayama, K.; et al. Roles of rho-associated kinase and oxidative stress in the pathogenesis of aortic stiffness. *J. Am. Coll. Cardiol.* **2007**, *49*, 698–705. [CrossRef] [PubMed]
30. Hackett, P.H.; Rennie, D. Rales, peripheral edema, retinal hemorrhage and acute mountain sickness. *Am. J. Med.* **1979**, *67*, 214–218. [CrossRef]
31. Bilo, G.; Caldara, G.; Styczkiewicz, K.; Revera, M.; Lombardi, C.; Giglio, A.; Zambon, A.; Corrao, G.; Faini, A.; Valentini, M.; et al. Effects of selective and nonselective beta-blockade on 24-h ambulatory blood pressure under hypobaric hypoxia at altitude. *J. Hypertens.* **2011**, *29*, 380–387. [CrossRef] [PubMed]
32. Palombo, C.; Kozakova, M.; Morizzo, C.; Gnesi, L.; Barsotti, M.C.; Spontoni, P.; Massart, F.; Salvi, P.; Balbarini, A.; Saggese, G.; et al. Circulating endothelial progenitor cells and large artery structure and function in young subjects with uncomplicated type 1 diabetes. *Cardiovasc. Diabetol.* **2011**, *10*, 88. [CrossRef] [PubMed]
33. Modesti, P.A.; Vanni, S.; Morabito, M.; Modesti, A.; Marchetta, M.; Gamberi, T.; Sofi, F.; Savia, G.; Mancia, G.; Gensini, G.F.; et al. Role of endothelin-1 in exposure to high altitude: Acute Mountain Sickness and Endothelin-1 (ACME-1) study. *Circulation* **2006**, *114*, 1410–1416. [CrossRef] [PubMed]
34. Bruno, R.M.; Cogo, A.; Ghiadoni, L.; Duo, E.; Pomidori, L.; Sharma, R.; Thapa, G.B.; Basnyat, B.; Bartesaghi, M.; Picano, E.; et al. Cardiovascular function in healthy Himalayan high-altitude dwellers. *Atherosclerosis* **2014**, *236*, 47–53. [CrossRef] [PubMed]
35. Parati, G.; Ochoa, J.E.; Torlasco, C.; Salvi, P.; Lombardi, C.; Bilo, G. Aging, High Altitude, and Blood Pressure: A Complex Relationship. *High Alt. Med. Biol.* **2015**, *16*, 97–109. [CrossRef] [PubMed]

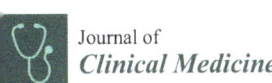

Article

Comparison between Carotid Distensibility-Based Vascular Age and Risk-Based Vascular Age in Middle-Aged Population Free of Cardiovascular Disease

Michaela Kozakova [1,2], Carmela Morizzo [3], Giuli Jamagidze [4], Dante Chiappino [4] and Carlo Palombo [3,*]

1. Department of Clinical and Experimental Medicine, University of Pisa, 56126 Pisa, Italy
2. Esaote SpA, 16152 Genova, Italy
3. Department of Surgical, Medical and Molecular Pathology and Critical Care Medicine, School of Medicine, University of Pisa, 56126 Pisa, Italy
4. Imaging Department, Fondazione Toscana G. Monasterio, 54038 Montignoso, Italy
* Correspondence: carlo.palombo@unipi.it; Tel.: +39-348-5840810

Abstract: The concept of vascular age (VA) was proposed to provide patients with an understandable explanation of cardiovascular (CV) risk and to improve the performance of prediction models. The present study compared risk-based VA derived from Framingham Risk Score (FRS) and Systematic Coronary Risk Estimation (SCORE) models with value-based VA derived from the measurement of the common carotid artery (CCA) distensibility coefficient (DC), and it assessed the impact of DC-based VA on risk reclassification. In 528 middle-aged individuals apparently free of CV disease, DC was measured by radiofrequency-based arterial wall tracking that was previously utilised to establish sex- and age-specific reference values in a healthy population. DC-based VA represented the median value (50th percentile) for given sex in the reference population. FRS-based and SCORE-based VA was calculated as recommended. We observed a good agreement between DC-based and FRS-based VA, with a mean difference of 0.46 ± 12.2 years ($p = 0.29$), while the mean difference between DC-based and SCORE-based VA was higher (3.07 ± 12.7 years, $p < 0.0001$). When only nondiabetic individuals free of antihypertensive therapy were considered (n = 341), the mean difference dropped to 0.70 ± 12.8 years ($p = 0.24$). Substitution of chronological age with DC-based VA in FRS and SCORE models led to a reclassification of 28% and 49% of individuals, respectively, to the higher risk category. Our data suggest that the SCORE prediction model, in which diabetes and antihypertensive treatment are not considered, should be used as a screening tool only in healthy individuals. The use of VA derived from CCA distensibility measurements could improve the performance of risk prediction models, even that of the FRS model, as it might integrate risk prediction with additional risk factors participating in vascular ageing, unique to each individual. Prospective studies are needed to validate the role of DC-based VA in risk prediction.

Keywords: vascular age; risk factors; carotid distension; primary prevention

1. Introduction

Atherothrombotic cardiovascular (CV) disease is the leading cause of morbidity and mortality worldwide, and, accordingly, effective and timely preventive interventions are required. The main goal of primary prevention is the identification of 'high-risk' individuals who would benefit from healthy lifestyle habits and more aggressive therapy. Constant adherence to medication and lifestyle interventions in high-risk individuals free of CV symptomatology depends in great part on motivation and, therefore, on an appropriate and effective explanation of the risk. The concept of vascular age (VA) was, therefore, introduced [1]. VA reflects the status of the vascular tree, and the comparison of individual VA with chronological age can provide a patient with a clear picture of risk.

There are two basic approaches for VA estimation, risk-based VA and value-based VA [2]. The first is based on existing risk models, as atherosclerotic and arteriosclerotic alterations of the vascular tree result from lifelong cumulative exposure to risk factors [3]. In this case, VA is calculated as the age of a person with the same predicted CV risk but with all risk factors within normal levels [4,5]. The second approach estimates VA from published sex- and age-specific percentiles of arterial wall thickness or stiffness obtained in healthy men and women [6–9].

Value-based VA has also been used to improve the predictive ability of risk models [10–12]. It is evident that degenerative changes in the arterial wall are caused not only by established CV risk factors but also by genetic predisposition, foetal programming and environmental factors. In fact, the existence of individuals with accelerated vascular ageing (early vascular ageing (EVA)) and individuals with delayed vascular ageing (supernormal vascular ageing (SUPERNOVA)) have been described [13,14]. Thus, replacing chronological age with VA derived from validated vascular biomarkers could incorporate into risk prediction algorithms additional risk factors participating in vascular ageing and unique to each person.

The aim of the present study was to compare risk-based VA derived from the two most frequently used risk models, the Framingham Risk Score (FRS) and the Systematic Coronary Risk Estimation (SCORE) model, with value-based VA derived from the measurement of common carotid artery (CCA) distensibility and also to assess the impact of carotid distensibility-derived VA on risk reclassification in a middle-aged population free of CV disease. The CCA distensibility coefficient (DC) was measured by the same radio-frequency-based device used to create sex- and age-specific reference values in a healthy population [8].

2. Materials and Methods

2.1. Study Population and Protocol

The study population consisted of 528 middle-aged individuals (45 to 65 years) free of overt CV disease referred for a primary prevention programme to the Clinic for Cardiometabolic Risk Prevention of the Department of Surgical and Medical Pathology, the University of Pisa, between December 2011 and January 2020. All individuals underwent an examination protocol that included medical history, anthropometry, brachial blood pressure (BP) measurements, a fasting blood test, ECG and a high-resolution carotid ultrasound. Diabetes mellitus was defined as fasting glucose ≥ 7.0 mmol/L or 2 h plasma glucose ≥ 11.1 mmol/L [15], hypercholesterolemia as total cholesterol >5.17 mmol/L and/or LDL-cholesterol >4.14 mmol/L and/or statin therapy, hypertriglyceridemia as fasting triglycerides >1.7 mmol/L and hypertension as systolic blood pressure >140 mmHg and/or diastolic blood pressure >90 mmHg [16].

2.2. Body Size and BP Measurement

Body weight (kg) and height (m) were measured, and body mass index (BMI, kg/m^2) was calculated. Waist circumference (cm) was measured as the narrowest circumference between the lower rib margin and anterior superior iliac crest. Brachial BP was measured at two different visits by a validated digital electronic tensiometer (Omron, model 705cp, Kyoto, Japan) in participants seated for at least 10 min, using regular or large adult cuffs according to the arm circumference. At both visits, two measurements were taken, separated by 2 min intervals, and the average was calculated. The average of two separate visits was used to estimate BP (mmHg).

2.3. Calculation of Vascular Age Based on FRS

FRS-based VA calculation was performed as indicated in the paper describing the risk prediction model for the calculation of a 10-year risk of CV disease [4]. The algorithm considers age, total cholesterol, high-density lipoprotein (HDL) cholesterol, brachial systolic BP, ongoing treatment of hypertension, smoking and diabetes status and provides, besides the estimation of a 10-year risk, the estimation of VA. VA represents the age of a person with the same risk but with all other risk factors at a normal level (nontreated systolic blood pressure of 125 mm Hg, total cholesterol of 180 mg/dL, HDL of 45 mg/dL, nonsmoker, nondiabetic). The highest VA value calculated by the FRS prediction model is >80 years; in the statistical analysis of this study, individuals having a VA of >80 years were considered to have a VA of 80. The difference between FRS-based VA and chronological age was calculated (ΔAge FRS). The risk was classified as low, intermediate or high when the 10-year risk of CV disease was <10%, 10–20% or >20%, respectively.

2.4. Calculation of Vascular Age Based on SCORE

SCORE-based VA used the same principle as the FRS-based VA calculation, i.e., it indicates the age of the subject with the same CV risk but with risk factors within normal ranges [5]. The SCORE risk prediction model calculates a 10-year risk of fatal CV disease; the algorithm is based on age, sex, brachial systolic BP, total and HDL cholesterol and smoking status and is different for European regions with low and high CV risk. The low-risk chart was used for Italy [17]. Individuals having a VA of >80 years were considered to have a VA of 80. The difference between SCORE-based VA and chronological age was calculated (ΔAge SCORE). The risk was classified as low, intermediate or high when the 10-year risk of fatal CV disease was <2%, 2–5% or >5%, respectively.

2.5. Common Carotid Artery Distension Coefficient and Vascular Age

Measurement of CCA distension was performed in the afternoon, 3 h after a light meal, in a quiet room with a stable temperature of 22°, after resting comfortably for at least 15 min in the supine position. All individuals were asked to abstain from cigarette smoking, caffeine and alcohol consumption and vigorous physical activity for 24 h.

Carotid ultrasound was performed on the right CCA using an ultrasound scanner equipped with a 10 MHz linear probe (MyLab 70, Esaote, Genova, Italy) and implemented with a previously validated radiofrequency-based tracking of the arterial wall (QAS®) that allows an automatic and real-time determination of CCA diameter and distension with a high spatial and temporal resolution. Briefly, longitudinal images of the right CCA with a clear definition of both carotid walls were obtained, and a rectangular ROI was placed at the CCA segment starting approximately 1 cm before the flow divider. Arterial distension was measured in 32 scanning lines positioned within the ROI (sampling rate of 550 Hz on 32 lines). From the real-time distension curves, the diastolic carotid diameter and carotid distension were automatically measured and a distension coefficient (DC) was calculated as follows: DC = (ΔA/A)/pulse pressure, where $A = \pi \times (\text{diastolic diameter}/2)^2$, $\Delta A = \pi \times [(\text{diastolic diameter} + \Delta\text{diameter})/2]^2 - \pi \times (\text{diastolic diameter}/2)^2$ and pulse pressure = systolic BP–diastolic BP [8]. Radiofrequency-derived measures represent an average over six consecutive cardiac beats. The mean of two acquisitions was used for statistical analysis. BP used in the calculation was measured at the left brachial artery (Omron, Kyoto, Japan) during each acquisition of the distension curves.

Intra- and interindividual variability of acquisitions was evaluated in 25 volunteers, including individuals with diabetes and hypertension. The acquisitions were performed twice, in two different sessions separated by 30 min, both by the same operator and by two different operators. Brachial PP was comparable between the different acquisitions ($p = 0.88$ and 0.69). Intra- and interindividual variability of CCA distension in two different acquisitions was expressed as a percentage of the absolute difference between the two acquisitions and was 7.5 ± 4.6 and $9.0 \pm 6.9\%$, respectively [18].

DC-based VA was obtained in tables/nomograms reporting the sex- and age-specific percentiles of CCA DC measured by the same radiofrequency-based system in 3601 healthy men and women [8]. Age corresponding to the 50th percentile (median) of DC for given sex was considered a DC-based VA. The maximum VA reported in DC tables/nomograms is 80 years; the individuals with a DC lower than the median corresponding to the age of 80 (therefore, having a VA of >80 years) were considered to have a VA of 80. Individuals with extremely high and extremely low DC were identified as those with DC higher than the 95th percentile and lower than the 5th percentile for given sex and age, respectively [19].

2.6. Statistical Analysis

Data are expressed as mean ± SD, and categorical data as percentages. Variables with skewed distribution are summarised as median [interquartile range] and were logarithmically transformed for parametric statistical analysis. Wilcoxon test was used to test the mean difference between DC-based VA and chronological age or VA derived from risk models. To assess the associations between VA obtained by different approaches, Spearman correlation coefficient r was calculated. Multiple linear regression analysis with backward stepwise removal was used to identify the independent associations of DC with established risk factors used in prediction models. Statistical tests were two-sided, and significance was set at a value of $p < 0.05$. Statistical analysis was performed by JMP software, version 3.1 (SAS Institute Inc., Cary, NC, USA).

3. Results

Characteristics of the study population, values of CCA DC and values of VA based on risk models and on carotid distensibility are reported in Table 1.

Table 1. Characteristics of study population.

	Mean ± SD/Median [IQR]/n(%)
Gender M F	266 (50) 262 (50)
Age (years)	58.3 ± 5.5
BMI (kg/m^2)	27.1 ± 4.7
Waist (cm)	96 ± 13
Systolic BP (mmHg)	132 ± 17
Diastolic BP (mmHg)	80 ± 10
Total cholesterol (mmol/L)	5.4 ± 0.9
HDL cholesterol (mmol/L)	1.6 ± 0.5
LDL cholesterol (mmol/L)	3.3 ± 0.8
Triglycerides (mmol/L)	1.1 [0.7]
Fasting glucose (mmol/L)	5.7 ± 1.4
Current smoker yes	116 (22)
Hypertension yes	152 (29)
Hypertension therapy yes	120 (23)
Hypercholesterolemia yes	297 (56)
Hypertriglyceridemia yes	106 (21)
T2DM yes	118 (22)
CCA DC (10^{-3} kPa^{-1})	14.0 ± 5.0
FRS-based VA (years)	65.5 ± 12.0
SCORE-based VA (years)	62.9 ± 7.9
CCA DC-based VA (years)	66.0 ± 13.8

The mean differences between DC-based VA and chronological age or risk-based VA are reported in Table 2. It is evident that DC-based VA was higher than chronological age. There was a good agreement between DC-based and FRS-based VA, with the mean difference being less than half a year. The mean difference between DC-based VA and SCORE-based VA was higher. However, when only nondiabetic individuals were considered ($n = 410$), the mean difference decreased to 1.35 ± 12.5 years ($p = 0.01$), and when individuals with ongoing hypertensive therapy were excluded, the mean difference in the remaining 341 individuals dropped to 0.70 ± 12.8 years ($p = 0.24$).

Table 2. Mean difference and correlation between DC-based vascular age, chronological age and risk-based vascular age and reclassification of risk with DC-based vascular age.

	Mean Difference (Years)	p	Spearman r	Reclassification n (%) ↑ Risk Category	↓ Risk Category
DC-based VA (years) vs.					
Chronological age (years)	7.71 ± 13.4	<0.0001	0.26		
FRS-based VA (years)	0.46 ± 12.2	0.29	0.56	150 (28)	26 (5)
SCORE-based VA (years)	3.07 ± 12.7	<0.0001	0.42	258 (49)	32 (6)
Risk Categories Low: Intermediate: High	Chronological Age; n (%)			DC-based VA; n (%)	
FRS	219 (41):172 (33):137 (26)			177 (34):129 (24):222 (42)	
SCORE	281 (53):195 (37):52 (10)			180 (34):95 (18):253 (48)	

Replacement of chronological age by DC-based VA in the FRS model resulted in the reclassification of 28% of individuals into a higher risk category, and the percentage of individuals in the high-risk category increased from 26% to 42%. In the SCORE model, this replacement resulted in the reclassification of 49% of individuals into a higher risk category, and the percentage of individuals in the high-risk category increased from 10% to 48% (Table 2).

Table 3 compares the arithmetic difference between risk-based VA and chronological age (ΔAge) together with established risk factors between individuals with extremely high (DC above the 95th percentile of the reference population) or low DC (DC below the 5th percentile of the reference population) and those with DC in the 5th to 95th percentile. Individuals with extremely low DC had FRS-based VA significantly higher than chronological age, while individuals with extremely high DC had FRS-based VA lower than chronological age. The former also had higher BP, prevalence of antihypertensive treatment and T2DM and lower HDL cholesterol, while the latter had lower BP, prevalence of antihypertensive treatment and T2DM and higher HDL cholesterol. The difference in ΔAge between DC percentiles was less prominent but still significant when chronological age was subtracted from SCORE-based VA.

Table 3. Arithmetic difference between risk-based vascular age and chronological age (ΔAge) and established risk factors according to percentiles of carotid distension coefficient in reference population.

	CCA DC (10^{-3} kPa^{-1})		
	<5th Percentile	5–95th Percentile	>95th Percentile
N (%)	62 (12)	448 (85)	18 (3)
ΔAge FRS (years)	15.8 ± 7.8 **	6.5 ± 10.4	−4.3 ± 8.7 **
ΔAge SCORE (years)	7.7 ± 5.3 **	4.4 ± 4.6	0.7 ± 3.1 **
Systolic BP (mmHg)	146 ± 17 **	130 ± 15	111 ± 7 **
HDL cholesterol (mmol/L)	1.3 ± 0.4 **	1.6 ± 0.4	1.8 ± 0.6 **
Total cholesterol (mmol/L)	5.2 ± 0.9	5.4 ± 0.9	6.1 ± 0.8 *
Hypertensive therapy yes (n (%))	24 (39) **	96 (21)	0 **
Smoking yes (n (%))	16 (25)	98 (22)	2 (11)
T2DM yes (n (%))	33 (53) **	84 (19)	1 (6)*

Statistical significance tested against values in the 5th–95th percentile; * $p < 0.05$; ** $p < 0.01$–0.0001.

Table 4 reports the independent correlates of CCA DC. CCA DC was independently associated with age, systolic BP, HDL cholesterol, ongoing treatment for hypertension and diabetes mellitus, and these risk factors explained 43% of its variability. None of other possible risk factors (BMI, waist circumference, plasma glucose, LDL-cholesterol and triglycerides) entered the model.

Table 4. Independent correlates of CCA distension coefficient.

	CCA DC (10^{-3} kPa^{-1})	
	β ± SE	p
Age (years)	−0.18 ± 0.03	<0.0001
Systolic BP (mmHg)	−0.48 ± 0.03	<0.0001
HDL cholesterol (mmol/L)	0.12 ± 0.03	0.001
Hypertensive treatment yes	−0.16 ± 0.04	<0.0005
Diabetes mellitus yes	−0.19 ± 0.04	<0.0001
Cumulative R^2	0.43	<0.0001

4. Discussion

The identification of individuals with an increased risk of CV disease is a foundation of primary prevention. According to the Guidelines of the European Society of Cardiology, in asymptomatic men >40 years of age and women >50 years of age, a systematic or opportunistic evaluation of CV risk should be considered, and in individuals at intermediate–high risk, a healthy lifestyle strategy and preventive pharmacological treatment should be adopted [20]. Recommendations include a healthy dietary pattern with limited consumption of red meat, soft drinks and alcohol, weight control, smoking cessation, the substitution of sedentary behaviour with regular physical activity, strict control of T2DM and hypertension and, eventually, statin and aspirin therapy. Sustained adherence to these often unpopular recommendations depends on appropriate communication with the patient and a clear illustration of individual risk. For this reason, a theory of VA was adopted, assuming that the demonstration that one's own arteries are older than chronological age is more convincing than a mathematical model calculating the chance of developing CV disease over the next 10 years [1,21].

VA can be estimated from risk prediction models (risk-based VA) as the age of a person with the same predicted CV risk but with all risk factors within normal ranges [4,5] or from vascular biomarkers of atherosclerosis and arteriosclerosis (value-based VA) as the age of a healthy person with the same value of measured vascular biomarker [2,6–9,22,23]. The most frequently used prediction algorithms are FRS and SCORE, and the most frequently used vascular biomarkers are carotid IMT and carotid–femoral pulse wave velocity (cfPWV) [10–12].

Arterial distensibility, in general, and carotid distensibility, in particular, have been proposed as possible biomarkers capable of improving CV risk prediction. A meta-analysis of nine longitudinal studies including 18 993 individuals has shown that carotid DC is a significant predictor of future CV events (pooled risk ratio 1.19 (1.06–1.35, 95%CI)) [24]. Therefore, in this study, we compared risk-based and DC-based VA and evaluated the impact of DC-based VA on risk reclassification in a large middle-aged population free of apparent CV disease but with various risk factors that may affect arterial compliance. We observed a good agreement between VA corresponding to the median value of DC in the healthy population and FRS-based VA. The mean difference was less than half a year. In contrast, the difference between DC-based and SCORE-based VA was 3 years (Table 2). This is not surprising, as the SCORE model does not take into account diabetes mellitus and antihypertensive treatment [17], which are important determinants of arterial stiffness and CV risk [25–27], and whose prevalence in our population was 22% and 23%, respectively. Indeed, when only nondiabetic individuals were considered, the mean difference decreased to 1.5 years, and when individuals with high BP treatment were also excluded, the mean difference dropped below 1 year. This observation indicates that the SCORE prediction model and SCORE-based VA should be used only in individuals free of diabetes and antihypertensive treatment, i.e., as a screening tool in an apparently healthy population.

A good agreement between DC-based and FRS-based VA reflects the fact that five out of seven risk factors considered in FRS [4] were independent determinants of DC, explaining 43% of DC variation (Table 4). The impact of established risk factors on carotid compliance was also evident in individuals with extremely low (EVA) or extremely high

(SUPERNOVA) carotid compliance for their sex and age. The former had significantly higher BP, prevalence of diabetes and hypertensive treatment and lower HDL cholesterol as compared with individuals in the 5th to 95th percentile of the reference population, while the latter had the opposite trend. As a consequence, individuals with EVA had FRS-based VA much higher than chronological age (mean difference 15.8 ± 7.8 years), and individuals with SUPERNOVA had FRS-based VA lower than chronological age (mean difference −4.3 ± 8.7 years).

Numerous investigators have suggested substituting chronological age in the risk prediction model with VA derived from vascular biomarkers of atherosclerosis and arteriosclerosis in order to include in the risk prediction the factors that may participate in CV risk but are not clearly related to established risk factors, such as genetic predisposition, socioeconomic status, physical inactivity or psychological stress. In previous studies, the incorporation of value-based VA derived from sex- and age-specific IMT and cfPWV nomograms into risk models [10–12] resulted in the reclassification of 10–51% of individuals into a higher risk category [2]. In our population, the substitution of chronological age with DC-based VA resulted in the reclassification of 28% to a higher category of the FRS model and 49% to a higher category of the SCORE model. The reassignment of nearly half of the study population to a higher SCORE risk category once again indicates that the SCORE algorithm may underestimate risk when used in a population with diabetes and hypertensive treatment. Indeed, 111 out of 258 reclassified individuals had diabetes and/or hypertensive therapy.

Despite a good agreement between DC-based and FRS-based VA, more than a quarter of the population was reassigned to a higher FRS category when DC-based VA replaced chronological age in the FRS algorithm. Since the established risk factors explained only 43% of the DC variance, it is likely that other factors not accounted for in the FRS model, such as family history, habitual physical activity or dietary habits, could modify carotid compliance [28–31]. Thus, the incorporation of DC-based VA could integrate additional risk factors into the prediction algorithm. Most importantly, the substitution of chronological age with DC-based VA increased the prevalence of high-risk individuals, that is, those requiring more aggressive preventive interventions, in both models.

Study Limitations

We did not use the latest SCORE risk prediction algorithm that calculates the 10-year risk of CV disease, as the VA for this new version was not yet established [32]. CV disease was excluded on the basis of clinical history and ECG; no provocative tests were performed. This was a cross-sectional study that did not allow to assess whether the reclassification with DC-based VA actually improved the prediction of CV events.

5. Conclusions

The present study indicates that the use of VA derived from the measurement of CCA distensibility might improve the performance of risk prediction models, especially the SCORE model, which does not account for the presence of diabetes and hypertensive treatment. Nevertheless, the replacement of chronological age by DC-based VA significantly increased the prevalence of high-risk individuals in the FRS model because the inclusion of VA could integrate risk prediction with additional risk factors unique to each individual. Prospective studies are needed to validate the true value of CCA DC-based VA for risk management in a population setting.

Author Contributions: Conceptualisation, C.P. and M.K.; methodology, M.K., C.P. and D.C.; formal analysis, M.K. and C.M.; investigation, C.M., G.J. and D.C.; data curation, C.M., G.J. and M.K.; writing—original draft preparation, M.K.; writing—review and editing, C.P. and D.C.; supervision, C.P. and D.C. All authors have read and agreed to the published version of the manuscript.

Funding: This research received no external funding.

Institutional Review Board Statement: The study protocol conformed to the ethical guidelines of the 1975 Declaration of Helsinki and was approved by the institutional ethics committee 'Comitato Etico di Area Vasta Nord Ovest' (reference number: 3146/2010).

Informed Consent Statement: All individuals gave their informed consent to participate.

Data Availability Statement: The data presented in this study are available on request from the corresponding author. The data are not publicly available due to privacy reasons.

Conflicts of Interest: M.K. is responsible for clinical studies in Esaote SpA.

References

1. Cuende, J.I. Vascular Age Versus Cardiovascular Risk: Clarifying Concepts. *Rev. Esp. Cardiol. Engl. Ed.* **2016**, *69*, 243–246 [CrossRef] [PubMed]
2. Groenewegen, K.A.; den Ruijter, H.M.; Pasterkamp, G.; Polak, J.F.; Bots, M.L.; Peters, S.A. Vascular age to determine cardiovascular disease risk: A systematic review of its concepts, definitions, and clinical applications. *Eur. J. Prev. Cardiol.* **2016**, *23*, 264–274 [CrossRef]
3. Kozakova, M.; Morizzo, C.; Guarino, D.; Federico, G.; Miccoli, M.; Giannattasio, C.; Palombo, C. The impact of age and risk factors on carotid and carotid-femoral pulse wave velocity. *J. Hypertens.* **2015**, *33*, 1446–1451. [CrossRef] [PubMed]
4. D'Agostino, R.B.; Vasan, R.S.; Pencina, M.J.; Wolf, P.A.; Cobain, M.; Massaro, J.M.; Kannel, W.B. General cardiovascular risk profile for use in primary care: The Framingham Heart Study. *Circulation* **2008**, *117*, 743–753. [CrossRef] [PubMed]
5. Cuende, J.I.; Cuende, N.; Calaveras-Lagartos, J. How to calculate vascular age with the SCORE project scales: A new method of cardiovascular risk evaluation. *Eur. Heart J.* **2010**, *31*, 2351–2358. [CrossRef] [PubMed]
6. Howard, G.; Sharrett, A.R.; Heiss, G.; Evans, G.W.; Chambless, L.E.; Riley, W.A.; Burke, G.L. Carotid artery intimal-medial thickness distribution in general populations as evaluated by B-mode ultrasound. ARIC Investigators. *Stroke* **1993**, *24*, 1297–1304 [CrossRef] [PubMed]
7. Reference Values for Arterial Stiffness' Collaboration. Determinants of pulse wave velocity in healthy people and in the presence of cardiovascular risk factors: 'Establishing normal and reference values'. *Eur. Heart J.* **2010**, *31*, 2338–2350. [CrossRef] [PubMed]
8. Engelen, L.; Bossuyt, J.; Ferreira, I.; van Bortel, L.M.; Reesink, K.D.; Segers, P.; Stehouwer, C.D.; Laurent, S.; Boutouyrie, P.; Reference Values for Arterial Measurements Collaboration. Reference values for local arterial stiffness. Part A: Carotid artery. *J. Hypertens.* **2015**, *33*, 1981–1996. [CrossRef]
9. Engelen, L.; Ferreira, I.; Stehouwer, C.D.; Boutouyrie, P.; Laurent, S.; Reference Values for Arterial Measurements Collaboration Reference intervals for common carotid intima-media thickness measured with echotracking: Relation with risk factors. *Eur. Heart J.* **2013**, *34*, 2368–2380. [CrossRef]
10. Gepner, A.D.; Keevil, J.G.; Wyman, R.A.; Korcarz, C.E.; Aeschlimann, S.E.; Busse, K.L.; Stein, J.H. Use of carotid intima-media thickness and vascular age to modify cardiovascular risk prediction. *J. Am. Soc. Echocardiogr.* **2006**, *19*, 1170–1174. [CrossRef]
11. Stein, J.H.; Fraizer, M.C.; Aeschlimann, S.E.; Nelson-Worel, J.; McBride, P.E.; Douglas, P.S. Vascular age: Integrating carotid intima-media thickness measurements with global coronary risk assessment. *Clin. Cardiol.* **2004**, *27*, 388–392. [CrossRef] [PubMed]
12. Łoboz-Rudnicka, M.; Jaroch, J.; Bociąga, Z.; Kruszyńska, E.; Ciecierzyńska, B.; Dziuba, M.; Dudek, K.; Uchmanowicz, I.; Łoboz-Grudzień, K. Relationship between vascular age and classic cardiovascular risk factors and arterial stiffness. *Cardiol. J.* **2013**, *20*, 394–401. [CrossRef] [PubMed]
13. Laurent, S.; Boutouyrie, P.; Cunha, P.G.; Lacolley, P.; Nilsson, P.M. Concept of extremes in vascular aging. *Hypertension* **2019**, *74*, 218–228. [CrossRef] [PubMed]
14. Nilsson, P.M.; Boutouyrie, P.; Laurent, S. Vascular aging: A tale of EVA and ADAM in cardiovascular risk assessment and prevention. *Hypertension* **2009**, *54*, 3–10.
15. World Health Organization. *Definition and Diagnosis of Diabetes Mellitus and Intermediate Hyperglycaemia: Report of a WHO/IDF Consultation*; WHO: Geneva, Switzerland, 2006.
16. Mancia, G.; Fagard, R.; Narkiewicz, K.; Redón, J.; Zanchetti, A.; Böhm, M.; Christiaens, T.; Cifkova, R.; De Backer, G.; Dominiczak, A.; et al. 2013 ESH/ESC Guidelines for the management of arterial hypertension: The Task Force for the management of arterial hypertension of the European Society of Hypertension (ESH) and of the European Society of Cardiology (ESC). *J. Hypertens.* **2013**, *31*, 1281–1357. [CrossRef]
17. Conroy, R.M.; Pyörälä, K.; Fitzgerald, A.P.; Sans, S.; Menotti, A.; De Backer, G.; De Bacquer, D.; Ducimetière, P.; Jousilahti, P.; Keil, U.; et al. Estimation of ten-year risk of fatal cardiovascular disease in Europe: The SCORE project. *Eur. Heart J.* **2003**, *24*, 987–1003. [CrossRef]
18. Palombo, C.; Kozakova, M.; Guraschi, N.; Bini, G.; Cesana, F.; Castoldi, G.; Stella, A.; Morizzo, C.; Giannattasio, C. Radiofrequency-based carotid wall tracking: A comparison between two different systems. *J. Hypertens.* **2012**, *30*, 1614–1619. [CrossRef]
19. Vasan, R.S. Biomarkers of cardiovascular disease: Molecular basis and practical considerations. *Circulation* **2006**, *113*, 2335–2362. [CrossRef]

20. Visseren, F.L.J.; Mach, F.; Smulders, Y.M.; Carballo, D.; Koskinas, K.C.; Bäck, M.; Benetos, A.; Biffi, A.; Boavida, J.M.; Capodanno, D.; et al. 2021 ESC Guidelines on cardiovascular disease prevention in clinical practice. *Eur. Heart J.* **2021**, *42*, 3227–3337. [CrossRef]
21. Weber, T.; Mayer, C.C. "Man is as old as his arteries" taken literally: In search of the best metric. *Hypertension* **2020**, *76*, 1425–1427. [CrossRef]
22. Gyöngyösi, H.; Kőrösi, B.; Batta, D.; Nemcsik-Bencze, Z.; László, A.; Tislér, A.; Cseprekál, O.; Torzsa, P.; Eörsi, D.; Nemcsik, J. Comparison of different cardiovascular risk score and pulse wave velocity-based methods for vascular age calculation. *Heart Lung Circ.* **2021**, *30*, 1744–1751. [CrossRef] [PubMed]
23. Climie, R.E.; Mayer, C.C.; Bruno, R.M.; Hametner, B. Addressing the unmet needs of measuring vascular ageing in clinical practice-European cooperation in science and technology action VascAgeNet. *Artery Res.* **2020**, *26*, 71–75. [CrossRef]
24. Yuan, C.; Wang, J.; Ying, M. Predictive value of carotid distensibility coefficient for cardiovascular diseases and all-cause mortality: A meta-analysis. *PLoS ONE* **2016**, *11*, e0152799. [CrossRef] [PubMed]
25. Asayama, K.; Satoh, M.; Murakami, Y.; Ohkubo, T.; Nagasawa, S.Y.; Tsuji, I.; Nakayama, T.; Okayama, A.; Miura, K.; Imai, Y.; et al. Cardiovascular risk with and without antihypertensive drug treatment in the Japanese general population: Participant-level meta-analysis. *Hypertension* **2014**, *63*, 1189–1197. [CrossRef] [PubMed]
26. Fuchs, F.D.; Whelton, P.K. High blood pressure and cardiovascular disease. *Hypertension* **2020**, *75*, 285–292. [CrossRef] [PubMed]
27. Stehouwer, C.D.; Henry, R.M.; Ferreira, I. Arterial stiffness in diabetes and the metabolic syndrome: A pathway to cardiovascular disease. *Diabetologia* **2008**, *51*, 527–539. [CrossRef]
28. Horváth, T.; Osztovits, J.; Pintér, A.; Littvay, L.; Cseh, D.; Tárnoki, A.D.; Tárnoki, D.L.; Jermendy, A.L.; Steinbach, R.; Métneki, J.; et al. Genetic impact dominates over environmental effects in development of carotid artery stiffness: A twin study. *Hypertens. Res.* **2014**, *37*, 88–93.
29. Riley, W.A.; Freedman, D.S.; Higgs, N.A.; Barnes, R.W.; Zinkgraf, S.A.; Berenson, G.S. Decreased arterial elasticity associated with cardiovascular disease risk factors in the young. Bogalusa Heart Study. *Arteriosclerosis* **1986**, *6*, 378–386. [CrossRef]
30. Kozakova, M.; Palombo, C.; Mhamdi, L.; Konrad, T.; Nilsson, P.; Staehr, P.B.; Paterni, M.; Balkau, B.; RISC Investigators. Habitual physical activity and vascular aging in a young to middle-age population at low cardiovascular risk. *Stroke* **2007**, *38*, 2549–2555. [CrossRef]
31. van de Laar, R.J.; Stehouwer, C.D.; van Bussel, B.C.; te Velde, S.J.; Prins, M.H.; Twisk, J.W.; Ferreira, I. Lower lifetime dietary fiber intake is associated with carotid artery stiffness: The Amsterdam Growth and Health Longitudinal Study. *Am. J. Clin. Nutr.* **2012**, *96*, 14–23. [CrossRef]
32. SCORE2 working group and ESC Cardiovascular risk collaboration. SCORE2 risk prediction algorithms: New models to estimate 10-year risk of cardiovascular disease in Europe. *Eur. Heart J.* **2021**, *42*, 2439–2454. [CrossRef] [PubMed]

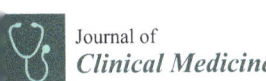

Article

The Correlation of Arterial Stiffness Parameters with Aging and Comorbidity Burden

Francesco Fantin [1,*], Anna Giani [1], Monica Trentin [1], Andrea P. Rossi [1], Elena Zoico [1], Gloria Mazzali [1], Rocco Micciolo [2] and Mauro Zamboni [3]

1. Section of Geriatric Medicine, Department of Medicine, University of Verona, 37126 Verona, Italy
2. Centre for Medical Sciences, Department of Psychology and Cognitive Sciences, University of Trento, 38122 Trento, Italy
3. Section of Geriatric Medicine, Department of Surgery, Dentistry, Pediatric and Gynecology, University of Verona, 37126 Verona, Italy
* Correspondence: francesco.fantin@univr.it; Tel.: +39-045-8122537; Fax: +39-045-8122043 (ext. 5291)

Abstract: The aim of the study was to evaluate the relationships between carotid-femoral pulse wave velocity (PVW-cf), cardio-ankle vascular index (CAVI) and CAVI0 (which is a mathematical elaboration of CAVI, theoretically less dependent on blood pressure), age and comorbidity burden. Furthermore, 183 patients (119 female, mean age 67.5 ± 14.3 years) referred to the Geriatric Ward and Outpatient Clinic at Verona University Hospital were included; demographic, clinical and blood analysis data were collected. Charlson Comorbidity Index (CCI), PVW-cf, CAVI and CAVI 0 were obtained. Significant correlations were found between CAVI, CAVI0, PVW-cf and both age ($r = 0.698$, $r = 0.717$, $r = 0.410$, respectively $p < 0.001$ for all) and CCI, ($r = 0.654$; $r = 0.658$; $r = 0.448$ respectively and $p < 0.001$ for all), still significant after adjustment for several variables. In a stepwise multiple regression model, considering several variables, CCI was the only predictor of PWV-cf, whereas age and CCI were significant predictors of both CAVI and CAVI 0. In conclusion, all arterial stiffness indexes are associated with CCI and aging; the latter correlation is more evident for CAVI and CAVI 0 than for PVW-cf. Arterial stiffness parameters can complement the characterization of patients affected by a remarkable comorbidity burden across aging; arterial stiffening might mirror the complexity of these individuals.

Keywords: CAVI; CAVI0; PWV; comorbidity; aging

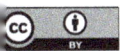

1. Introduction

Vascular aging is associated with arterial wall remodeling, with progressive stiffening and reduced compliance; arterial stiffness is an independent predictor of cardiovascular morbidity and mortality [1]. It is therefore of remarkable importance to evaluate arterial stiffness in older individuals and in those adult patients who, owing to the presence of vascular and metabolic comorbidities, display high cardiovascular risk. Carotid-femoral pulse wave velocity (PVW-cf) and cardio-ankle vascular index (CAVI) are two common and feasible techniques aimed at detecting signs of vascular stiffening. As compared to PWV-cf, CAVI can evaluate arterial stiffness from a larger proportion of the arterial tree and is considered less dependent on blood pressure at the time of measurement [2,3]. Thus, although pulse wave analysis is considered the gold standard technique to evaluate vascular stiffness [4,5], CAVI can provide a more comprehensive assessment of arterial stiffness [3]. Furthermore, in order to further relieve the dependence of CAVI by blood pressure, in 2016 the mathematical expression of CAVI was elaborated and CAVI 0 was then suggested [6–8], and the association between CAVI and CAVI 0 has been widely demonstrated [9,10].

A massive number of pathological conditions have been shown to be related to increased arterial stiffening. For instance, PVW-cf is known to be associated to aging [11], cardiovascular risk factors [1] and metabolic syndrome [12]. On the other hand, increased CAVI is described in older subjects [13,14], in hypertensive patients [15,16], in the presence of vascular calcification and inflammation [17], in diabetic individuals and with concomitant metabolic diseases, [18,19], and in the presence of dyslipidemia [20,21]. Furthermore weight loss is associated with CAVI reduction [22], and a positive association is described between CAVI and the presence of epicardial and visceral adipose tissue [23]. Increased CAVI is a predictor of cardiovascular events [24] and it is also associated to coronary artery disease [13], cerebral ischemia [25] and carotid arteries plaques [26].

Interestingly, although several comorbidities, as considered per se, are shown to be related to increased stiffness, less is known about the possible effect of the comprehensive comorbidity burden. The role of arterial stiffening in the characterization of complex patients with relevant comorbidity burden, considered across aging, is yet to be deeply explored; however, it may shed light on riveting pathophysiological issues. Furthermore, particular attention should be paid to cardiovascular comorbidities and risk factors, given their direct involvement in arterial structures. The aim of the study was to examine the correlation between arterial stiffness indexes, comorbidities and cardiovascular risk factors in a group of adults and older adults.

2. Materials and Methods

The study population included 183 subjects, 119 females and 64 males, hospitalized at Geriatric Clinic of Verona University Hospital or referred to Outpatient Clinic (medical nutrition or arterial hypertension, of any age). Exclusion criteria were: (I) limb amputation or history of surgical treatment to aorta, carotids, or femoral arteries; (II) severe peripheral arterial disease or proximal arterial stenosis; (III) atrial fibrillation or other major arrhythmias. A detailed clinical history, with particular mention to cardiovascular diseases and risk factors, and physical examination were recorded for each patient. To evaluate the comorbidity burden, Charlson comorbidity Index (CCI) was calculated for each patient, using anamnestic patient-reported data.

The study was approved by the Ethical Committee of the University of Verona. All participants gave informed consent to be involved in the research study.

2.1. Anthropometric Variables

With the subject barefoot and wearing light indoor clothing, body weight was measured to the nearest 0.1 kg (Salus scale, Milan, Italy), and height to the nearest 0.5 cm using a stadiometer (Salus stadiometer, Milan, Italy); whenever patients could not assume the erect position, the last anamnestic height was recoded. BMI was calculated as body weight adjusted by stature (kg/m^2).

2.2. Blood Pressure and Arterial Stiffness Measurements

CAVI, blood pressure and heart rate were measured and mean arterial pressure (MAP) and pulse pressure (PP) were calculated using VaSera-1000 (Fukuda-Denshi Company, LTD, Tokyo, Japan), as per the manufacturer's recommendations. BP cuffs were placed simultaneously on the four limbs and inflated two by two (right and left side) to increase the accuracy of measurements. ECG was obtained by two electrodes placed on both arms; to obtain phonocardiography, a microphone was placed on the sternum (second rib space). This device calculates CAVI, on the basis of the Bramwell–Hill Formula [27,28], measuring heart-ankle PWV by the following equation:

$$CAVI = a * \left(\ln \frac{P_s}{P_d} * \frac{PWV^2 * 2\rho}{P_s - P_d} \right) + b$$

where a and b are constants, ρ is considered the blood density, P_s stands for systolic blood pressure (SBP), and P_d stands for diastolic blood pressure (DBP). By means of this device, heart-ankle PWV (haPWV) was calculated as the ratio between aortic valve to ankle length (automatically derived by software) and the time T taken by pulse wave to run this distance (T = tb + tba, tb = time from the second heart sound to the dicrotic notch at the brachial pulse wave form, tba = time from brachial to ankle pulse waves) [29]. CAVI 0 was derived by proper electronic calculator [30] following the formula:

$$\text{CAVI 0} = \frac{\text{CAVI} - b}{a} * \frac{\frac{P_s}{P_d} - 1}{\ln\left(\frac{P_s}{P_d}\right)} - \ln\left(\frac{P_s}{P_{ref}}\right)$$

and considering Pref as a standard pressure of 100 mmHg.

2.3. Pulse Wave Velocity

The pulse wave analysis was performed noninvasively using a portable device called PulsePen (Diatecne, Milan, Italy) [31], and its software to obtain central aortic pressure values, an assessment of arterial pulse wave contours, an estimation of reflection waves and measurements of PWV. We previously provided a detailed description of PWA calculation, in previous studies [12,32]; we obtained carotid-femoral PWV (PWV-cf), which is considered representative of elastic arteries [33]. As recommended by consensus documents [34], the carotid-femoral distance was multiplied by a correction factor of 0.8.

Biochemical Analysis

Venous blood samples were obtained after the subjects fasted overnight. Plasma glucose was measured with a glucose analyzer (Beckman Instruments Inc, Palo Alto, CA, USA). Cholesterol and triacylglycerol concentrations were determined with an automated enzymatic method (Autoanalyzer; Technicon, Tarrytown, NY, USA). High-density-lipoprotein (HDL) cholesterol was measured by using the method of Warnick and Albers. LDL cholesterol was calculated using the Friedwald formula [35]. Creatinine was measured by a modular analyzer (Roche Cobas 8000; Monza, Italy); eGFR was calculated by Cockroft–Gault formula.

2.4. Statistical Analyses

Results are shown as mean value ± standard deviation (SD). Variables not normally distributed were log-transformed before analysis. Pearson correlation coefficient was used to estimate correlations between variables. Independent samples t-tests were used to compare baseline characteristics of female and male patients. Analysis of variance (ANOVA) was performed when comparing continuous data, after stratifying the population upon age classes and comorbidities and to evaluate the effect of independent variables included in regression models.

A significance threshold level of 0.05 was used throughout the study. All statistical analyses were performed using SPSS 23.0 version for Windows (IBM, Armonk, NY, USA).

3. Results

The study population included 183 individuals, mean age 67.5 ± 14.3 years, 65% (n = 119) female. The main characteristics of the study population are listed in Table 1.

Table 1. Main characteristics of the study population.

	Total (n = 183)	Male (n = 64)	Female (n = 119)	p Value
Age (years)	67.54 ± 14.25	70.13 ± 14.43	66.14 ± 14.02	0.075
Body weight (kg)	77.06 ± 18.01	81.30 ± 18.90	74.78 ± 17.17	0.023
BMI (kg/m^2)	28.92 ± 5.85	27.77 ± 5.65	29.54 ± 5.88	0.048
Glucose level (mg/dL)	100.08 ± 26.26	104.74 ± 30.95	97.41 ± 22.89	0.104
Total Cholesterol (mg/dL)	179.43 ± 46.92	164.16 ± 46.19	187.74 ± 45.39	0.001
HDL Cholesterol (mg/dL)	50.81 ± 17.02	46.75 ± 16.18	52.95 ± 17.14	0.02

Table 1. Cont.

	Total (n = 183)	Male (n = 64)	Female (n = 119)	p Value
LDL Cholesterol (mg/dL)	105.23 ± 40.80	93.38 ± 40.26	111.43 ± 39.88	0.007
Triglycerides (mg/dL)	132.35 ± 67.13	132.84 ± 71.81	132.07 ± 64.68	0.944
Creatinine (mg/dl)	0.95 ± 0.44	1.09 ± 0.52	0.87 ± 0.36	0.001
GFR (ml/min/1.73 m^2)	83.59 ± 36.90	85.15 ± 44.14	82.74 ± 32.52	0.675
SBP (mmHg)	138.84 ± 17.09	134.83 ± 16.40	140.99 ± 17.13	0.018
DBP (mmHg)	81.22 ± 10.85	80.81 ± 12.83	81.44 ± 9.67	0.711
PP (mmHg)	57.72 ± 13.940	53.86 ± 11.48	59.79 ± 14.73	0.003
MAP (mmHg)	110.03 ± 12.58	107.82 ± 13.54	111.21 ± 11.93	0.095
CAVI	8.92 ± 2.09	9.58 ± 2.23	8.56 ± 1.94	0.003
CAVI 0	14.93 ± 6.16	16.20 ± 6.48	14.24 ± 5.89	0.047
PWV-cf (m/s)	9.58 ± 4.36	9.39 ± 3.45	9.69 ± 4.79	0.636
Number of diseases	5.42 ± 2.41	5.45 ± 2.34	5.39 ± 2.45	0.875
CCI	3.30 ± 2.24	3.72 ± 2.31	3.07 ± 2.18	0.066

BMI: body mass index, HDL: high density lipoprotein; LDL: low density lipoprotein; GFR: glomerular filtration rate; SBP: systolic blood pressure; DBP: diastolic blood pressure; PP: pulse pressure; MAP: mean arterial pressure; CAVI: cardio-ankle vascular index; PWV-cf: pulse wave velocity carotid-femoral; CCI: Charlson Comorbidity Index.

3.1. Univariate Analysis

As shown by univariate analysis (Table 2), all arterial stiffness indexes display a positive relationship with age (CAVI r = 0.698, CAVI 0 r = 0.717, PWV-cf r 0.410, $p < 0.001$ for all of them). Furthermore, CAVI, CAVI 0 and PWV-cf resulted correlated to higher comorbidities, as measured by CCI (CAVI r = 0.654, $p < 0.001$; CAVI 0 r = 0.658, $p < 0.001$; PWV r = 0.448 and $p < 0.001$). Both CAVI and CAVI 0 showed a significant inverse relation with DBP (r = −0.296 and r = −0.389, respectively, $p < 0.001$ for both), MAP (r = −0.209, $p = 0.005$ and r = −0.274, $p < 0.001$, respectively) and a positive relation with PP (r = 0.165, $p = 0.025$ and r = 0.219, $p = 0.003$, respectively).

Table 2. Univariate Correlations between CAVI, CAVI0, PWV-cf and the main clinical variables.

	CAVI	CAVI 0	PWV-cf
Age	0.698 ***	0.717 ***	0.410 **
Glucose level	0.166 *	0.166 *	0.152
Total Cholesterol	−0.446 ***	−0.430 ***	−0.203 **
HDL Cholesterol	−0.187 *	−0.213 **	−0.173 *
LDL Cholesterol	−0.474 ***	−0.479 ***	−0.237 **
Triglycerides	0.036	0.070	0.139
GFR	−0.535 ***	−0.521 ***	−0.213 **
CCI	0.654 ***	0.658 ***	0.448 ***
SBP	−0.060	−0.074	−0.017
DBP	−0.296 ***	−0.389 ***	−0.146 **
MAP	−0.209 **	−0.274 ***	−0.097
PP	0.165 *	0.219 **	0.108
CAVI	1	0.955 ***	0.430 ***
CAVI 0	0.955 ***	1	0.438 ***
PWV-cf	0.430 ***	0.438 ***	1

* $p < 0.05$, ** $p < 0.01$, *** $p < 0.001$. HDL: high density lipoprotein; LDL: low density lipoprotein; GFR: glomerular filtration rate; CCI: Charlson Comorbidity Index; SBP: systolic blood pressure; DBP: diastolic blood pressure; MAP: mean arterial pressure; PP: pulse pressure; CAVI: cardio-ankle vascular index; PWV-cf: pulse wave velocity carotid-femoral.

Moreover, CAVI 0 is directly correlated to CAVI (r = 0.955, $p < 0.001$) and both CAVI and CAVI 0 relate to PVW-cf (r = 0.430 and r = 0.438 respectively, $p < 0.001$ for both).

3.2. Subgroup Analysis: Cardiovascular Comorbidities and Risk Factors

As outlined by subgroup analyses, patients with hypertension diagnosis, as compared to patients without, had increased arterial stiffness indexes (mean PWV-cf 10.05 ± 4.67 vs. 8.63 ± 3.36, $p = 0.017$; mean CAVI 9.25 ± 2.13 vs. 8.19 ± 1.85, $p = 0.001$; mean CAVI 0 15.82 ± 6.57 vs. 12.95 ± 4.58, $p = 0.003$). Mean CAVI, CAVI 0 and PVW-cf were also increased in diabetic patients, when compared to normoglycemic subjects (mean PWV-cf 12.53 ± 5.42 vs. 9.013 ± 3.96, $p < 0.001$; mean CAVI 10.15 ± 2.50 vs. 8.64 ± 1.91, $p < 0.001$; mean CAVI 0 18.27 ± 7.31 vs. 14.11 ± 5.30, $p < 0.001$). Furthermore, the subgroup of patients with previous CV events, as compared to subjects without, had increased CAVI and CAVI 0, whilst PVW-cf was not significantly different between groups (mean CAVI 10.82 ± 2.46 vs. 8.65 ± 1.90, $p < 0.001$; mean CAVI 0 20.13 ± 7.52 vs. 14.18 ± 5.58, $p < 0.001$). When stratifying the study population upon CCI, as CCI increased, we outlined a progressive increase in CAVI (Figure 1A), CAVI 0 (Figure 1B), and PVW-cf (Figure 1C), which remained significant after adjustment for age, sex, MAP and GFR.

3.3. Regression Analysis: Arterial Stiffness Predictors

Stepwise multiple regression models were performed (Table 3) in order to evaluate the combined effect of independent variables on arterial stiffness parameters. In the first model PWV-cf was considered as a dependent variable; among several independent variables (age, GFR, MAP, CCI, LDL and triglycerides) only CCI resulted as significant predictor of PWV-cf ($p < 0.001$), accounting for 20.5% of its variance. Interestingly, when considering CAVI as dependent variable, and age, GFR, MAP, CCI, LDL and triglycerides as independent variables, both age and CCI resulted to be significant predictors ($p < 0.001$ and $p = 0.012$, respectively), explaining almost 53% of CAVI variance. Likewise, as shown in the third model which considered CAVI 0 as dependent variable and again age, GFR, MAP, CCI, LDL and triglycerides as independent variables, age and CCI ($p < 0.001$ and $p = 0.010$, respectively) could predict CAVI 0, accounting for 55.8% of its variance.

Table 3. Stepwise regression analysis, considering PWV-cf, CAVI, and CAVI 0 respectively as dependent variables, and age, glomerular filtration rate, mean arterial pressure, Charlson Comorbidity Index, LDL-Cholesterol and Triglycerides as independent variables.

Dependent Variables	Independent Variables	β ± Standard Error	p Value	R^2
PWV-cf				
	CCI	0.924 ± 0.144	<0.001	0.205
CAVI				
	Age	0.076 ± 0.014	<0.001	
	CCI	0.238 ± 0.094	0.012	0.528
CAVI 0				
	Age	0.226 ± 0.039	<0.001	
	CCI	0.680 ± 0.259	0.010	0.558

CCI: Charlson Comorbidity Index; CAVI: cardio-ankle vascular index; PWV-cf: pulse wave velocity carotid-femoral.

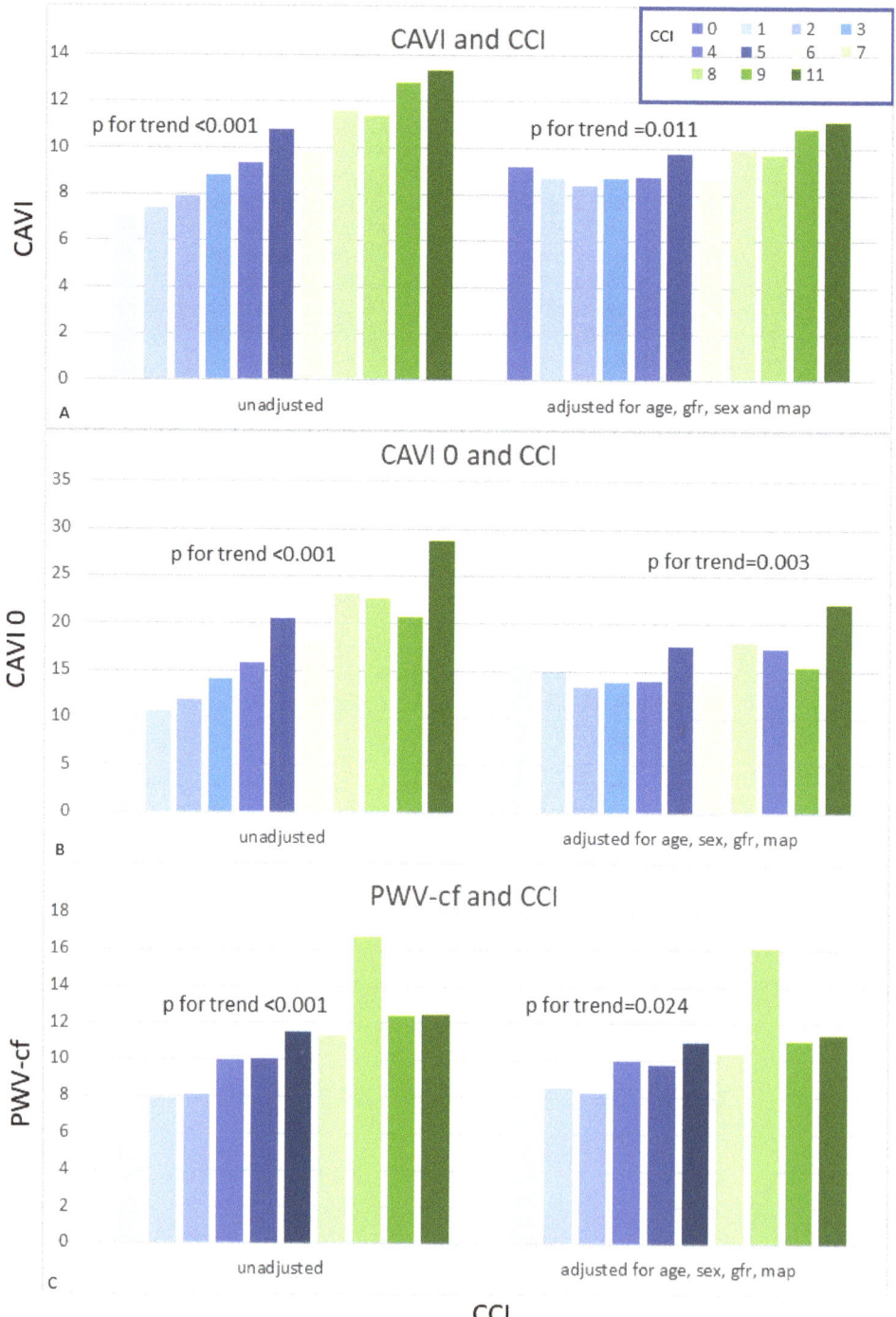

Figure 1. CAVI (**A**), CAVI 0 (**B**) and PWV-cf (**C**) values stratified by Charlson Comorbidity Index Columns represent increasing values of cci; on y axes arterial stiffness parameters are displayed.

4. Discussion

The present study shows significant positive correlations between all parameters of arterial stiffness and CV risk factors, comorbidities, and aging. The positive correlation with age is stronger for CAVI and CAVI 0 than PVW-cf. Moreover, our data confirm and complement previous knowledge showing that age and comorbidity can predict arterial stiffness parameters.

We could demonstrate a positive relationship between CAVI, CAVI 0, PVW-cf and the main CV risk factors, even after adjustment for age, sex, MAP and GFR. In line with previous evidence [36], in our population all the arterial stiffness indexes resulted increased in hypertensive patients, reflecting the vascular remodeling, characterized by wall stiffening typical of this condition. In particular, we outlined a significant increase in CAVI among hypertensive subjects, which is consistent with the results of Nagayama and colleagues [16], who demonstrated increased CAVI values in a cohort of 2300 individuals, describing a sharper increase after the SBP threshold of 140 mmHg.

As is predictable considering vascular involvement in the diabetes mellitus course [37], we described increased arterial stiffness indexes among diabetic patients and among subjects with impaired fasting glucose levels, as compared to normoglycemic individuals. These results are in line with previous finding regarding both PVW-cf [37] and CAVI [18,38]; the latter was found increased in diabetic patients, showing however a progressive decrease after 8 weeks of glucose lowering therapy, consistent with HbA1c reduction [18]. Moreover, we found a significant correlation between all the arterial stiffness indexes and metabolic syndrome components, confirming previous evidence [12,39,40], and corroborating the hypothesis of increased arterial stiffening as a crucial change in the presence of metabolic disorders or metabolic syndrome.

We further outlined increased CAVI and CAVI 0 in patients with previous CV events, still in line with several studies that described increased CAVI in subjects with known coronary artery disease and cerebral ischemia [25,41–43]. Altogether, our and other results suggest that different vascular diseases, affecting different segments of the arterial tree, share the common finding of increased arterial stiffness. Our findings actually complement previous observations because they show that the heterogeneity of the vessels involved may be more accurate by testing CAVI, instead of PVW-cf, since the first is more representative of a large proportion of the arterial tree [3].

Although several conditions are known to be associated to worse values of CAVI and PVW-cf, the possible association with the comprehensive comorbidities burden is not entirely explored. In this regard, although less is known about increased comorbidity index, CAVI has already been depicted as increased among frail individuals; thus, our results confirm and complement previous evidence by Xue and colleagues who described higher CAVI values in elderly frail patients (relaying on Fried's frailty definition) [44]. Noteworthily, moving one step further, we observed a positive relationship between all the arterial stiffness indexes and both comorbidities number and CCI, still significant after adjustment for age, sex, MAP and GFR. The pathophysiological background of this finding might rely on the vascular remodeling, which occurs during healthy aging [45], and pathological conditions [1]. Certainly, arterial stiffening is the common denominator of several diseases included in the CCI calculation, and therefore a double-sided relation might be inferred: first, arterial wall stiffening in otherwise healthy aging subjects might increase the risk of developing a huge number of vascular-associated conditions. On the other hand, presenting relevant comorbidities (primarily involving or not the vascular system) might promote a complex network of tissue remodeling processes, leading to arterial wall stiffening. Thus, more than a single disease, the comprehensive burden of multiple co-existing conditions might contribute to widespread and increased vascular stiffening. According to the latter interpretation, we could demonstrate that considering arterial stiffness parameters as dependent variables, the comorbidity burden described by CCI is a strong predictor of all the arterial stiffness indexes, and along with age it can explain a consistent percentage of CAVI and CAVI 0 variance. Arterial stiffness might thus be considered as part of the expression of a multidimensional decline; in particular we found that CAVI, as compared to PVW-cf, was more strongly related to the comorbidity burden, and, once more, a possible explanation lies in the wider proportion of arterial segments that is simultaneously investigated by CAVI, therefore including a broad spectrum of pathological conditions.

According to consolidated knowledge [45], our study confirms a significant association between aging and arterial stiffness: each arterial stiffness index displays significant relation with age; the strength of the association is higher for CAVI and CAVI 0, as compared to PVW-cf. Furthermore, on top of several variables, age is shown to be a significant predictor of CAVI and CAVI 0, yet not of PWV-cf. The remarkable relationship between age and CAVI was previously demonstrated by Shirai et al. [46], who described increased CAVI in elderly subjects as a possible expression of age-related arterial wall sclerosis. Although PVW-cf is still considered as the primary arterial stiffness evaluation technique for outcome prediction [47], CAVI could be also considered as a more reliable index in the elderly, due to its lower dependence from blood pressure [48].

A few limitations of the study should be recognized: this is a cross-sectional study, and therefore we were not allowed to test the power of arterial stiffness indexes in predicating long term cardiovascular risk. Our study was predominantly performed in female patients and given the increased prevalence of cardiovascular diseases in the male population, we need to test our hypothesis in a more represented male population. Further, information regarding medical therapy was not available, but we acknowledge that the possible effect of different medications on arterial stiffness may be of interest. As concerns arterial stiffness parameters, we acknowledge that the augmentation index, which is deemed to be an important parameter, was not significant in our findings, and therefore excluded from the results.

In conclusion, our study, conducted on a relatively wide and heterogeneous cohort of patients, demonstrated that PVW-cf, CAVI and CAVI 0 are associated to CV risk factors and higher comorbidity burden, even after adjustment for several variables. Furthermore, our data outline a strong correlation between arterial stiffness indexes and age. Our findings might complement the pathophysiological understanding of the cardiovascular impairment in subjects with older age and remarkable comorbidity burden. Therefore, in the clinical setting, arterial stiffness evaluation, which is a feasible and easily available technique, may complement the characterization of complex patients.

Author Contributions: Conceptualization, F.F. and M.Z.; methodology, F.F., A.G., M.T., A.P.R. and E.Z.; formal analysis, R.M. and F.F.; investigation, F.F., A.G. and G.M.; data curation, F.F., A.G. and R.M.; writing—original draft preparation, F.F., A.G. and E.Z.; writing—review and editing, F.F. and M.Z.; supervision, M.Z. All authors have read and agreed to the published version of the manuscript.

Funding: This research received no external funding.

Institutional Review Board Statement: Approval Code: CE 191CESC University Hospital, Verona, approval Date: 11 February 2015.

Informed Consent Statement: Informed consent was obtained from all subjects involved in the study.

Data Availability Statement: The data presented in this study are available on request from the corresponding author.

Conflicts of Interest: The authors declare no conflict of interest.

References

1. Vlachopoulos, C.; Xaplanteris, P.; Aboyans, V.; Brodmann, M.; Cífková, R.; Cosentino, F.; De Carlo, M.; Gallino, A.; Landmesser, U.; Laurent, S.; et al. The role of vascular biomarkers for primary and secondary prevention. A position paper from the European Society of Cardiology Working Group on peripheral circulation. Endorsed by the Association for Research into Arterial Structure and Physiology (ARTERY) Society. *Atherosclerosis* **2015**, *241*, 507–532. [CrossRef] [PubMed]
2. Shirai, K.; Song, M.; Suzuki, J.; Kurosu, T.; Oyama, T.; Nagayama, D.; Miyashita, Y.; Yamamura, S.; Takahashi, M. Contradictory Effects of β1- and α1-Aderenergic Receptor Blockers on Cardio-Ankle Vascular Stiffness Index (CAVI). *J. Atheroscler. Thromb.* **2011**, *18*, 49–55. [CrossRef] [PubMed]
3. Asmar, R. Principles and usefulness of the cardio-ankle vascular index (CAVI): A new global arterial stiffness index. *Eur. Heart J. Suppl.* **2017**, *19*, B4–B10. [CrossRef]
4. Van Popele, N.M.; Grobbee, D.E.; Bots, M.L.; Asmar, R.; Topouchian, J.; Reneman, R.S.; Hoeks, A.P.G.; Van Der Kuip, D.A.M.; Hofman, A.; Witteman, J.C.M. Association between arterial stiffness and atherosclerosis: The Rotterdam study. *Stroke* **2001**, *32*, 454–460. [CrossRef]
5. Asmar, R.; Benetos, A.; Topouchian, J.; Laurent, P.; Pannier, B.; Brisac, A.M.; Target, R.; Levy, B.I. Assessment of arterial distensibility by automatic pulse wave velocity measurement: Validation and clinical application studies. *Hypertension* **1995**, *26*, 485–490. [CrossRef]
6. Takahashi, K.; Yamamoto, T.; Tsuda, S.; Okabe, F.; Shimose, T.; Tsuji, Y.; Suzuki, K.; Otsuka, K.; Takata, M.; Shimizu, K.; et al. Coefficients in the CAVI Equation and the Comparison between CAVI with and without the Coefficients Using Clinical Data. *J. Atheroscler. Thromb.* **2019**, *26*, 465–475. [CrossRef] [PubMed]
7. Spronck, B.; Avolio, A.P.; Tan, I.; Butlin, M.; Reesink, K.D.; Delhaas, T. Arterial stiffness index beta and cardio-ankle vascular index inherently depend on blood pressure but can be readily corrected. *J. Hypertens.* **2017**, *35*, 98–104. [CrossRef] [PubMed]
8. Spronck, B.; Mestanik, M.; Tonhajzerova, I.; Jurko, A.; Jurko, T.; Avolio, A.P.; Butlin, M. Direct means of obtaining CAVI 0—A corrected cardio-ankle vascular stiffness index (CAVI)—from conventional CAVI measurements or their underlying variables. *Physiol. Meas.* **2017**, *38*, N128–N137. [CrossRef]
9. Shirai, K.; Suzuki, K.; Tsuda, S.; Shimizu, K.; Takata, M.; Yamamoto, T.; Maruyama, M.; Takahashi, K. Comparison of Cardio–Ankle Vascular Index (CAVI) and CAVI0 in Large Healthy and Hypertensive Populations. *J. Atheroscler. Thromb.* **2019**, *26*, 603–615. [CrossRef]
10. Saiki, A.; Ohira, M.; Yamaguchi, T.; Nagayama, D.; Shimizu, N.; Shirai, K.; Tatsuno, I. New Horizons of Arterial Stiffness Developed Using Cardio-Ankle Vascular Index (CAVI). *J. Atheroscler. Thromb.* **2020**, *27*, 732–748. [CrossRef]
11. Fantin, F.; Disegna, E.; Manzato, G.; Comellato, G.; Zoico, E.; Rossi, A.P.; Mazzali, G. Adipokines and Arterial Stiffness in the Elderly. *Vasc. Health Risk Manag.* **2020**, *16*, 535–543. [CrossRef] [PubMed]
12. Fantin, F.; Giani, A.; Gasparini, L.; Rossi, A.P.; Zoico, E.; Mazzali, G.; Zamboni, M. Impaired subendocardial perfusion in patients with metabolic syndrome. *Diabetes Vasc. Dis. Res.* **2021**, *18*, 147916412110471. [CrossRef] [PubMed]
13. Nakamura, K.; Tomaru, T.; Yamamura, S.; Miyashita, Y.; Shirai, K.; Noike, H. Cardio-Ankle Vascular Index is a Candidate Predictor of Coronary Atherosclerosis. *Circ. J.* **2007**, *72*, 598–604. [CrossRef]
14. Namekata, T.; Suzuki, K.; Ishizuka, N.; Shirai, K. Establishing baseline criteria of cardio-ankle vascular index as a new indicator of arteriosclerosis: A cross-sectional study. *BMC Cardiovasc. Disord.* **2011**, *11*, 51. [CrossRef]
15. Kiuchi, S.; Kawasaki, M.; Hirashima, O.; Hisatake, S.; Kabuki, T.; Yamazaki, J.; Ikeda, T. Addition of a renin-angiotensin-aldosterone system inhibitor to a calcium channel blocker ameliorates arterial stiffness. *Clin. Pharmacol. Adv. Appl.* **2015**, *7*, 97. [CrossRef] [PubMed]
16. Nagayama, D.; Watanabe, Y.; Saiki, A.; Shirai, K.; Tatsuno, I. Difference in positive relation between cardio-ankle vascular index (CAVI) and each of four blood pressure indices in real-world Japanese population. *J. Hum. Hypertens.* **2019**, *33*, 210–217. [CrossRef] [PubMed]
17. Uzui, H.; Morishita, T.; Nakano, A.; Amaya, N.; Fukuoka, Y.; Ishida, K.; Arakawa, K.; Lee, J.-D.; Tada, H. Effects of Combination Therapy with Olmesartan and Azelnidipine on Serum Osteoprotegerin in Patients with Hypertension. *J. Cardiovasc. Pharmacol. Ther.* **2014**, *19*, 304–309. [CrossRef]
18. Ibata, J.; Sasaki, H.; Hanabusa, T.; Wakasaki, H.; Furuta, H.; Nishi, M.; Akamizu, T.; Nanjo, K. Increased arterial stiffness is closely associated with hyperglycemia and improved by glycemic control in diabetic patients. *J. Diabetes Investig.* **2013**, *4*, 82–87. [CrossRef]
19. Tsuboi, A.; Ito, C.; Fujikawa, R.; Yamamoto, H.; Kihara, Y. Association between the Postprandial Glucose Levels and Arterial Stiffness Measured According to the Cardio-ankle Vascular Index in Non-diabetic Subjects. *Intern. Med.* **2015**, *54*, 1961–1969. [CrossRef]
20. Dobsak, P.; Soska, V.; Sochor, O.; Jarkovsky, J.; Novakova, M.; Homolka, M.; Soucek, M.; Palanova, P.; Lopez-Jimenez, F.; Shirai, K. Increased Cardio-ankle Vascular Index in Hyperlipidemic Patients without Diabetes or Hypertension. *J. Atheroscler. Thromb.* **2015**, *22*, 272–283. [CrossRef]
21. Nagayama, D.; Watanabe, Y.; Saiki, A.; Shirai, K.; Tatsuno, I. Lipid Parameters are Independently Associated with Cardio–Ankle Vascular Index (CAVI) in Healthy Japanese Subjects. *J. Atheroscler. Thromb.* **2018**, *25*, 621–633. [CrossRef] [PubMed]

22. Satoh, N.; Shimatsu, A.; Kato, Y.; Araki, R.; Koyama, K.; Okajima, T.; Tanabe, M.; Ooishi, M.; Kotani, K.; Ogawa, Y. Evaluation of the Cardio-Ankle Vascular Index, a New Indicator of Arterial Stiffness Independent of Blood Pressure, in Obesity and Metabolic Syndrome. *Hypertens. Res.* **2008**, *31*, 1921–1930. [CrossRef] [PubMed]
23. Kawada, T.; Andou, T.; Fukumitsu, M. Relationship between cardio-ankle vascular index and components of metabolic syndrome in combination with sex and age. *Diabetes Metab. Syndr. Clin. Res. Rev.* **2014**, *8*, 242–244. [CrossRef]
24. Kirigaya, J.; Iwahashi, N.; Tahakashi, H.; Minamimoto, Y.; Gohbara, M.; Abe, T.; Akiyama, E.; Okada, K.; Matsuzawa, Y.; Maejima, N.; et al. Impact of Cardio-Ankle Vascular Index on Long-Term Outcome in Patients with Acute Coronary Syndrome. *J. Atheroscler. Thromb.* **2020**, *27*, 657–668. [CrossRef] [PubMed]
25. Suzuki, J.; Sakakibara, R.; Tomaru, T.; Tateno, F.; Kishi, M.; Ogawa, E.; Kurosu, T.; Shirai, K. Stroke and Cardio-ankle Vascular Stiffness Index. *J. Stroke Cerebrovasc. Dis.* **2013**, *22*, 171–175. [CrossRef]
26. Kim, K.J.; Lee, B.-W.; Kim, H.; Shin, J.Y.; Kang, E.S.; Cha, B.S.; Lee, E.J.; Lim, S.-K.; Lee, H.C. Associations between Cardio-Ankle Vascular Index and Microvascular Complications in Type 2 Diabetes Mellitus Patients. *J. Atheroscler. Thromb.* **2011**, *18*, 328–336. [CrossRef] [PubMed]
27. Bramwell, J.C.; Hill, A. Velocity of transmission of the pulse-wave. *Lancet* **1922**, *199*, 891–892. [CrossRef]
28. Saiki, A.; Sato, Y.; Watanabe, R.; Watanabe, Y.; Imamura, H.; Yamaguchi, T.; Ban, N.; Kawana, H.; Nagumo, A.; Nagayama, D.; et al. The Role of a Novel Arterial Stiffness Parameter, Cardio-Ankle Vascular Index (CAVI), as a Surrogate Marker for Cardiovascular Diseases. *J. Atheroscler. Thromb.* **2016**, *23*, 155–168. [CrossRef]
29. Hayashi, K.; Yamamoto, T.; Takahara, A.; Shirai, K. Clinical assessment of arterial stiffness with cardio-ankle vascular index. *J. Hypertens.* **2015**, *33*, 1742–1757. [CrossRef]
30. Spronck, B.; Mestanik, M.; Tonhajzerova, I.; Jurko, A.; Tan, I.; Butlin, M.; Avolio, A.P. Easy conversion of cardio-ankle vascular index into CAVI. *J. Hypertens.* **2019**, *37*, 1913–1914. [CrossRef]
31. Salvi, P.; Lio, G.; Labat, C.; Ricci, E.; Pannier, B.; Benetos, A. Validation of a new non-invasive portable tonometer for determining arterial pressure wave and pulse wave velocity: The PulsePen device. *J. Hypertens.* **2004**, *22*, 2285–2293. [CrossRef] [PubMed]
32. Fantin, F.; Giani, A.; Macchi, F.; Amadio, G.; Rossi, A.P.; Zoico, E.; Mazzali, G.; Zamboni, M. Relationships between subendocardial perfusion impairment, arterial stiffness and orthostatic hypotension in hospitalized elderly individuals. *J. Hypertens.* **2021**, *39*, 2379–2387. [CrossRef] [PubMed]
33. McVeigh, G.E.; Bratteli, C.W.; Morgan, D.J.; Alinder, C.M.; Glasser, S.P.; Finkelstein, S.M.; Cohn, J.N. Age-related abnormalities in arterial compliance identified by pressure pulse contour analysis: Aging and arterial compliance. *Hypertension* **1999**, *33*, 1392–1398. [CrossRef] [PubMed]
34. Van Bortel, L.M.; Laurent, S.; Boutouyrie, P.; Chowienczyk, P.; Cruickshank, J.K.; De Backer, T.; Filipovsky, J.; Huybrechts, S.; Mattace-Raso, F.U.S.; Protogerou, A.D.; et al. Expert consensus document on the measurement of aortic stiffness in daily practice using carotid-femoral pulse wave velocity. *J. Hypertens.* **2012**, *30*, 445–448. [CrossRef]
35. Friedewald, W.T.; Levy, R.I.; Fredrickson, D.S. Estimation of the concentration of low-density lipoprotein cholesterol in plasma, without use of the preparative ultracentrifuge. *Clin. Chem.* **1972**, *18*, 499–502. [CrossRef]
36. Wang, H.; Liu, J.; Zhao, H.; Fu, X.; Shang, G.; Zhou, Y.; Yu, X.; Zhao, X.; Wang, G.; Shi, H. Arterial stiffness evaluation by cardio-ankle vascular index in hypertension and diabetes mellitus subjects. *J. Am. Soc. Hypertens.* **2013**, *7*, 426–431. [CrossRef]
37. Choi, S.-Y.; Oh, B.-H.; Bae Park, J.; Choi, D.-J.; Rhee, M.-Y.; Park, S. Age-Associated Increase in Arterial Stiffness Measured According to the Cardio-Ankle Vascular Index without Blood Pressure Changes in Healthy Adults. *J. Atheroscler. Thromb.* **2013**, *20*, 911–923. [CrossRef]
38. Gómez-Marcos, M.Á.; Recio-Rodríguez, J.I.; Patino-Alonso, M.C.; Agudo-Conde, C.; Gómez-Sánchez, L.; Gomez-Sanchez, M.; Rodríguez-Sanchez, E.; Maderuelo-Fernandez, J.A.; García-Ortiz, L. Cardio-ankle vascular index is associated with cardiovascular target organ damage and vascular structure and function in patients with diabetes or metabolic syndrome, LOD-DIABETES study: A case series report. *Cardiovasc. Diabetol.* **2015**, *14*, 7. [CrossRef]
39. Di Pino, A.; Alagona, C.; Piro, S.; Calanna, S.; Spadaro, L.; Palermo, F.; Urbano, F.; Purrello, F.; Rabuazzo, A.M. Separate impact of metabolic syndrome and altered glucose tolerance on early markers of vascular injuries. *Atherosclerosis* **2012**, *223*, 458–462. [CrossRef]
40. Topouchian, J.; Labat, C.; Gautier, S.; Bäck, M.; Achimastos, A.; Blacher, J.; Cwynar, M.; De La Sierra, A.; Pall, D.; Fantin, F.; et al. Effects of metabolic syndrome on arterial function in different age groups: The Advanced Approach to Arterial Stiffness study. *J. Hypertens.* **2018**, *36*, 824–833. [CrossRef]
41. Tabara, Y.; Setoh, K.; Kawaguchi, T.; Takahashi, Y.; Kosugi, S.; Nakayama, T.; Matsuda, F. Factors affecting longitudinal changes in cardio–ankle vascular index in a large general population. *J. Hypertens.* **2018**, *36*, 1147–1153. [CrossRef] [PubMed]
42. Tonhajzerova, I.; Mestanikova, A.; Jurko, A.; Grendar, M.; Langer, P.; Ondrejka, I.; Jurko, T.; Hrtanek, I.; Cesnekova, D.; Mestanik, M. Arterial stiffness and haemodynamic regulation in adolescent anorexia nervosa versus obesity. *Appl. Physiol. Nutr. Metab.* **2020**, *45*, 81–90. [CrossRef] [PubMed]
43. Izuhara, M.; Shioji, K.; Kadota, S.; Baba, O.; Takeuchi, Y.; Uegaito, T.; Mutsuo, S.; Matsuda, M. Relationship of Cardio-Ankle Vascular Index (CAVI) to Carotid and Coronary Arteriosclerosis. *Circ. J.* **2008**, *72*, 1762–1767. [CrossRef] [PubMed]
44. Xue, Q.; Qin, M.; Jia, J.; Liu, J.; Wang, Y. Association between frailty and the cardio-ankle vascular index. *Clin. Interv. Aging* **2019**, *14*, 735–742. [CrossRef] [PubMed]

5. Vallée, A. Arterial Stiffness Determinants for Primary Cardiovascular Prevention among Healthy Participants. *J. Clin. Med.* **2022**, *11*, 2512. [CrossRef] [PubMed]
6. Shirai, K. Analysis of vascular function using the cardio–ankle vascular index (CAVI). *Hypertens. Res.* **2011**, *34*, 684–685. [CrossRef]
7. Spronck, B.; Obeid, M.J.; Paravathaneni, M.; Gadela, N.V.; Singh, G.; Magro, C.A.; Kulkarni, V.; Kondaveety, S.; Gade, K.C.; Bhuva, R.; et al. Predictive Ability of Pressure-Corrected Arterial Stiffness Indices: Comparison of Pulse Wave Velocity, Cardio-Ankle Vascular Index (CAVI), and $CAVI_0$. *Am. J. Hypertens.* **2022**, *35*, 272–280. [CrossRef]
8. Shirai, K.; Utino, J.; Otsuka, K.; Takata, M. A Novel Blood Pressure-independent Arterial Wall Stiffness Parameter; Cardio-Ankle Vascular Index (CAVI). *J. Atheroscler. Thromb.* **2006**, *13*, 101–107. [CrossRef]

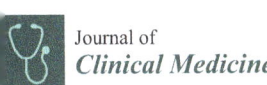

Article

Detectable Bias between Vascular Ultrasound Echo-Tracking Systems: Relevance Depends on Application

Afrah E. F. Malik [1], Alessandro Giudici [1,2], Koen W. F. van der Laan [1], Jos Op 't Roodt [3], Werner H. Mess [4], Tammo Delhaas [1], Bart Spronck [1,5] and Koen D. Reesink [1,*]

[1] Department of Biomedical Engineering, CARIM School for Cardiovascular Diseases, Maastricht University, Universiteitssingel 50, 6229 ER Maastricht, The Netherlands
[2] GROW School for Oncology and Reproduction, Maastricht University, Universiteitssingel 50, 6229 ER Maastricht, The Netherlands
[3] Department of Internal Medicine, CARIM School for Cardiovascular Diseases, Maastricht University, Universiteitssingel 50, 6229 ER Maastricht, The Netherlands
[4] Department of Clinical Neurophysiology, CARIM School for Cardiovascular Diseases, Maastricht University, Universiteitssingel 50, 6229 ER Maastricht, The Netherlands
[5] Macquarie Medical School, Faculty of Medicine, Health and Human Sciences, Macquarie University, 75 Talavera Rd., Sydney, NSW 2109, Australia
* Correspondence: k.reesink@maastrichtuniversity.nl; Tel.: +31-6-4216-1888

Abstract: The Esaote MyLab70 ultrasound system has been extensively used to evaluate arterial properties. Since it is reaching end-of-service-life, ongoing studies are forced to seek an alternative, with some opting for the Esaote MyLabOne. Biases might exist between the two systems, which, if uncorrected, could potentially lead to the misinterpretation of results. This study aims to evaluate a potential bias between the two devices. Moreover, by comparing two identical MyLabOne systems, this study also aims to investigate whether biases estimated between the MyLabOne and MyLab70 employed in this study could be generalized to any other pair of similar scanners. Using a phantom set-up, we performed $n = 60$ measurements to compare MyLab70 to MyLabOne and $n = 40$ measurements to compare the two MyLabOne systems. Comparisons were performed to measure diameter, wall thickness, and distension. Both comparisons led to significant biases for the diameter (relative bias: −0.27% and −0.30% for the inter- and intra-scanner model, respectively, $p < 0.05$) and wall thickness (relative bias: 0.38% and −1.23% for inter- and intra-scanner model, respectively $p < 0.05$), but not for distension (relative bias: 0.48% and −0.12% for inter- and intra-scanner model, respectively, $p > 0.05$). The biases estimated here cannot be generalized to any other pair of similar scanners. Therefore, longitudinal studies with large sample sizes switching between scanners should perform a preliminary comparison to evaluate potential biases between their devices. Furthermore, caution is warranted when using biases reported in similar comparative studies. Further work should evaluate the presence and relevance of similar biases in human data.

Keywords: echo-tracking; vascular ultrasound; arterial properties; arterial stiffness

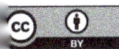

1. Introduction

Arterial properties, such as diameter, wall thickness, and distension, are extensively investigated in the literature [1–6], considering the valuable information they provide about cardiovascular health. Moreover, they are used to quantify arterial stiffness: an independent predictor of cardiovascular diseases [7]. Local arterial stiffness can be characterized by the distensibility coefficient and Young's elastic modulus, among other indices. These indices require the assessment of the instantaneous diameter change and wall thickness by means of ultrasound echo-tracking [8–10].

Efforts made by prof. Hoeks and his group [2,11,12] represent seminal endeavors for the utilisation of ultrasound echo-tracking in the field of large artery (patho-)physiology.

Their efforts mainly focused on analysing radiofrequency (RF) signals to estimate arterial distensibility. Hoeks' group developed the necessary software and hardware (ART.LAB) to be integrated ultimately with the MyLab70 (Esaote Europe B.V. Maastricht, the Netherlands) and to present a top-class research-oriented echo-tracking system. In the past two decades the MyLab70/ART.LAB combo has been used extensively in expert centers to quantify arterial elastic and geometrical properties, predominantly in a research context [13–15]. At the same time, ultrasound manufacturers continued to incorporate such technology into commercial devices with the objective of bringing the technology to clinical practice. Today the MyLab70/ART.LAB has reached its end-of-service-life, forcing ongoing longitudinal epidemiological and interventional studies to switch to another scanner, which, because of technical differences, may not necessarily provide identical results. For instance, the Maastricht Study opted for the MyLabOne with RFQAS and RFIMT functionalities, plus a radiofrequency output license (Esaote) [14], with technology based on the original radiofrequency tracking [2]. The newer system represents a portable, integrated, and more affordable substitute to MyLab70/ART.LAB. The two systems, however, have different technical characteristics, and hence, their use at two-time points of a longitudinal study might result in a bias in the follow-up measurement. Not considering or correcting for such an ultrasound system-related bias may lead to misinterpretation of results and, thereby, erroneous conclusions.

The primary aim of the present study was to compare MyLabOne- and MyLab70-based echo-tracking systems to assess potential bias in quantifying diameter, wall thickness, and distension. In addition, we explored if such biases might also arise when comparing two MyLabOne systems with identical specifications. We conducted the comparative measurements in two steps, using a phantom set-up and three ultrasound systems: MyLabOne I, MyLab70, and MyLabOne II. First, we compared MyLab70 and MyLabOne I. We refer to this comparison as inter-scanner model comparison. Next, we estimated the biases between MyLabOne I and MyLabOne II. We refer to this comparison as intra-scanner model comparison. To confirm that the inter- and intra-system model biases estimated in this study are not spurious but that they originate from real intra- and inter-system model differences, we also performed an intra-device comparison. To this end, we assessed the differences between two measurement sets performed with MyLabOne I.

2. Materials and Methods

2.1. Ultrasound Scanners

Measurements in this study were performed using three different ultrasound systems: MyLabOne I, MyLabOne II, and MyLab70. A summary of the specifications of these systems is shown in Table 1. MyLab70 was equipped with a linear array transducer operating at 7.5 MHz and had a practical axial resolution of 0.125 mm. MyLabOne systems were equipped with linear array transducers operating at 10 MHz. The systems had a practical axial resolution of approximately 0.120 mm. All three systems were operating in fast B-mode, with high frame rates of 498 and 524 for MyLab70 and the MyLabOne systems, respectively. These high frame rates are achieved by generating multiple M-lines separated by 0.98 mm in the longitudinal direction of the probe. The number of M-lines is, however, different between the two scanners: $n = 19$ for MyLab70 and $n = 14$ for MyLabOne. In addition, all three scanners enabled the recording of raw radiofrequency signals sampled at 50 MHz for MyLab70 and 33 MHz for MyLabOne.

Table 1. Specifications of echo-tracking systems used in the study.

	MyLab70	MyLabOne I & II
Operating frequency (MHz)	7.5	10
RF sampling frequency (MHz)	50	33
Frame rate (fps)	498	524
No. of M-lines	19	14
Practical * axial resolution (mm)	0.125	0.120
Approx. cost	120 k	25 k
RF wall tracking	ART.LAB	RF module
RF output format	.r70	.zrf

RF—radiofrequency; * Practical here refers to the resolution estimated and based on the actual bandwidth measured from received RF signals in contrast to theoretical axial resolution.

2.2. Phantom Configuration

To perform the inter- and intra-ultrasound system model comparisons to estimate scanner biases for assessing diameter, wall thickness, and distension, a two-part phantom set-up was used (Figure 1). The first part consisted of a static silicone tube with an outer diameter of 12.4 mm and a wall thickness of 1 mm. This part was used to estimate biases between the ultrasound system pairs for diameter and wall thickness. The second part consisted of an eccentric wheel connected to a motor via a rod, which was inserted in the wheel 300 µm off centre. Thus, measuring the instantaneous location of the top surface of the wheel results in a sinusoidal distension waveform with a peak-to-peak amplitude of 600 µm. A silicone slab was mounted above the wheel to mimic the artery near wall. This near wall was held in a fixed position; hence, it did not contribute to the simulated vessel distension. The phantom set-up and the transducer lens were immersed in tap water at room temperature to enable ultrasound propagation.

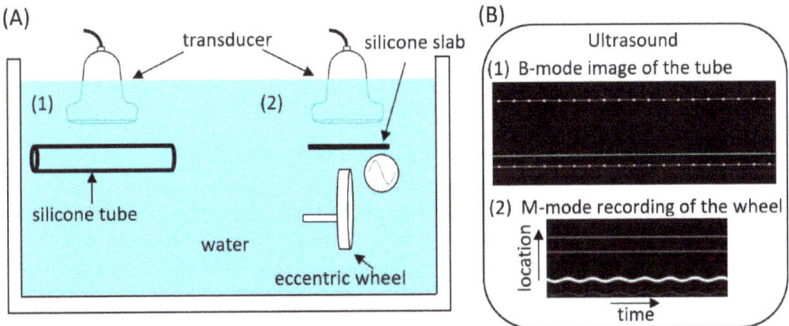

Figure 1. Study set-up for ultrasound system bias estimation (**A**) and how it appeared in the ultrasound measurements (**B**). Two-part phantom set-up consisting of a silicone tube (1), used to assess inter- and intra-scanner biases in diameter and wall thickness, and an eccentric wheel with a silicone slab mounted on top of it (2), used to assess the bias in distension. (B.1): Example of a B-mode image for the silicone tube. The white dot markers indicate the outer tube-water echo interfaces (appearing as horizontal white lines) of the near (top) and far (bottom) walls of the silicone tube used to measure the diameter. The green line indicates the inner tube-water echo interface of the far wall, which, together with the far wall outer echo interface, was used to measure wall thickness. (B.2): Example of an M-mode acquisition of the wheel 'distension'. The white sinusoidal line reflects the motion of the wheel surface, while the two less echogenic parallel reflections above the undulating line indicate the silicone slab.

2.3. Data Acquisition

To compare MyLabOne I and MyLab70, we obtained $n = 60$ repeated RF acquisitions for both scanners. Post hoc analysis using data from the previously mentioned comparison revealed that after about 40 repeated measurements, the bias and confidence intervals (CI) remained relatively constant for all examined variables indicating that $n = 40$ repeated measurements were sufficient to provide a reliable estimate of the bias. Therefore, for the intra-device model comparison, we performed $n = 40$ repeated measurements using MyLabOne I and MyLabOne II for diameter and wall thickness. Moreover, we inferred from the inter-device comparison that part of the distension recordings might be lost potentially due to uncontrolled saturation; hence, $n = 60$ repeated distension measurements were performed for the intra-device model case. The MyLabOne I measurement set available for the inter-scanner model comparison was also used to perform an intra-device comparison. For all the studied variables, two groups were created by dividing this measurement set into two groups based on the order of performing the measurement (even and odd). Individual acquisitions were performed by repositioning the ultrasound probe at random distances (ranging between 1 and 3 cm) from the tube and the wheel. This was conducted to simulate in vivo situations due to the fact that the depth from the skin to the carotid artery varies between different individuals.

2.4. Data Processing

The diameter was defined as the distance between the near and far wall outer silicone-water reflections and is indicated by white dotted lines in Figure 1B.1. Wall thickness was defined as the distance in the far wall between the inner and outer silicone-water reflections. Both diameter and wall thickness were estimated based on longitudinal acquisitions covering 19 and 14 equidistant M-lines for Mylab70 and MyLabOne, respectively. On the contrary, cross-sectional acquisitions of the wheel motion were performed to estimate distension. Since the wheel thickness was 4 mm and the distance between the ultrasound M-lines was approximately 1 mm, only a few M-lines covered the wheel. Therefore, we estimated the distension based on a single M-line with the most wheel coverage [9]. This was deduced based on the brightness of the corresponding B-mode of the line, indicating a strong wheel reflection. RF signals were processed in MATLAB (MATLAB R2020b; The MathWorks, Natick, MA, USA) using proprietary wall-tracking software that was previously described in [2,12,16].

2.5. Statistical Analyses

RF recordings were acquired for at least five seconds for all scanners. Biases were quantified as means ± 95% CI and are reported in absolute and relative terms. For all three considered variables, the absolute bias was calculated as the difference between the average of estimates obtained with MyLabOne I and MyLab70 (i.e., MyLabOne I- minus MyLab70-derived values) and between those obtained with MyLabOne I and MyLabOne II (i.e., MyLabOne I- minus MyLabOne II-derived values) for the inter-device and intra-device comparisons, respectively, and tested with an independent sample Student's t-test. The relative bias was defined as the absolute bias normalized with respect to the mean value of both systems. Precision was assessed by the estimates' standard deviation (SD) and compared with F-test. Statistical analyses were performed using SPSS version 27 (SPSS, Chicago, IL, USA). A two-sided p-value <0.05 was considered statistically significant.

3. Results

3.1. MyLabOne I vs. MyLab70

Post hoc, 21 MyLabOne I distension recordings were excluded due to the uncontrolled saturation in the corresponding RF complex [17].

The diameter obtained with MyLabOne I was significantly lower than that obtained with MyLab70 (12.3830 vs. 12.4170 mm, $p = 0.001$), corresponding to a relative bias of −0.27%. However, the precision of the diameter measurements defined as the SD was similar for the two scanners (0.0533 vs. 0.0527 mm, $p = 0.542$). Compared to MyLab70, MyLabOne I resulted in a significantly higher wall thickness (1.0019 vs. 0.9981 mm, $p = 0.004$) which translated into a relative bias of 0.38%. Further, MyLabOne I yielded a significantly higher standard deviation for wall thickness (0.0079 vs. 0.0062 mm, $p < 0.001$). The SD obtained with MyLabOne I for distension was significantly higher than that achieved with MyLab70 (17.8 vs. 12.1 µm, $p = 0.047$). However, we found no significant difference between the two scanners for distension (617.0 vs. 614.1 µm, $p = 0.333$) (Table 2 and Figure 2).

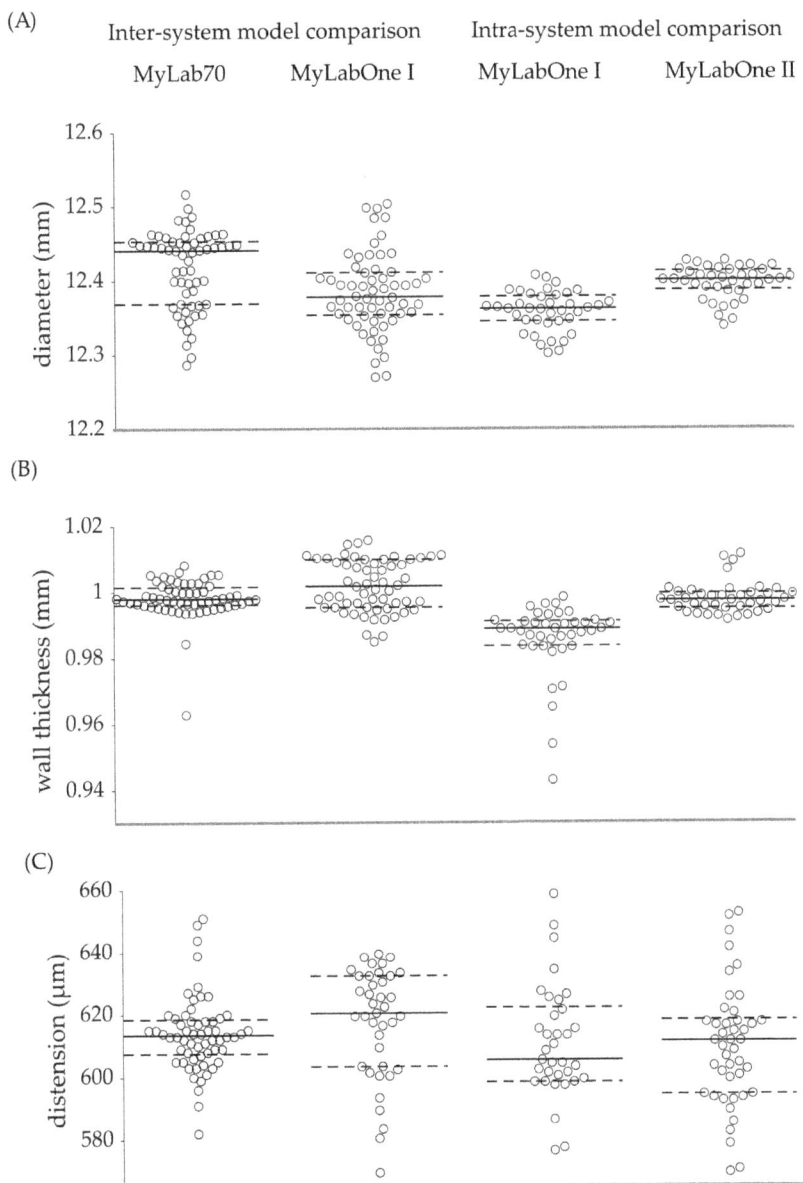

Figure 2. Overview of absolute values of all repeated measurements performed for the inter- and intra-scanner model comparisons. Measurements were performed with MyLab70, MyLabOne I, and MyLabOne II for diameter (**A**), wall thickness (**B**), and distension (**C**). Solid lines indicate the medians and dashed lines indicate the 25th and 75th percentiles.

Table 2. Diameter, wall thickness, and distension as determined by MyLabOne I, MyLab70, and MyLabOne II for the inter- and intra-device model and the intra-device comparisons.

Inter-system model comparison				Bias (95% CI)		
				Absolute	Relative (%)	p
		MyLabOne I	MyLab70			
Diameter (mm)	n	60	60			
	Mean	12.3830	12.4170	−0.0339 (−0.0530 to −0.0147)	−0.27 (−0.43 to −0.12)	0.001
	SD	0.0533	0.0527			0.542
Wall thickness (mm)	n	60	60			
	Mean	1.0019	0.9981	0.0038 (0.0013 to 0.0064)	0.38 (0.13 to 0.63)	0.004
	SD	0.0079	0.0062			<0.001
Distension (μm)	n	39	60			
	Mean	617.0	614.1	2.9 (−3.0 to 8.8)	0.48 (−0.56 to 1.51)	0.333
	SD	17.8	12.1			0.047
Intra-system model comparison						
		MyLabOne I	MyLabOne II			
Diameter (mm)	n	40	40			
	Mean	12.3569	12.3945	−0.0376 (−0.0484 to −0.0268)	−0.30 (−0.39 to −0.22)	<0.001
	SD	0.0222	0.0267			0.343
Wall thickness (mm)	n	40	40			
	Mean	0.9855	0.9976	−0.0121 (−0.0159 to −0.0084)	−1.23 (−1.60 to −0.85)	<0.001
	SD	0.0110	0.0048			0.013
Distension (μm)	n	37	45			
	Mean	609.5	610.2	−0.7 (−11.0 to 9.6)	−0.12 (−1.81 to 1.52)	0.892
	SD	25.5	21.4			0.591
Intra-device comparison						
		MyLabOne I 1st set	MyLabOne I 2nd set			
Diameter (mm)	n	30	30			
	Mean	12.3824	12.3837	−0.0012 (−0.0284 to 0.0260)	−0.01 (−0.23 to 0.21)	0.929
	SD	0.0500	0.0573			0.257
Wall thickness (mm)	n	30	30			
	Mean	1.0006	1.0032	−0.0026 (−0.0066 to 0.0013)	−0.26 (−0.66 to 0.13)	0.198
	SD	0.0086	0.0070			0.364
Distension (μm)	n	20	19			
	Mean	615.2	618.8	−3.6 (−14.8 to 7.6)	−0.59 (−2.41 to 1.23)	0.529
	SD	18.9	16.8			0.697

SD—standard deviation; CI—confidence intervals.

3.2. MyLabOne I vs. MyLabOne II

Of the distension measurements performed for the intra-scanner model comparison, $n = 23$ were excluded for MyLabOne I and $n = 15$ were excluded for MyLabOne II due to uncontrolled saturation in the corresponding RF complex.

The comparison of the two MyLabOne systems yielded significantly different diameter estimates (12.3569 vs. 12.3945 mm, $p < 0.001$), corresponding to a relative bias of -0.30%. However, the two systems yielded similar SDs (0.0222 vs. 0.0267 mm, $p = 0.343$) for diameter. The two systems resulted in significantly different wall thickness measurements (0.9855 vs. 0.9976 mm, $p < 0.001$), translating into a relative bias of -1.23%. Further, the two scanners yielded significantly different SDs of the wall thickness (0.0110 vs. 0.0048 mm, $p = 0.013$). We found no significant difference between the distension estimates obtained with the two scanners (609.5 vs. 610.2 µm, $p = 0.892$). Similarly, there was no significant difference between the SDs of the distension estimates obtained with the two systems (25.5 vs. 21.4 µm, $p = 0.591$) (Table 2 and Figure 2).

3.3. MyLabOne I vs. MyLabOne I

The results of this comparison are shown in Table 2. The intra-device comparison yielded statistically non-significant differences for diameter (difference -0.0012 mm, $p = 0.929$), wall thickness (difference $= -0.0026$ mm, $p = 0.198$), and distension (difference -3.6 µm, $p = 0.529$). Similarly, the two measurement sets of MyLabOne I resulted in statistically non-significant SDs for all the examined variables ($p > 0.05$). Because of the considerable intercurrent time between the two available MyLabOne I measurement sets (i.e., one set for the inter- and one for the intra- system model comparisons) as well as the lack of consistency in measurement conditions/set-up status, we refrained from intra-device comparison based on the two available MyLabOne I measurement sets.

4. Discussion

Using a phantom set-up, this study assessed the inter- and intra-scanner biases between MyLabOne I- and MyLab70-based echo-tracking systems for measuring arterial diameter, wall thickness, and distension. Our results show detectable biases for diameter and wall thickness but not for distension. This held true for the comparison between the MyLab70 and a MyLabOne I system, as well as for the comparison between two MyLabOne systems. Biases were in the same order of magnitude in both comparisons. All biases were very small with respect to the values reported in the literature for studies comparing two echo-tracking systems (Table 3) [1,3,4]. Based on our results, research studies should adhere to one device unless switching is necessary. Whenever replacement is unavoidable, a comparison between the two systems should be performed to establish the amount of bias, even if the devices have the same vendor and model.

To the best of our knowledge, this is the first study to compare MyLabOne and MyLab70, as well as two MyLabOne systems with identical specifications. MyLab70 and MyLabOne share several common features. Indeed, they are both RF-based echo-tracking systems designed and manufactured by the same manufacturer. In addition, the two systems employ conceptually similar RF tracking approaches [2]. As shown in Table 3, the biases between MyLabOne and MyLab70 for all the examined variables were lower than the values reported by similar studies comparing two different devices/models. This indicates that MyLabOne is a good substitute for MyLab70.

To ensure that the non-significant bias found in the case of the distension was not due to insufficient statistical power, we performed a post hoc power analysis. This analysis was performed using G*Power version 3.1.9.4: an open-source statistical power analysis tool available at https://www.gpower.hhu.de (accessed on 23 June 2021) [18]. The power analysis showed that a sample size of 39 would enable us to detect an effect size greater than 0.64 (power 80% and a two-sided $\alpha = 0.05$). Note that based on our study design, we would, thus, be able to detect a bias greater than 64% of the device's precision.

Table 3. Studies found in the literature that compare two different ultrasound devices for measuring arterial diameter, wall thickness, and distension.

Variable	Study	Type of Data	Compared Devices	n	Absolute Bias	Relative Bias (%)
Diameter (mm)	Bozec et al., 2020 [1]	Carotid artery	Wall tracking system (WTS) and ART.LAB	188	0.119	1.8
	Palombo et al., 2012 [4]	Carotid artery	Two RF-based systems	105	0.263	3.4
	Morganti et al., 2005 [3]	Carotid artery	Multigate Doppler system against commercially available ultrasound device	37	0.05	0.7
	This study, 2022	**Phantom set-up**	**Esaote MyLabOne I and MyLab70**	**60**	**0.0339**	**0.27**
Wall thickness (mm)	Bozec et al., 2020 [1]	Carotid artery	WTS and ART.LAB	186	0.046	6.1
	This study, 2022	**Phantom set-up**	**Esaote MyLabOne I and MyLab70**	**60**	**0.0038**	**0.38**
Distension (μm)	Bozec et al., 2020 [1]	Carotid artery	WTS and ART.LAB	181	23	4.3
	Palombo et al., 2012 [4]	Carotid artery	Two RF-based systems	105	91	22
	Morganti et al., 2005 [3]	Carotid artery	Multigate Doppler system against commercially available ultrasound device	37	34	6.8
	This study, 2022	**Phantom set-up**	**Esaote MyLabOne I and MyLab70**	**39 and 60**	**2.9**	**0.48**

Bold texts highlight the current study.

Biases between MyLabOne I and MyLab70 systems for all examined variables did not exceed 0.5%, which appears clinically irrelevant for personalized risk stratification and diagnosis (e.g., in the context of cardiovascular risk assessment). However, the findings presented in this study may have direct implications for research studies, particularly follow-up designs. By alleviating the effect of device-related biases on the outcomes of these studies, the findings presented here have an indirect clinical relevance. For such studies, an appraisal of the relevance of the bias depends on multiple factors, with the sample size/statistical power being the most important. For instance, for the same value of the bias, a low population variability would lead to significant results with a small sample size, while larger variability requires a larger sample size for the results to be relevant.

Let one consider the lowest sample size ($n_{\min}$) beyond which the estimated biases would be considered relevant. In other words, studies with a sample size exceeding $n_{\min}$ should consider the effect of the inter-/intra-scanner bias in their analysis and interpretation. Figure 3 shows the results of our calculations of $n_{\min}$ for a range of population variabilities. Based on the results presented in Figure 3, research studies are recommended to consider their population variability/statistical power when evaluating the relevance of the biases detectable between MyLabOne and MyLab70 systems.

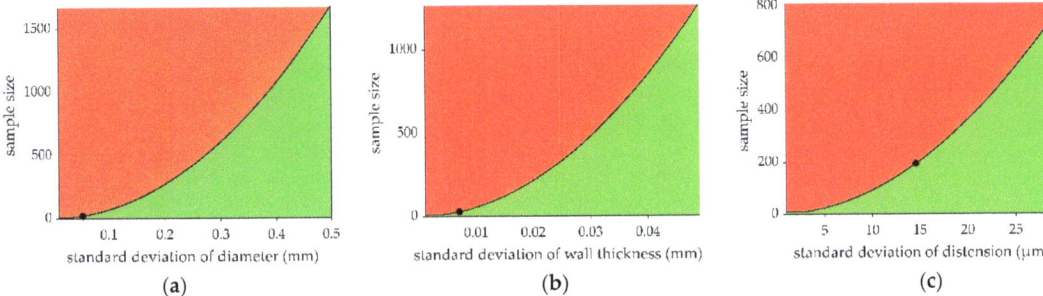

Figure 3. Lowest sample size (n_{min}) for estimated biases to be considered relevant. n_{min} is estimated using several values of standard deviation for (**a**) diameter, (**b**) wall thickness, and (**c**) distension. We assumed that variability within research studies conducted in humans could be expected to be larger than that observed here using a phantom and, hence, considered a range of variabilities (defined with SD) in quantifying n_{min}. The black line represents n_{min} as a function of SD, while the red area represents sample sizes for which estimated biases are considered significant. Black dots represent n_{min} for a significant bias calculated using the SDs observed in this study, and they correspond to 21, 28, and 193 samples for diameter (**a**), wall thickness (**b**), and distension (**c**), respectively.

This study found differences between two identical-on-paper systems (MyLabOne I and MyLabOne II) for diameter, and wall thickness, indicating that the results found here for the inter-scanner comparison could not be generalized to any other pair of similar scanners. These findings also imply that caution is warranted when using systematic biases reported in similar comparative studies. A potential explanation for the intra-scanner model differences relates to the different operational periods between our two systems and the supposed 'wear' effect on data quality. Another possible explanation relates to the uncertainty in the manufacturing process, which is determined by the adopted tolerance, and the admissible variation in the end product.

The intra-device comparison was performed to check if the differences found in the cases of the inter- and intra- system model comparisons were spurious, originating from factors such as study set-up, environmental conditions, and wear effect or if they were real, originating from inter- and intra- system model differences. Intra-device differences for all the studied variables were not statistically significant (Table 2), confirming that the significant differences found in the cases of inter- and intra-scanner model comparisons originated from real device/device model differences. Compared to inter- and intra- system model differences, intra-device differences were smaller for diameter and wall thickness and larger for distension. We believe that the difference found in the case of distension was caused by the relative uncertainty of the distension estimate.

For studies switching between devices, a similar phantom set-up and approach could be used to calibrate the new system against the old one to avoid any effect that a systematic bias between the two systems could have on the study outcomes. Phantom set-ups are controllable and provide repeatable estimates; hence, they are superior to human data for calibration purposes. By using a phantom, one mitigates additional uncertainty in bias estimates originating from human data variability.

This study has several possible limitations: (1) Some distension recordings were excluded due to saturation in the RF complex. This problem was experienced with the MyLabOne systems but not with MyLab70. The eccentric wheel used in the phantom set-up was made of a strong reflector; hence, with certain gain settings, the peaks of the incoming RF signal may exceed the dynamic range (16 bit or 96 dB) of the scanner. While adjusting the gain setting was possible with MyLab70 during the RF acquisitions, this option was not available for MyLabOne, explaining the occurrence of saturation issues. (2) The set-up used here consisted of homogeneous materials, and diameter and wall thickness measurements were performed under static conditions. Tissue inhomogeneity and vessel wall motion might alter bias estimates under in vivo situations. (3) In vivo arterial diameter and wall thickness (defined as intima-media thickness) are typically smaller than those of the phantom tube. Hence, the effect of the ultrasound scanners limited axial resolution may be expected to be more pronounced during in vivo settings.

5. Conclusions

The present study found detectable inter- and intra-scanner model biases for diameter and wall thickness measurements but not for distension measurements. The existence of a detectable bias between two identical systems/models indicates that the biases estimated in the present study cannot be generalized to any other pair of scanners. Therefore, studies with large sample sizes and particularly those with longitudinal designs, in which a change in or an exchange of scanners is necessary, should check for the presence of biases between devices following our approach. Further work should evaluate the presence and relevance of biases in (existing) human studies.

Author Contributions: A.E.F.M. and K.D.R.: conceptualization. A.E.F.M., K.D.R., W.H.M., A.G., B.S and T.D.: methodology. A.E.F.M., K.D.R., A.G. and B.S.: data analysis. A.E.F.M.: data processing A.E.F.M. and K.D.R.: writing—original draft preparation. A.E.F.M., K.D.R., W.H.M., A.G., B.S., K.W.F.v.d.L., J.O.'t.R. and T.D.: writing—review and editing. T.D., W.H.M. and K.D.R.: supervision All authors have read and agreed to the published version of the manuscript.

Funding: A.E.F.M. was supported by the European Union-funded Horizon 2020 project InSiDe (no. 871547). B.S. was supported by the European Union's Horizon 2020 research and innovation program (no. 793805).

Data Availability Statement: Data will be made available upon request to the corresponding author

Acknowledgments: The authors would like to thank Arnold P. G. Hoeks for developing the Distension software code that was used to analyse the RF recordings in this study.

Conflicts of Interest: The authors declare no conflict of interest.

References

1. Bozec, E.; Girerd, N.; Ferreira, J.P.; Latar, I.; Zannad, F.; Rossignol, P. Reproducibility in echotracking assessment of local carotid stiffness, diameter and thickness in a population-based study (The STANISLAS Cohort Study). *Artery Res.* **2020**, *26*, 5–12. [CrossRef]
2. Hoeks, A.; Brands, P.; Smeets, F.; Reneman, R. Assessment of the distensibility of superficial arteries. *Ultrasound Med. Biol.* **1990**, *16*, 121–128. [CrossRef] [PubMed]
3. Morganti, T.; Ricci, S.; Vittone, F.; Palombo, C.; Tortoli, P. Clinical validation of common carotid artery wall distension assessment based on multigate Doppler processing. *Ultrasound Med. Biol.* **2005**, *31*, 937–945. [CrossRef] [PubMed]
4. Palombo, C.; Kozakova, M.; Guraschi, N.; Bini, G.; Cesana, F.; Castoldi, G.; Stella, A.; Morizzo, C.; Giannattasio, C. Radiofrequency-based carotid wall tracking: A comparison between two different systems. *J. Hypertens.* **2012**, *30*, 1614–1619. [CrossRef] [PubMed]
5. Baldassarre, D.; Hamsten, A.; Veglia, F.; De Faire, U.; Humphries, S.E.; Smit, A.J.; Giral, P.; Kurl, S.; Rauramaa, R.; Mannarino, E. Measurements of carotid intima-media thickness and of interadventitia common carotid diameter improve prediction of cardiovascular events: Results of the IMPROVE (Carotid Intima Media Thickness [IMT] and IMT-Progression as Predictors of Vascular Events in a High Risk European Population) study. *J. Am. Coll. Cardiol.* **2012**, *60*, 1489–1499. [PubMed]
6. Jensen-Urstad, K.; Jensen-Urstad, M.; Johansson, J. Carotid artery diameter correlates with risk factors for cardiovascular disease in a population of 55-year-old subjects. *Stroke* **1999**, *30*, 1572–1576. [CrossRef] [PubMed]
7. Laurent, S.; Boutouyrie, P.; Asmar, R.; Gautier, I.; Laloux, B.; Guize, L.; Ducimetiere, P.; Benetos, A. Aortic stiffness is an independent predictor of all-cause and cardiovascular mortality in hypertensive patients. *Hypertension* **2001**, *37*, 1236–1241. [CrossRef] [PubMed]
8. Engelen, L.; Bossuyt, J.; Ferreira, I.; van Bortel, L.M.; Reesink, K.D.; Segers, P.; Stehouwer, C.D.; Laurent, S.; Boutouyrie, P.; Collaboration, R.V.f.A.M. Reference values for local arterial stiffness. Part A: Carotid artery. *J. Hypertens.* **2015**, *33*, 1981–1996. [CrossRef] [PubMed]
9. Malik, A.E.; Delhaas, T.; Spronck, B.; Henry, R.; Joseph, J.; Stehouwer, C.D.; Mess, W.H.; Reesink, K.D. Single M-Line is as reliable as multiple M-line ultrasound for carotid artery screening. *Front. Physiol.* **2021**, *2265*, 787083. [CrossRef] [PubMed]
10. Reneman, R.S.; Meinders, J.M.; Hoeks, A.P. Non-invasive ultrasound in arterial wall dynamics in humans: What have we learned and what remains to be solved. *Eur. Heart J.* **2005**, *26*, 960–966. [CrossRef] [PubMed]

1. Brands, P.J.; Hoeks, A.P.; Willigers, J.; Willekes, C.; Reneman, R.S. An integrated system for the non-invasive assessment of vessel wall and hemodynamic properties of large arteries by means of ultrasound. *Eur. J. Ultrasound* **1999**, *9*, 257–266. [CrossRef] [PubMed]
2. Hoeks, A.P.; Willekes, C.; Boutouyrie, P.; Brands, P.J.; Willigers, J.M.; Reneman, R.S. Automated detection of local artery wall thickness based on M-line signal processing. *Ultrasound Med. Biol.* **1997**, *23*, 1017–1023. [CrossRef] [PubMed]
3. Kozakova, M.; Morizzo, C.; La Carrubba, S.; Fabiani, I.; Della Latta, D.; Jamagidze, J.; Chiappino, D.; Di Bello, V.; Palombo, C. Associations between common carotid artery diameter, Framingham risk score and cardiovascular events. *Nutr. Metab. Cardiovasc. Dis.* **2017**, *27*, 329–334. [CrossRef] [PubMed]
4. Schram, M.T.; Sep, S.J.; van der Kallen, C.J.; Dagnelie, P.C.; Koster, A.; Schaper, N.; Henry, R.; Stehouwer, C.D. The Maastricht Study: An extensive phenotyping study on determinants of type 2 diabetes, its complications and its comorbidities. *Eur. J. Epidemiol.* **2014**, *29*, 439–451. [CrossRef] [PubMed]
5. Spronck, B.; Heusinkveld, M.H.; Vanmolkot, F.H.; Op't Roodt, J.; Hermeling, E.; Delhaas, T.; Kroon, A.A.; Reesink, K.D. Pressure-dependence of arterial stiffness: Potential clinical implications. *J. Hypertens.* **2015**, *33*, 330–338. [CrossRef] [PubMed]
6. Brands, P.J.; Hoeks, A.P.; Ledoux, L.A.; Reneman, R.S. A radio frequency domain complex cross-correlation model to estimate blood flow velocity and tissue motion by means of ultrasound. *Ultrasound Med. Biol.* **1997**, *23*, 911–920. [CrossRef] [PubMed]
7. Rossi, A.C.; Brands, P.J.; Hoeks, A.P. Nonlinear processing in B-mode ultrasound affects carotid diameter assessment. *Ultrasound Med. Biol.* **2009**, *35*, 736–747. [CrossRef] [PubMed]
8. Faul, F.; Erdfelder, E.; Buchner, A.; Lang, A.-G. Statistical power analyses using G* Power 3.1: Tests for correlation and regression analyses. *Behav. Res. Methods* **2009**, *41*, 1149–1160. [CrossRef] [PubMed]

Disclaimer/Publisher's Note: The statements, opinions and data contained in all publications are solely those of the individual author(s) and contributor(s) and not of MDPI and/or the editor(s). MDPI and/or the editor(s) disclaim responsibility for any injury to people or property resulting from any ideas, methods, instructions or products referred to in the content.

MDPI
St. Alban-Anlage 66
4052 Basel
Switzerland
www.mdpi.com

Journal of Clinical Medicine Editorial Office
E-mail: jcm@mdpi.com
www.mdpi.com/journal/jcm

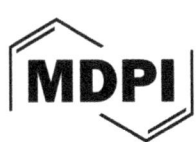

Disclaimer/Publisher's Note: The statements, opinions and data contained in all publications are solely those of the individual author(s) and contributor(s) and not of MDPI and/or the editor(s). MDPI and/or the editor(s) disclaim responsibility for any injury to people or property resulting from any ideas, methods, instructions or products referred to in the content.

www.ingramcontent.com/pod-product-compliance
Lightning Source LLC
LaVergne TN
LVHW070711100526
838202LV00013B/1070